M. Angermaier
Auricular Acupuncture

Acknowledgements

First and foremost my thanks go to the editor Christl Kiener who was also responsible for some of the German editions of this textbook. Very early on we both had the idea of translating this title into English, especially because of the book's success in Germany as an 'instruction manual' for auricular acupuncture. Since its first publication in 1999 it is now in its 5th edition.

I would also very much like to thank the translator and foreign language assistant Johanna Schuster. She did an excellent job in translating this very specialized aspect of medicine. Many terms used in auricular acupuncture are as yet not defined to an international standard. Translating them required great sensitivity and understanding of the German and Chinese terms.

I would also like to give my thanks to the typesetter, Kadja Gericke, for her invaluable support and contributions to this project.

And finally I would like to thank my wife Barbara Angermaier for her continuous support and for creating an environment that allows me to spend so much time and energy on all my projects. Without all her help neither the German edition nor this English translation would have been possible.

Last but not least my thanks go to each and everyone who was involved in creating this English edition!

Note

Terminology

This textbook lists all auricular points currently used by the French, the Chinese as well as the Vienna School. Points of the Chinese School are named in English. In cases where no translation exists the Chinese terminology has been used. The numbers traditionally used for points of the Chinese School are set in brackets after the name of the point. In cases where points of the Chinese and French School respectively are located in the same place but have different names they are listed with a slash; the French name first and the Chinese name second.

Key to Illustration Symbols

Auricular points of the French School are shown in red, those of the Chinese School in black.

- ● Point on the anterior aspect of the ear
- ● French and Chinese point
- ◑ Partially hidden point
- ⋮ Hidden point
- ⬡ Point on the inner side of the ear

- ▬ Point located on an edge
- ▢ Area
- ➚ Point in the Sympathetic Groove
- ▬ Point on the Hormonal Line

Manfred Angermaier

Auricular Acupuncture
A Clinical Handbook

Including All French and Chinese Auricular Points

Translated by Johanna Schuster

KIENER Munich 2014

Original edition

Manfred Angermaier: Leitfaden Ohrakupunktur

5th edition 2011, Elsevier Urban & Fischer Verlag, München,

ISBN 978-3-437-55424-7

© 2011: Elsevier GmbH, Urban & Fischer, Munich. All rights reserved.

Notice

Neither the Publisher nor the Author assume any responsibility for any loss or injury and/or damage to persons or poperty arising out of or related to any use of the material contained in this book. It is the responsibility of the treating practicitioner, relying on independent expertise and knowledge of the patient to determine the best treatment and method of application for the patient.

Bibliographic information published by the Deutsche Nationalbibliothek

The Deutsche Nationalbibliothek lists this publication in the Deutsche Nationalbibliografie; detailed bibliographic data are available in the Internet at http://www.d-nb.de.

A CIP catalogue record for this book is available from the British Library.

All rights reserved

1st Edition 2014

© KIENER, München/Germany

14 15 16 17   5 4 3 2 1

Translation from German and copy-editing: Johanna Schuster, Foyers/Scotland

Production: Kadja Gericke, Arnstorf/Germany

Printing and binding: Stürtz GmbH, Würzburg/Germany

Photographs/Drawings: Manfred Angermaier, Bergen/Germany; Henriette Rintelen, Velbert/Germany

Ear drawings: Societas Medicinae Sinensis (SMS), München/Germany; Grafik: Ulrike Brugger, München/Germany; Margarete Baumgartner, Wasserburg am Inn/Germany

Cover photographs: Manfred Angermaier, Bergen/Germany

Cover design: SpieszDesign, Neu-Ulm/Germany

Printed in Germany

ISBN 978-3-943324-29-7

www.kiener-press.com

KIENER

Preface

For more than 20 years auricular acupuncture has been a focal point of my interest. During and also following my seven-year training as surgeon at a hospital in Munich I dedicated myself to the study of Chinese Medicine; participating in training courses organized by the various German professional organizations whose aim is to establish Chinese Medicine in Europe. The society I am now most involved with is the SMS (Societas Medicinae Sinensis) whose chairman and founder member, Prof. Dr. Carl-Hermann Hempen, is also responsible for a new training course in Chinese Medicine at the Technical University of Munich. As a member of his team I teach auricular acupuncture. I am also a member of the examination board of the Medical Association of Bavaria.

In addition to teaching I have a private practice in Bergen (Chiemgau/Bavaria) the main focus of which is Chinese Medicine with an emphasis on auricular acupuncture. After several moves the clinic has been firmly established in its current location since 1998 and also allows me to work in conjunction with some osteopaths, notably Svenja Dresen. My wife, Barbara Angermaier, a naturopath, is also a partner in this clinic, specializing in self-experience work as well as working with clients with psychological problems. In addition, we offer courses in yoga, qi gong and Feldenkrais to educate our clients how to best maintain their health.

Overall, it is our aim to offer an integral way of keeping body and soul in balance. More detailed information is available on my website www.ohrakupunktur.de. It also contains information about forthcoming courses, conferences, and lectures.

I hope that this book which contains all my knowledge about auricular acupuncture will provide practitioners with insights into this particular aspect of acupuncture.

Bergen, January, 2014
Dr. med. Manfred Angermaier

Table of Contents

1 Introduction

1.1 Historical Overview

1.1.1 Origins of Auricular Acupuncture

- In China, the first mention of auricular acupuncture in literature is in the 1st century BC. The *Huangdi Neijing* (The Inner Classic of the Yellow Emperor) mentions connections between the auricle and certain areas of the body. Twenty anterior and posterior auricular points were known by the time of the *Tang* dynasty (618–907 AD).

- In Persia and Egypt auricular acupuncture was already in use for pain relief and contraception 2000 years ago.

- In the 4th century *Hippocrates* recognized that it was possible to treat ailments via the ear. He tried to cure impotence through bloodletting on the ear.

- In Europe, references about the use of auricular acupuncture date back to only the 17th century. In the famous painting 'Garden of Earthly Delights' by *Hieronymus Bosch* correspondences between the auricle and various areas of the body are recognizable in the symbolic depiction of hell.

- In 1637 *Zacatus Lusitanus* describes the cauterisation of a part of the ear for the treatment of sciatica, while in 1717 *Valsalva* outlines the same procedure for tooth ache.

- Following a report by Dr. Luciana Bastia (France) about the treatment of sciatica by means of cauterisation in the 19th century there are further publications about similar successful treatment by other physicians. At the same time similar developments take place in Italy (Prof Ignaz Colla, Parma) and in America (Dr Rülker, Cincinnati).

In contrast to body acupuncture, auricular acupuncture was not further developed in China in the following centuries. It was only after the publications of the French physician Paul Nogier in 1957 that auricular acupuncture once again became the focus of interest for doctors of traditional Chinese medicine. Nogier's discoveries soon reached China and led to the development of the Chinese school of auricular acupuncture.

1.1.2 French School

Auricular acupuncture has been systematically researched only since 1950 – initially by Paul Nogier. He had noticed scars on the ears of some of his Arabic patients. They had been cauterized in the area of the antihelix as a form of treatment for lower back pain or sciatica, resulting in pain relief within minutes to a few hours. At first, Nogier tried cauterisation himself but later replaced this method by inserting needles, which also led to positive results without causing permanent scars. It took him a further three years to recognise the relationship between the spine and its inverse projection on the antihelix.

Subsequently, Nogier discovered that all organs of the human body are represented on the ear. In 1956, at a lecture given in Marseille, he presented this new treatment method under the name 'auriculothérapie'. This lecture was translated into German by Gerhard Bachmann and published in 1957 in the 'Deutsche Zeitschrift für Akupunktur'.

In 1968 Nogier accidentally discovered a change in the quality of the pulse when examining locations on the ear corresponding to pathological areas of the patient's body. A systematic investigation of this phenomenon showed that stimulating disturbed areas of the ear resulted in a characteristic change of the pulse. Nogier interpreted this reaction as a polysynaptic reflex and referred to it as 'réflexe auriculocardiaque' (RAC). This phenomenon solved the problem of detecting relevant ear points. It was the decisive breakthrough for the development of an objective and safe method for the location and treatment of 'pathological' ear points.

1.1.3 Chinese and Vienna School

Chinese School

In 1958 Yeh Hsiao-Lin published Nogier's discoveries in Shanghai. Chinese doctors realised that it was possible to integrate auricular acupuncture into Traditional Chinese Medicine. Henceforth, auricular acupuncture has been increasingly utilised in addition to body acupuncture. Previously, the few auricular points known for millennia had been of minor significance. They were mainly considered in the context of body acupuncture rather than a self-contained therapeutic system.

Following Nogier's publication of his map of auricular points in 1969 and 1977, an auricular map, based on Nogier's map, was published in China, also in 1977. On this map the ear lobe was divided into nine zones. This division is also used on the auricular maps in this book thus taking into account the Chinese influence on auricular acupuncture. In Europe, the validation and further development of auricular acupuncture advanced more quickly than in China. There, the early insights were adhered to for longer while these were quickly modified in Europe. Furthermore, RAC-palpation as a method for point location was not used in China. For these reasons diverging locations developed for the same auricular points.

Vienna School

The Vienna School, headed by Prof Johannes Bischko and his disciples (including Dr Kurt König and Dr Ingrid Wancura), is the main representative of the Chinese School in Europe. They, too, do not use RAC-palpation, but locate points topographically. Given the high variation in ear anatomy, there are limits to the accuracy of this method, in particular since various ear points are often located only a few millimetres apart.

1.2 Effects of Auricular Acupuncture

1.2.1 Explanatory Models

For the physiological effects of auricular acupuncture there exist, to date, only explanatory models. In essence, there are two hypotheses; one with a physiological, the other with an energetic approach.

Physiological approach

The physiological approach explains the physical reactions to acupuncture by means of existing physiological structures, such as the nervous systems or nociceptors. This explanation is comparable to neural therapy. The effect of acupuncture could therefore be seen as a reflex to external stimulation (needle insertion). Several scientific studies were conducted to prove this hypothesis, for example by Dr Gernot Pauser (Beeinflussung der Schmerzempfindung, des Schmerzgefühls und der vegetativen Lage unter Akupunktur-„Analgesie". [The influence of acupuncture-'analgesia' on the sensation and experiencing of pain, and the autonomic nervous system.] Wiener Klassische Wochenschrift 1975; 87[19]:25–28). While these studies provided evidence that stimulating skin receptors does indeed result in a physiological reaction it remains doubtful whether this proof is sufficient to embrace the effect of acupuncture.

Energetic approach

The second model assumes that, in addition to the lymphatic and nervous system, the human body contains an invisible energetic system. This seems to be a fair assumption as acupuncture points, both on the ear (only in pathological conditions) and on the body, can be measured due to their different skin resistance compared to adjacent areas. Auricular acupuncture is considered as having a stabilising effect on the body's energetic system and is thus able to support the body's regulatory powers. It is further assumed to have a stimulating effect on the energetic system, e.g. to resolve blockages. However, it should be noted that while needling many points broadens the therapeutic range, the integration of the information provided by each point is weaker as the energy is divided up. By limiting an acupuncture treatment to only a few points, their effects are more powerful since more energy is available for each point.

The fact that the anatomically clearly defined body and ear acupuncture points can be objectively measured indicates the existence of an energetic system in the human body. However, clear scientific evidence is still missing to date.

1.2.2 Indications

Pain therapy (› 7.1–7.2)

Indicated for acute and chronic pain (› 7.1–7.2). Auricular acupuncture
- cuts down on analgesic medication
- can be used as adjunctive therapy with conventional treatments (e.g. for tumours, dental treatment etc.)

Cardiovascular disorders (› 8.1)

- As adjunctive therapy to conventional treatments (e.g. following myocardial infarction) or, initially, in combination with conventional medication (e.g. hypertension › 8.1.1)
- Reduction of medication and therefore avoidance of side effects (e.g. impotence as side effect of β-blockers)

Respiratory disorders (› 8.2)

- Curative treatment is possible with acupuncture even when conventional medicine has to resort to invasive interventions (e.g. surgery) to improve the condition (e.g. polyps, sinusitis › 8.2.4)
- Reduction of medication and therefore avoidance of side effects (e.g. cortisone for bronchial asthma › 8.2.1)

Gastrointestinal disorders (› 8.3)

- Curative treatment is possible with acupuncture even for advanced stages when conventional medicine can offer only permanent medication to improve the condition (e.g. Crohn's disease › 8.3.11)

- Reduction of medication and therefore avoidance of side effects (e.g. immunosuppressants for ulcerative colitis › 8.3.10, antacids for gastritis › 8.3.2)

Urogenital disorders (› 8.4)

- Curative treatment is possible with acupuncture even when conventional medicine can offer only permanent medication to improve the condition (e.g. urinary incontinence › 8.4.2).
- Reduction of medication and therefore avoidance of side effects (e.g. antibiotics for urinary tract infections › 8.4.1).

Skin disorders (› 8.5)

- Reduction of medication and therefore avoidance of side effects (e.g. immunosuppressants/cortisone for atopic eczema › 8.5.1).
- Increased resistance against disease-causing environmental factors

Allergic disorders (› 8.6)

- Curative treatment is possible with acupuncture while conventional medicine can offer only permanent medication or lengthy desensitisation to improve the condition (e.g. hay fever › 8.6.1)
- Reduction of medication and therefore avoidance of side effects (e.g. cortisone for allergic rashes › 8.6.2)
- Increased resistance against disease-causing environmental factors

Eye disorders (› 8.7)

- Curative therapy is possible and can replace conventional pharmacotherapy
- Slows down the progression of the disease process

Addiction (› 8.8)

- Effective only if the patient wishes to break free from his/her addiction; the success rate increases with maximum patient compliance.
- In the United States drug-dependent offenders may be given the choice between acupuncture treatments and imprisonment.
- A research study by Uwe Vertheim of the acupuncture project 'Palette 4' in Hamburg demonstrated a significant reduction of drug consumption, especially of cocaine and alcohol, as well as an overall improvement in wellbeing (March 1999).

Metabolic (› 8.9) and hormonal disorders (› 8.10)

- Curative therapy with acupuncture is possible even if conventional medicine can offer only permanent medication to improve the condition (e.g. early stages of type-II diabetes › 8.9.1, menopausal disorders › 8.10.3, premenstrual syndrome › 8.10.1).
- Reduction of medication is possible (e.g. antidiabetic medication)
- Changed laboratory parameters can be normalised

Neurological disorders (› 8.11) and disorders of the autonomic nervous system (› 8.12)

- Curative therapy for 'impaired wellbeing'
- Curative therapy with acupuncture is possible, even if conventional medicine can offer only permanent medication (e.g. for insomnia › 8.12.1)

Psychological disorders (› 8.13)

- Curative therapy with acupuncture is possible, even if conventional medication and psychotherapy (duration depends on the diagnosis) tend to be successful (e.g. depression › 8.13.1).

Anxiety (› 8.14)

- Curative therapy with acupuncture is possible, even if conventional medication and psychotherapy (duration depends on the diagnosis) tend to be successful.

1.2.3 Contraindications

Absolute contraindications

- **Localized inflammation of the ear:** Needling inflamed areas of the skin risks the transmission of germs and may cause (peri)chondritis. Since some auricular points are located very close together even a localised inflammation may result in numerous points becoming contraindicated for acupuncture. In such cases the other ear can be treated instead (based on RAC-palpation › 3.1.4). Unaffected areas of a partially inflamed ear can still be used for auricular acupuncture.
- **Scars on the external ear:** Scar tissue is contraindicated for auricular acupuncture. Scars distorting or pulling on the surrounding tissue may hinder auricular acupuncture as expected point locations may have been displaced. In these cases RAC-palpation is of particular importance.
- **Ear damage:** If parts of the ear are missing, the points represented there are lost for auricular acupuncture. This also applies to holes associated with ear rings or piercings (› 5.9.3 and › 5.9.4).
- **Absolute indication for surgery:** If, upon examining a patient, there are indications for surgery (e.g. highly acute appendicitis › 8.3.5) the patient has to be referred immediately for adequate treatment. In such cases any attempt to provide auricular acupuncture would be irresponsible.
- **Acute (life-threatening) disorders:** Any patient with a condition requiring intensive medical care (e.g. allergic oedema, asthma attack, hypertonic crisis) has to be referred for treatment with conventional medicine (e.g. cortisone in cases of allergies), even if just for legal reasons.
- **Congenital disorders:** These disorders do not respond to auricular acupuncture, in some cases symptoms can even become worse. This can, for example, occur in adrenogenital syndrome with altered steroid biosynthesis. Acupuncture can lead to an increased synthesis of steroid precursors and therefore androgenisation.

Relative contraindications

- **Pregnancy:** During pregnancy acupuncture points have to be chosen very carefully in case of any tendency to miscarry. Stimulating points should not be used (e.g. hormonal points › 6.6), while stabilising points are beneficial (e.g. Point Zero › 6.10.3, Laterality Point › 6.8.5).
- **Patient rejection:** Consciously dismissing acupuncture can block the body's energetic system to the extent that it cannot be accessed, and information provided by the acupuncture treatment can therefore not be integrated. Treating with acupuncture against the patient's wishes or without his/her consent (e.g. in the treatment of addiction) will have no effect and is therefore contraindicated. However, not believing in the effectiveness of acupuncture does not present an obstacle to treatment since, similar to conventional medicine, acupuncture is effective without 'believing' in it.

1.2.4 Complications/Interactions

Complications

On rare occasions the following can occur:
- **Needle collapse:** *Prevention* › 5.10.2; The patient should always lie down for treatment with auricular acupuncture.
- **Local inflammation** of an area that was needled: generally occurs about 3 days after an acupuncture treatment. It should not be confused with a reddening after needling (› 3.2.3). *Action:* antiseptic cream.
- **(Peri)chondritis:** *Action:* local antiseptics (e.g. Rivanol, Braunol) or poultices with chloramine solution; if required antibiotics and referal to a physician; **caution**: stop auricular acupuncture treatments until the affected area has healed completely!

Interactions

Negative interactions

Auricular acupuncture has a stabilising effect possibly on the body's energetic system and supports physiological processes in the human body. Any concurrent therapy suppressing physiological processes will interfere with acupuncture and vice versa.

In combination with acupuncture the following drugs may result in a temporary exacerbation of symptoms (› 5.9.1 Concurrent medication):
- Cortisone
- Immunosuppressants
- Antibiotics

Despite this, auricular acupuncture is still beneficial in such cases to possibly eventually discontinue these drugs. However, it requires considerable experience to manage a possible worsening of the condition and to keep it within reasonable limits.

Positive interactions

Body acupuncture and herbal medicine as part of Traditional Chinese Medicine (TCM) perfectly complement auricular acupuncture. Sometimes this combination will be necessary for optimal treatment results. When providing treatments with auricular acupuncture it is therefore of great value to have some knowledge of TCM. Auricular acupuncture is easier and quicker to learn than TCM and thus a good way to get started. The wide range of TCM treatments can then be continuously added to one's repertoire.

The following alternative and complementary therapies can be combined with auricular acupuncture without any concerns:

- Anthroposophical medicine
- Breathing therapy
- Detoxification (cupping, blood letting, leech therapy etc.)
- Autogenic training
- Bach flower remedies
- Autohemotherapy
- Enzyme therapy
- Homoeopathy
- Manual therapies
- Osteopathy
- Lifestyle regulation therapy
- Physical therapies
- Western herbal medicine
- Reflexology
- Oxygen/ozone therapy
- Microbiological therapy
- Vitamin therapy
- Live cell therapy

Generally, a combination of many of these therapies with auricular acupuncture and TCM does not further enhance the treatment effect, neither does it shorten the treatment course. The motto 'the more, the better' does not apply in this case since the body's ability to respond to set stimuli is limited.

2 Clinical Equipment and Practice Management

2.1 Tips for Everyday Clinical Work

Attention to those aspects that help the patient to relax can significantly enhance the therapeutic effect of auricular acupuncture and TCM.

2.1.1 Treatment Rooms

- **Atmosphere:** A personal atmosphere – the patient should already feel comfortable in the waiting room. Decorative features such as pictures and flowers as well as a welcoming cup of tea all have a positive effect.
- **Layout:** Ideal are three treatment rooms per practitioner in order to facilitate a smooth flow. This allows the patient to rest with inserted needles for at least 20 minutes. Ideally walk-through rooms should not be used as treatments rooms.
- **Lighting:** Daylight is best for optimal tongue diagnosis. If artificial light has to be used ideal is indirect, bright lighting as this does not blind the patient and promotes relaxation.

2.1.2 Clinic Hours

It is advisable to use an appointment-based system as acupuncture treatments tend to be lengthy but calculable. Long waiting times (more than 15 minutes) related to organisational matters should be avoided. Unforeseen circumstances or emergencies leading to delays have, of course, to be taken into consideration.

If possible, patients should be able to contact the practitioner on weekends and public holidays (e.g. voicemail and call back) or a weekend cover should be organised with colleagues. This gives the patient the confidence to be treated in an emergency and not having to rely on conventional medicine. It also allows the therapeutic approach to remain unaffected (e.g. trying to avoid cortisone).

2.1.3 Clinic Organisation

- **Appointment time:** The patient should be advised to come at least 5 minutes prior to the actual appointment time
- **Initial consultation:** At least 30 minutes; comprises the medical history (› 5.1) including both the conventional medical history as well as aspects of TCM; review of preliminary findings brought along by the client
- **Patient information:** At the first appointment the auricular acupuncture treatments should be discussed in some detail. Any questions should be answered and the treatment process should be explained to allay any fears of this potentially unknown therapy.
- **Initial examination:** Generally a systematic and complete examination of the whole body (› 5.2.1) including TCM-parameters (especially tongue and pulse diagnosis) as well as RAC-palpation (› 3.1.4)
- **Needling** (› 3.2): Patients should always be treated lying down to prevent cardiovascular reactions (e.g. dizziness, fainting). In addition, lying down will further relax the patient.

- **Needle removal** (› 3.2.5): The needles are retained for at least 20 minutes; they are removed by the practitioner or an assistant.
- **Follow-up examinations:** Known pathological findings must be monitored while new findings have to be taken into consideration; tongue and pulse diagnosis have to be repeated at each session; RAC-findings of all needled points to date have to be re-examined while relevant points pertaining to new symptoms have to be checked.

The therapist cannot delegate the following activities:
- Taking of the medical history
- Physical examination
- Needling

2.1.4 Marketing

Due to increasing competition as well as the growing number of therapies on offer it is becoming more and more important to clearly present and define one's own skills (scope of practice).

- **Patient marketing:** mainly word of mouth; advertising is generally not as effective.
- **Clinic location:** For a specialised practice, such as for auricular acupuncture, a central location does not tend to be relevant. It is much more important to provide a stress-free access route, parking, and a relaxing environment.
- **Target group selection:** During the initial stages of practice development it is sensible to offer a wide spectrum (e.g. treatments for a wide range of disorders, addressing all age ranges); specialisations, such as in auricular acupuncture, will follow naturally based on therapeutic results.
- **Range of therapies:** A wide range of therapies (e.g. auricular acupuncture **and** homoeopathy **and** osteopathy **and** conventional medicine) is certainly desirable but not realistic since each method alone requires intensive training, experience in clinical application as well as continuous professional development. **Caution:** Don't diversify too much, it's better to expand core competencies! Due to the different diagnostic principles and partially conflicting treatment approaches using Chinese and Western medicine side-by-side makes only limited sense. However, a good knowledge of conventional medicine is an indispensable basis for the assessment of disease and for recognising the limits of auricular acupuncture/TCM.

Rules and Regulations

As rules and regulations regarding signage, advertising, professional stationery, as well as practice logos vary from country to country describing these in more detail is well beyond the scope of this book. The same applies to fee structures, billing, and dealing with insurance companies.

Requirements for a successful acupuncture practice:
- In-depth knowledge of conventional medicine
- Specialisation (e.g. auricular acupuncture)
- Verifiable in-depth training in auricular acupuncture/TCM
- Compassionate approach to clients, taking sufficient time for clients
- Well-managed practice with short waiting times

- Fair fee structure
- A pleasant and comfortable atmosphere (e.g. based on *feng shui*) and appropriate service (e.g. drinks available in the waiting area).

2.1.5 Documentation

The documentation required by the legislator, local authorities, and/or professional organisations varies from country to country. Below is a sample, which may have to be modified based on regional requirements.

The patient documentation is carried out on a separate page from the patient record. Alternatively, all points used can be marked in a print of an ear (or an ear stamp › 2.4.6). Example:

Ms Gaby Sunshine (Date of Birth: 30 May 1968)

16/02/1999

Main complaint: acute myalgia of the spine for 2 days

RHS: PGE$_1$, L4, Muscle Relaxation (98a), Diazepam

LHS: Atlanto-occipital Joint, C7, T8, Thymus

20/02/1999

Main complaint: following acupuncture symptom-free, after 2 days again pain in the cervical and lumbar spine, but less than before

RHS: L4, Diazepam

LHS: C7, Thalamus (26a)

2.2 Tools for Point Location

2.2.1 Stirrup Probe

This is a stirrup-shaped metal wire or a tool with a plastic edge (approximately 5 mm long) attached to a guide handle. Variation: also available with the stirrup integrated into the handle of a spring-loaded probe (› 2.2.3, › fig. 2.4-1).

- **Method:** notches in the auricular cartilage are easily palpable by sliding with light pressure over the cartilage with the flat wire or the plastic surface
- **Application:** used for the location of objective auricular landmarks palpable as notches: Atlanto-occipital Joint, transition cervical/thoracic spine, transition thoracic/lumbar spine (› 6.1.1, Point Zero (› 6.10.3)
- **Evaluation:** useful tool for beginners facilitating confident location of notches and certain points which serve as landmarks for locating further ear points
- **Maintenance:** none

 An improvised stirrup probe can easily be made from a paper clip by bending open the long wire on its side and using it as a guide handle. The short straight end is used for palpation.

2.2.2 Electrical Tools for Point Location

- **Method**: These tools measure the electrical skin resistance. Irritated projection zones/points present with an altered skin resistance compared to adjacent areas. The potential difference is measured by means of a metal pin with a tip with a diameter of 0.3 mm, which is brought into contact with the suspected ear point, and (in most devices) an integrated reference probe. To close the circuit, and depending on the type of detector, either the patient's hand has to be placed on an electrode plate or, (if the reference electrode is integrated in the handle of the device) the practitioner has to touch the patient's ear lobe with his/her hand. Suspicious skin areas are displayed either visually or acoustically depending on the make of the detector. **Caution**: Before the examination, the device has to be calibrated to the patient's skin resistance; in modern devices this adjustment is automatic.
- **Application:** commonly used method; suitable for beginners to confirm points which have been detected by RAC-palpation (› 3.1.4)
- **Evaluation:** advocated by many authors as a suitable point location method besides RAC; disadvantages: hidden points are difficult to measure; depending on the adjustment of the sensitivity false positive or false negative values are possible; suitable for checking pathological points determined by RAC-palpation.
- **Maintenance:** regular monitoring of the device by the manufacturer

2.2.3 Spring-loaded Probe

This comprises a metal pin mounted on a spring and is used to check the pressure sensitivity of auricular points (› fig. 2.4-1).
- **Principle:** this point location method dates back to the beginnings of auricular acupuncture (mechanical point detection, › 3.1.1). Rule of thumb: the more active (that is the more pathological) a point, the more pressure-sensitive it will be
- **Application:** to confirm points detected by RAC-palpation (› 3.1.4), useful for beginners
- **Evaluation:** Today, this method is considered not suitable for clinical practice as it is time-consuming and not very meaningful due to the subjective nature of the patient's feedback ('after a thorough examination the whole ear hurts')
- **Maintenance:** The spring function should be checked before each examination

2.3 Examination Hammers

2.3.1 3-Volt Hammer

Plastic hammer with two steel poles; › fig. 2.4-1.
- **Principle:** The potential difference of 3V between the two steel poles is maintained by an AA battery. **Caution**: A short circuit between the two poles (e.g. by contact with the opposing pole of a second hammer) must be avoided at all costs!
- **Application:** Points with an altered skin resistance will trigger a RAC. To find points

with reduced skin resistance (approximately 90 % of points, › 3.1.4) the area to be examined is touched or scanned (at a distance of a few millimetres) with the positive pole. The same procedure is carried out for points with increased skin resistance (approximately 10 % of points, › 3.1.4) but the negative pole is used instead. Pathological or irritated points will elicit a RAC-response.

- **Evaluation:** provides significantly stronger stimulation than the black-white hammer, and somewhat weaker stimulation than the gold-silver-hammer; most widely used type of hammer due to the best cost-benefit ratio
- **Maintenance:** regular (weekly) checks of the voltage with a voltmeter are necessary if the maximum RAC-response is to be achieved. **Caution:** If the battery is flat the hammer will still trigger an – albeit significantly weaker – RAC-response due to the self potential of the steel pin

2.3.2 Gold-Silver Hammer

The hammer head is formed by a gold pin and a silver pin which are separated from the handle by a non-conducting material (e.g. wood), › fig. 2.4-1. This type of hammer was originally used by Nogier (› 1.1.2) for RAC-palpation

- **Principle:** the gold and the silver pin are separated by (non-conducting) wood, resulting in a voltage build-up between the gold and the silver
- **Application:** Points with an altered skin resistance will trigger a RAC. To find points with reduced skin resistance (approximately 90 % of points, › 3.1.4) the area to be examined is touched or scanned (at a distance of a few millimetres) with the positive pole. The same procedure is carried out for points with increased skin resistance (10 % of points, › 3.1.4) but the negative pole is used instead. Pathological or irritated points will elicit a RAC-response.
- **Evaluation:** provides a stronger stimulus than the 3V or the black-white hammer. Disadvantage: expensive, basically the price depends on the price of gold
- **Maintenance:** checking the voltage not necessary
- **Caution:** Gold-silver hammers must not get wet to prevent a voltage drop
- **Special note:** Gold-silver hammers are not available by acupuncture suppliers. They are bespoke tools made by a goldsmith or dental technician (generally the cheaper option).

2.3.3 Black-White Hammer

A plastic hammer with a white and black plastic pin on opposite sides (› fig. 2.4-1).

- **Principle:** based on the assumption that ear points are energetically influenced by the different wave lengths of the colours black and white.
- **Application:** Points with an altered skin resistance will trigger a RAC (› 3.1.4). To find points with reduced skin resistance (approximately 90 % of points, › 3.1.4) the area to be examined is touched or scanned (at a distance of a few millimetres) with the positive pole. The same procedure is carried out for points with increased skin resistance (approximately 10 % of points, › 3.1.4) but the negative pole is used instead. Pathological or irritated points will elicit a RAC-response.

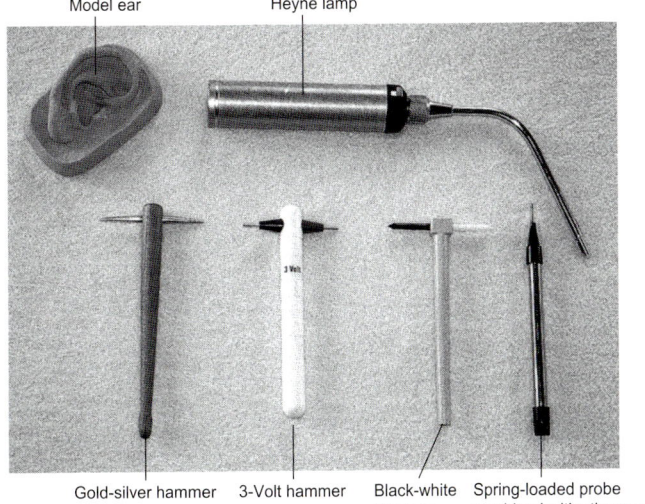

Fig. 2.4-1 Tools used in auricular acupuncture

- **Evaluation:** provides a significantly weaker stimulus than the 3V hammer or the gold-silver hammer, therefore not recommended for beginners. Advantage: inexpensive
- **Maintenance:** none

2.4 Other Tools

2.4.1 Heyne-Lamp

Light source with point light bundling (low dispersion), battery operated, also is used for ENT examinations, › fig. 2.4-1.
- **Principle:** The light stimulus causes a change of the arterial pulse curve (artificial RAC › 3.1.4)
- **Application:** for standardised RAC-activation in each patient before starting ear point diagnosis; it provides the practitioner with a sense of the individual differences in RAC quality; stronger response when stimulating more sensitive skin areas (e.g. face).
- **Evaluation:** useful for beginners; may be replaced by a flashlight with a focussed light beam as this is a significantly cheaper option
- **Maintenance:** regular change of batteries

2.4.2 9-Volt Rod

A bipolar metal rod, approximately 20 cm long with a diameter of 2.5 cm. The potential difference between the poles is usually 9V but there are also devices with a higher voltage.
- **Principle:** The patient's energetic field can be influenced by holding the rod with either the positive or negative pole in his/her hand

- **Method:** Amplifies pathological points (which can be measured by changes in the electrical skin resistance); corresponds roughly to the gold-silver hammer. By touching certain locations on the ear with different substances (histamine, Cytoxan, vitamin C, prostaglandin, and ginseng) while at the same time amplifying the energetic field (by the patient holding the positive terminal of the 9V rod in the hand contralateral to the examined ear), it is possible to establish a hierarchy of interference field points according to their severity.
- **Evaluation:** Establishing a hierarchy of pathological points according to their severity is irrelevant to the therapeutic results; the device is therefore more of diagnostic value.
- **Maintenance:** Regular (weekly) checks of the voltage with a voltmeter necessary. The device is operated with several AA batteries with a lifespan of several years, as long as a short-circuit between the two poles is avoided (e.g. by touching it with the opposing pole of a second rod).

2.4.3 Patient Grounding

- **Principle:** A metal clip which is attached to the patient's ear lobe is connected by a wire to the ground in an electric outlet.
- **Method:** Reduces electrical potentials which could trigger artificial RAC-reactions (› 3.1.4)
- **Evaluation:** of consideration for beginners in order to reduce artificial RAC-reactions
- **Maintenance:** none

2.4.4 Marker Pen

- **Method:** to mark pathological points following point location to facilitate precise needle insertion
- **Choice of pen:** coloured felt-tip pens (ideally green as this provides the best contrast) with a fine point are the pen of choice; best are waterproof pens as they are more resistant to contact with sebum. **Caution: always** remove the marked points with an alcohol swab before needling (› 3.2.1, disinfection), otherwise there will be permanent 'tattoos'!

2.4.5 Model Ear

Replica of a human ear for training purposes, › fig. 2.4-1.
- **Material:** usually rubber as this corresponds well to the consistency of the human ear; practice needling leaves no permanent marks
- **Application:**
  - **demonstrating** needling and point location
  - **patient information**, in particular when using semi-permanent needles that have to be stimulated by the patient
  - **training purposes:** useful for beginners practising point location but also for demonstrating the relative location of points on the anterior aspect of the ear compared to points on its posterior aspect; e.g. shoulder (› 6.2.1, › 6.11.2) and elbow (› 6.2.1, › 6.11.2)

2.4.6 Ear Stamp

A stamp representing the gross anatomical structures of the ear.
- **Application:** documentation of each treatment by marking the points needled on the stamped image; it is essential to label all the points since points located close to each other cannot be distinguished by marking alone.

2.5 Needles

2.5.1 Stainless Steel Disposable Needles

As a general rule, the intensity of the pain is largely independent of the needle gauge.
- **Material:** disposable stainless steel needles are preferable to gold and silver needles as they combine the advantages of both (material overview, table › 2.5-1).
- **Length:** approximately 35 mm; longer needles are available but not recommended. Disadvantage: inaccurate placement due to the greater distance between the tip and the handle of the needle, difficulty of placing several needles close together in the confined space of the ear
- **Gauge:** 0.3–1.0 mm, usually recommended are 0.4–0.7 mm as this is a suitable gauge even for hidden locations (not flexible!). **Caution:** the smaller the gauge, the more accurately the needles have to be placed
- **Needling technique:** › 3.2

2.5.2 Semi-permanent Needles

Semi-permanent needles remain inserted beyond the actual treatment session.
- **Duration:** 7 days to a maximum of 2 weeks; based on experience the therapeutic effect diminishes significantly after approximately one week. Also, some needles fall out prematurely despite proper insertion, a typical phenomenon in points with stagnant energy, or after successful therapy of the complaint (if symptoms persist, needling should be repeated after 2–3 days).
- **Indications:** The use of semi-permanent needles is controversial; according to some authors the effect corresponds to that of needling during the actual treatment while the risk of infection is higher due to skin germs in the vicinity of the insertion site; often favoured by patients due to the psychological aspect ('taking the therapy home'); mainly used in addiction treatment (› 8.8), for interference fields (› 5.7), and for chronic disorders
- **Contraindications:** children (due to greater pain than disposable needles)
- **Complications:** infection; mechanical irritation, e.g. during sleep
- **Needle types:** generally ASP semi-permanent needles; less commonly Pyonex needles, Chinese seeds, and stainless steel press pellets
- **Needle technique:** › 3.2

ASP Semi-permanent Needles

A semi-permanent needle implanted by means of a guiding device with a plunger

- **Length:** approximately 3 mm, tip 2 mm
- **Diameter:** cone-shaped, on the base approximately 0.7 mm
- **Advantages:** The guiding device can be used to scan the ear for RAC-reactions (›
  3.1.4). Embedded in the needle guide is a magnet for stimulating the semi-permanent needle; the stimulation can also be carried out at home by the patient; this feature
  makes semi-permanent ASP needles particularly useful for addiction therapy (needling technique › 3.2.2); ASP semi-permanent needles are also available in gold.
- **Disadvantage:** due to the cone-shaped tip more painful insertion than Pyonex semi-
  permanent needles
- **Application:** once the accurate location has been determined by RAC-palpation the
  guiding device with the needle is pressed onto the ear, and the guiding device is then
  removed; a plaster supplied with the needle can be applied.
- **Needling technique:** › 3.2

Pyonex™ Press Tack Needles

Semi-permanent needle ending in a small, flat spiral which is attached to a plaster.

- **Length:** 1.5–1.8 mm
- **Diameter:** approximately 0.3 mm
- **Advantage:** thinner than ASP semi-permanent needles; due to the smoothly tapered
  tip less painful insertion than ASP needles
- **Disadvantage:** difficult to insert in precisely the right place, especially with hidden
  points
- **Needling technique:** › 3.2
- **Application:** press onto the ear the tape to which the press tack is attached

Permanent Implants

Permanent needles implanted directly and invisibly under the skin at pathological areas of
the ear.

- **Length:** approximately 2.9 mm +/− 0.2 mm
- **Diameter**: approximately 0.8 mm
- **Bio-resolvable material:** transparent, absorption time approximately 18 months, e.g.
  Templax quint (pentangle), Templax (cone)
- **Non-resolvable material**: medical titanium, e.g. Implax (cone)
- **Advantage:** more intense effect than other acupuncture techniques, e.g. for tinnitus,
  Parkinson's disease
- **Disadvantage:** granuloma formation cannot be excluded
- **Needling technique:** inserted by pressing a guide tube into subcutaneous tissue, simi-
  lar to the insertion of ASP semi-permanent needles (see above)

Chinese Seeds

Chinese version of semi-permanent needles; generally vaccaria seeds (cow soapwort seeds) are used.

- **Advantage:** additional hyperaemic effect; well suited for self-massage; useful for needle-phobic patients, environmentally friendly
- **Disadvantage:** difficult to place in the precise spot, for this reason inferior to the needles described above

Press balls

Small stainless steel balls; magnetic versions are available (allegedly stronger therapeutic effect).

- **Advantage:** well-suited for self-massage; useful for needle-phobic patients
- **Disadvantage:** difficult to place in the precise spot, for this reason inferior to the needles described above
- **Indication:** treatment of addiction

 As Chinese seeds and press balls are difficult to place in precisely the correct spot they are inferior to the semi-permanent needles described above. They can therefore not be recommended for a differentiated therapy.

2.5.3 Needle Material

In contrast to body acupuncture, auricular acupuncture cannot achieve a tonifying or sedating effect based on needling technique. These effects are more likely elicited by the material of the needle. The sole use of stainless steel needles seems justified as they generally have a balancing effect. The use of gold and silver needles therefore offers no significant advantage. For historical reasons and for the sake of completeness the different usage is shown in the following table:

Tab. 2.5-1 Needle material

Material	Gold	Silver	Stainless Steel
Properties	• tonifying • augments energy • stimulating	• sedating • drains energy	• depending on the ear point either tonifying or sedating*
Special features	• contraindicated for ear points that are to be sedated (e.g. Anti-Aggression, Diazepam etc.)	• contraindicated for ear points that are to be tonified (e.g. analgesic points, organ points)	• suitable for all ear points
Needle type	• disposable and semi-permanent needles (generally gold-plated)	• disposable and semi-permanent needles (generally silver-plated)	• disposable and semi-permanent needles

* In cases of deficiency, the point is tonified; in cases of excess it is sedated. In case of the latter, there can be bleeding upon needle removal (› 3.2.3).

2.5.4 Needle Disposal

All needles have to be disposed in accordance with the relevant regulations of the local authority, state, and/or professional organisation.

3 Methods and Techniques

Patients will find it reassuring and will feel more confident if the practitioner explains every step of the examination and treatment at the first appointment.

3.1 Point Location

The best environment for safe and reliable point location is a treatment room without technical equipment, providing a relaxing atmosphere (tranquillity, some ornaments, flowers) for both, therapist and patient.

 All pathological points should be located before needling since needling of the first point may change all other points. Pathological points may reinforce each other and are therefore easier to locate before the start of the actual treatment.

3.1.1 Mechanical Point Location

This is the oldest method for locating pathological ear points; correlating findings on the ear with existing disease patterns formed the basis for the auricular topography.
- **Principle:** systematic palpation of the entire surface of the ear with a probe (› 2.2.3). Important: constant and unchanging pressure! Points that are tender in comparison to their environment are classified as pathological and require treatment.
- **Advantage:** easy to use
- **Disadvantage:**
  - painful and inaccurate; findings depend, among other things, on the patient's sensitivity to pain
  - detailed examination of the ear or repeated checking of a particular point are not possible due to the painful nature of this method
  - difficulty in differentiating painful points located close to each other

This method is not suitable for a comprehensive examination of the whole ear but is useful for verifying results obtained by other point location methods.

3.1.2 'Very-Point-Technique'

This technique developed by J Gleditsch represents a further development of the mechanical point location method. It was initially developed as part of mouth acupuncture for locating pathological points on the oral mucosa since direct palpation is hardly possible in the damp environment of the oral cavity. Today this technique is also used in auricular acupuncture as a direct method.
- **Principle:** Auricular areas suspected to be pathological are scanned with an acupuncture needle for increased sensitivity by very lightly tapping or very gently brushing over the surface. Points with increased pain sensitivity and reduced skin turgor (the 'very point' after Gleditsch) can be needled without any resistance of the tissue.
- **Advantage:** quick and elegant method since it does not require a change of equipment between point location and needling
- **Disadvantage:** risk of injury during scanning if the technique is not adequately performed

Needling a pathological point may influence other pathological points/areas that have not been located yet, changing both their quality and their size. Sometimes points may no longer be found. For these reasons point location and actual needling should ideally be separate processes. However, this is not possible with the 'very point-technique'.

3.1.3 Electrical Point Location

- **Principle:** Compared to adjacent skin areas, pathological ear points exhibit an increased electrical skin resistance. In around 90 % of points the resistance is reduced while in around 10 % of points it is increased. Special point detectors (› 2.2.2) were developed to measure electrical skin resistance. Depending on the type of change in electrical resistance these detectors distinguish between silver points (increased resistance) and gold points (decreased resistance). A number of different models are available. When selecting a detector the following general rule applies: the simpler the construction and the more functional the design, the easier it will be to use in clinical practice.

- **Method:** Patient in relaxed supine position; the therapist's arms are resting on the treatment couch, while the fingers of the examining hand are resting at the level of the mastoid; if the detector has a grounding electrode, the patient has to hold this in his/her hand; if there is no grounding electrode the therapist has to touch the patient with the other hand. *Calibration*: The patient's individual skin resistance should be calibrated on an inconspicuous area (e.g. Point Zero); longer examinations may require recalibration. **Caution**: Failing to calibrate the detector or improper calibration may result in incorrect measurements! *Point location*: Based on the medical history relevant points are scanned with the tip of the detector. The device will respond to a pathological point with either an acoustic or optic signal.

 Different areas of the ear may present with a different skin resistance: the area adjacent to a suspected point should therefore be recalibrated.

- **Advantages:** standardised, objective method; suitable for beginners
- **Disadvantages:** The devices can be awkward to handle and are often expensive; false negative or false positive results depending on the sensitivity of the detector; due to being unwieldy they are not suitable for a complete examination of the ear and therefore not useful for everyday clinical practice. Covered points are difficult to evaluate.

3.1.4 Réflexe Auriculocardiaque (RAC)

Synonym: Vascular autonomic signal (VAS). The 'réflexe auriculocardiaque' refers to a change in pulse quality (amplitude and time shift, no change in frequency) caused by the stimulation of a pathological ear point with a diagnostic device (› 2.3, examination hammer).

- **Historical background:** In 1968, the French physician Paul Nogier discovered by accident a change in the pulse when examining auricular locations corresponding to pathological areas of the body. A systematic investigation of this phenomenon showed that during stimulation of altered ear zones the arterial pulse wave (e.g. radial pulse) showed a characteristic change. Nogier interpreted this reaction as a polysynaptic reflex and introduced the term 'réflexe auriculocardiaque' (RAC).

- **Theory:** Pathological auricular acupuncture points show an altered electrical skin resistance. In around 90 % of cases the resistance is reduced, while in around 10 % of cases it is increased. If points with an altered electrical resistance are brought into contact (skin contact or a small distance from the skin) with an electrical current (e.g. self potential of a metal or battery voltage) or a colour stimulus (black, white), this will trigger a sympathetic stimulation in the body. This causes the closure of arteriovenous shunts which in turn results in a short-term increase of blood in the arterial system, triggering the so-called RAC.

Requirements for RAC-palpation

- **Selecting an ear probe:** Despite the plethora of devices available only a few basic tools are necessary. Much more important than specific tools is the sensitivity and experience of the therapist, which no tool can replace. The only essential tool for RAC-palpation is an ear probe(› 2.3). Whether any further devices are considered necessary has to remain the judgement of the therapist.
- **Selecting an artery:** As the sympathetic reaction affects the entire vascular system, any artery can be used to assess the change in pulse quality. Traditionally, the radial artery is used since the therapist tends to be seated behind the patient. Alternatively, the carotid artery can be used if there is shoulder pain or in elderly patients with less mobile upper arms, as well as in patients with large forearms or a hardly palpable arterial pulse. As the quality of the pulse may vary simply due to the differences in diameter it is recommended to use only one artery, especially for beginners.

RAC-palpation: method

- Patient in a supine position, therapist seated behind the patient's head.
- The therapist takes the patient's pulse (ideally the arterial pulse, in exceptional cases the carotid pulse) with the thumb of the non-dominant hand (left hand in right-handed persons, right hand in left-handed persons).
- At the same time the therapist scans first the patient's dominant ear with an ear probe, followed by the non-dominant ear (e.g. in right-handed patients first the right ear, then the left ear); maximum distance to the surface of the skin: 5 mm; the skin may be touched.
- **Selecting auricular points to be tested:** The selection of relevant points is based on the patient's main complaint, his/her medical history as well as the physical examination (point recommendations › 7.1–7.5 und › 8.1–8.15)
- **Palpating finger:** Compared to the other fingers, the thumb has the highest number of sensitive receptors and is therefore most suited for perceiving changes in the pulse. Although the therapist's own pulse can feel disturbing in the beginning, after some practice one generally does not perceive it anymore.
- **Two methods for taking the pulse:**
  - The tip of the thumb is placed on the artery against its flow (classical method): this method has the advantage that the pulse wave contacts the thumb on its most sensitive area (tip) and is therefore easier to feel (› Fig. 3.1-1).
  - The tip of the thumb is placed on the artery at an angle of 90° to the arterial flow; this method has the advantage that the patient's arm does not have to be overextended towards posterior as much (› Fig. 3.1-2).

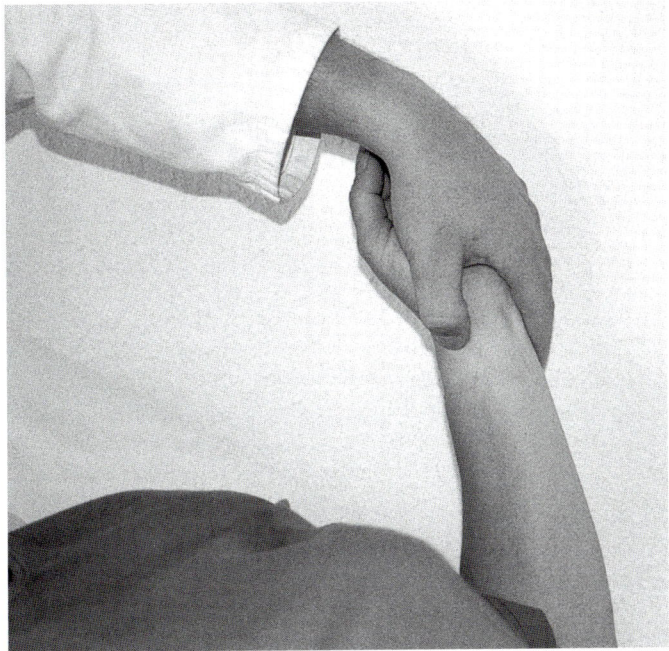

Fig. 3.1-1 Taking the pulse, method a. The pulse wave travels towards the thumb

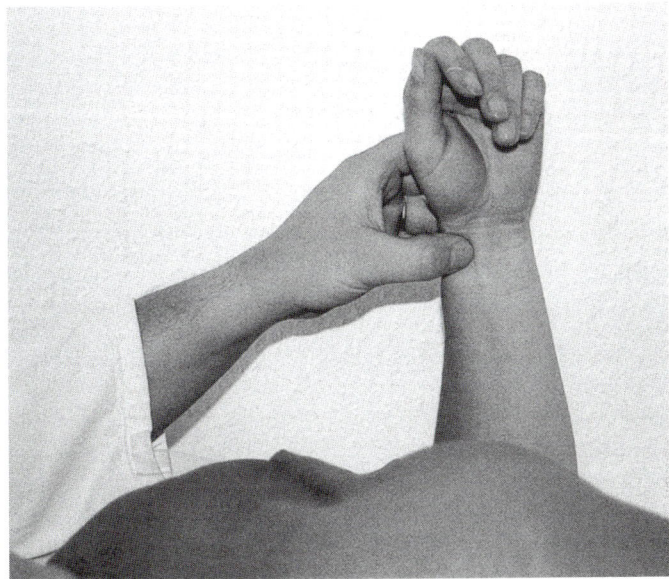

Fig. 3.1-2 Taking the pulse, method b. The pulse wave travels transversely past the thumb

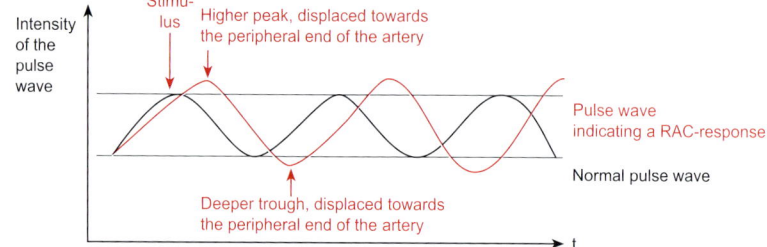

Fig. 3.1-3   RAC: Change of the waveform.

- If a pathological ear point is stimulated the therapist will feel a change in the quality of the pulse. *Characteristic phenomenon*: The typical RAC-reaction can be felt as an increase of blood volume in the palpated artery (generally the radial artery). While the pulse rate itself does not increase the amplitude is higher. Since each peak is followed by a trough, a deeper trough develops briefly (› Fig. 3.1-3). By focusing on the peak of the wave the therapist will feel a fuller pulse approaching his/her finger, while by concentrating on the trough, he/she will feel the pulse receding (referred to as negative RAC). Both sensations describe the same phenomenon.

RAC-reaction at pathological ear points

The RAC in reaction to the stimulation of pathological ear points has the following quality:
- A significantly fuller pulse for at least 3–7 beats.
- The RAC-reaction can be reproduced by repeating the same stimulus.

Artificial RAC-reaction at non-pathological points

Non-pathological ear points as well as any skin area will elicit a RAC-response when stimulated by touch (e.g. with a probe › 2.3) or a light source with a punctiform beam (› 2.4.1). However, this differs from the RAC-response of stimulated pathological points:
- A significantly fuller pulse for a maximum of 1–3 beats
- The RAC response cannot be reproduced reliably but it can be triggered by simply touching the skin or other external stimuli (e.g. light source with punctiform beam)

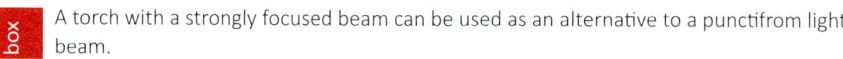

box A torch with a strongly focused beam can be used as an alternative to a punctifrom light beam.

Factors affecting the RAC-response

Various factors can influence the quality of the RAC-response. These have to be considered when interpreting the test results.
- **Sensitivity of each individual patient:** The sensitivity threshold as well as the range of the reactivity necessary for triggering a RAC and changing the waveform before and after the stimulus vary from patient to patient. Beginners should therefore carry out a 'self-calibration' in the patient before the actual RAC-palpation. This is achieved by triggering an artificial RAC for several times (e.g. with a light stimulus [› 2.4.1] on the face).
- **Size of the artery:** Larger arteries (e.g. carotid artery), by their nature, carry a larger amount of blood. A change in volume caused by a RAC will result in the pulse feeling somewhat stronger.

- **Quality of the pulse:** If a pulse is strong, e.g. due to hypertension, a change in the volume of the artery can be felt more easily.
- **Location of the vessel:** The more superficial and the less embedded in tissue (adipose, muscle, and connective tissue) the more distinctive will be the pulse and its changes during a RAC-response.
- **Observation by the therapist:** Depending on whether the therapist places the focus on the peak or the trough of the pulse wave, he/she will perceive the RAC response as a fuller or a more receding pulse.
- **Pathological pulse:** In particular atrial fibrillation with irregular conduction of impulses as well as ectopic beats result in a variable fullness of the pulse, even without stimulation of auricular points. This can mimic a RAC response. Considerable experience is required to differentiate between a pathological pulse and an actual RAC response.

> **box** Locating points by RAC-palpation is an objective method which can be reproduced in the same way by several practitioners independent of each other. However, the prerequisite is a professional training, sensitivity, sufficient practice, and consideration of interfering factors.

3.2 Needling

> **box** The points relevant for treatment are selected and needled by RAC-palpation. Both French and Chinese points are equally effective, and, depending on findings, can be combined with each other. By the same token the combination of auricular and body acupuncture is always advisable and often necessary for optimal treatment results. 'Moxibustion' (warming the needle with a lighter/match) can be used for points which should be tonified. Since this method does not tend to significantly improve the treatment effect it is not recommended here, especially since there is a substantial risk of singeing hair in the proximity of the ear.

The preparations and diagnostic process allow the therapist to establish a rapport with the patient. Once the pathological points have been determined the acupuncture treatment can eventually be carried out. After disinfecting the relevant areas the dominant ear is needled first, followed by the non-dominant ear (> 5.4.1). This standardised treatment procedure helps to avoid location mistakes related to dominance. For example, the point Barbiturate (> 6.7.1) is located only on the non-dominant ear, that is on the left ear in right-handed persons and on the right ear in left-handed persons. If the non-dominant ear is always examined second, it is easy to avoid needling the wrong (dominant) ear.

> **box** Acupuncture always causes a microtrauma in the surrounding tissue. After removing the needle, healing processes in the body (migration of leukocytes, new growth of connective tissue etc.) result in a continued stimulation of the point for days. The one-off puncture of a point has therefore the same effect as a semi-permanent needle which becomes ineffective after about one week (provided it does not fall out before) as the body adapts to the stimulus.

3.2.1 Disinfection

After marking the points with a marker pen (› 2.4.4) they are wiped with a swab (soaked with a disinfecting agent) before needling. This prevents 'tattooing' the ear and disinfects the surface.

Marking the points provides an overview of the ear before needling it. This is particularly helpful when treating both ears in several patients one after the other as it can be difficult to remember all the relevant points prior to needling.

 Prior to needling, the coloured points have to be wiped off with a disinfecting solution to avoid point-shaped 'tattoos' by inserting the needle into the coloured dots.

3.2.2 Needling Techniques

Disposable needles

- **Hand position for needling:** the needle is held by the handle with the thumb and forefinger of the dominant hand (pincer grasp)
- **Insertion:** with a quick turning movement; the quicker the insertion the less pain will be felt by the patient
- **Insertion depth:** approximately 2–3 mm; depending on the location the needle tip will generally reach soft tissue (e.g. perichondrium, subcutaneous tissue), more rarely also cartilage (e.g. on the antihelix). **Caution**: due to the higher risk of infection a trauma to the cartilage should be avoided! The ear should not be punctured since a connection between the anterior and posterior ear creates an energetic short circuit and weakens the effect of acupuncture. This does not apply to the pincer technique (needling a point with two separate needles on the corresponding anterior and posterior points) which increases the effect of acupuncture on the point.

Semi-permanent needles

ASP semi-permanent needles (› 2.5.3)

- **Hand position for needling:** The needle is held by the handle with the thumb and forefinger of the dominant hand (pincer grasp).
- **Insertion:** The needle with the guide tube (injector) is pressed into the tissue; the injector is then pushed back and the handle removed; the enclosed adhesive plaster is attached over the needle.
- **Depth:** approximately 2 mm; depending on the location the needle tip will generally reach soft tissue (e.g. perichondrium, subcutaneous tissue), more rarely also cartilage (e.g. on the antihelix). **Caution**: due to the higher risk of infection a trauma to the cartilage should be avoided!
- **Special feature:** The injector, which contains a small magnet, can be given to the patient for added stimulation (instruction: turn the magnet over the semi-permanent needle, e.g. for withdrawal › 8.8).

Pyonex semi-permanent needles (› 2.5.3)

- **Hand position for needling:** The needle, including the adhesive plaster, is guided with thumb and forefinger of the dominant hand.

- **Insertion:** The needle is pressed perpendicularly into the auricular tissue, the plaster will automatically cover the insertion site. **Caution:** More painful than disposable needles as it is not possible to turn Pyonex needles during insertion.

- **Depth:** Approximately 2 mm; depending on the location the needle tip will generally reach soft tissue (e.g. perichondrium, subcutaneous tissue), more rarely also cartilage (e.g. on the antihelix). **Caution**: due to the higher risk of infection a trauma to the cartilage should be avoided!

- **Special feature:** Precise placement is difficult as these needles cannot be easily guided, especially when needling hidden ear points

3.2.3 Accompanying Signs and Symptoms

Pain

The pain sensation experienced with auricular acupuncture shows considerable individual differences, ranging from 'insignificant' to 'hardly bearable'. Most patients describe auricular acupuncture as 'unpleasant but perfectly tolerable'.

- **Initial pain:** most common form of pain, especially during puncturing of the skin or upon reaching the cartilage with the needle tip; the intensity of the pain can be reduced by turning the needle during insertion (› 3.2.3)

- **Pain during needle retention:** rare; occasionally a distending pain as an expression of the increased activity of the point; the more active (i.e. the more pathological) a point is, the more it will be sensitive to pain.

- **Pain during needle removal:** very rare

- **Pain after needle removal:** very rarely the pain will persist after needle removal; sometimes it may last for several days as a sign of increased activity of the point

Generally, all forms of pain occur independently of the needle gauge (0.3–0.8 mm).

Erythema of the insertion site

- Typically, this occurs within seconds after needle insertion; does not occur always or in every patient (among other factors it is dependent on the sensitivity of the skin). **Caution:** a reddening of the skin immediately after acupuncture should not be confused with an inflammatory reaction (e.g. infectious chondritis or mechanical irritation; › 1.2.3, Complications). This occurs at the earliest 3–4 days after the treatment.

- A reddening of the skin indicates an 'energetic reaction'. This is a perfectly desired effect and certainly not an inflammatory response.

- The more pathological the point (the more it requires treatment), the more pronounced will be the reaction. **Caution:** Do not remove the needle early just because of a reddening around the insertion site!

If a needle falls out

- Even well-inserted needles may fall out during needle retention. These needles do not have to be re-inserted as they would fall out again.

- If a needle falls out this does not mean that the treatment is less effective. The small injury caused by the insertion represents a therapeutic stimulus which can persist for a few days after the treatment (similar to the needles retained for the normal duration of approximately 20 minutes).

- Assumed mechanism: an increase in the 'energetic pressure' pushes the needle out.

Bleeding upon needle removal

- Needle removal may cause slight oozing of blood or even blood spurting one to several centimetres.
- Bleeding occurs independent of the depth of insertion which, in any case, is only a few millimetres.
- Bleeding indicates balancing of the excess energetic pressure at the needled point. As the blood vessels in the ear are very small and the needles very thin and hardly injury-causing, spurting bleeding cannot be explained by hitting a vessel alone.
- If the bleeding cannot reach the surface a small haematoma will develop. While this, too, releases the 'energetic pressure' of the ear point, it can be somewhat painful and visually unpleasant for a few days.

> **box** The bleeding should be stopped with a swab only after a few seconds. The point should be allowed to bleed out sufficiently!

3.2.4 Needle Retention

- **Disposable needles** should be retained for at least 20 minutes. The patient should remain in a lying position during this time.
- **Semi-permanent needles** should be retained until they drop out on their own accord. This occurs generally within one week; otherwise they should be removed after one week (with tweezers). At that point they will be no longer effective due to the body's adaptation to the stimulus.

3.2.5 Needle Removal

- **Technique:** The needle is simply pulled out; a swab should be held ready in case of any bleeding; however, bleeding upon needle removal is not considered a negative side effect, it rather indicates a release of an 'energetic stagnation'; it is recommended to count the removed needles and compare the number with the treatment protocol.
- **Procedure**: Carried out by the therapist or his/her assistant (if delegating needle removal to an assistant the acupuncturist must still be present and available in the clinic; the assistant has to be fully trained and the acupuncturist should always check the procedure has been carried out correctly). Each needle has to be removed individually and placed into a sharps container to minimise the risk of injury during needle removal.
- **Complications:** needle collapse (> 5.10.2), bleeding (> 3.2.3) needle stick (> 5.10.1)
- **Disposal:** All needles have to be placed in specific sharps containers (> 2.5.4).

> **box** Needle removal is generally a painless and unproblematic procedure.

4 Auricular Laser Treatments

4.1 Introduction

4.1.1 Historical Background

Light treatments are about as old as the origins of acupuncture. The first experiments with sun light were carried out by Hippocrates (460–370 BC) and Galen (131–201 AD). In both Chinese and Arabic culture there were therapeutic approaches with red light therapy which was noted and further developed in Europe in the 19th century. In the 30s of last century experiments were carried out with fluorescent light emitting a wave length of 632.8 nm. This frequency is used today by red lasers (› 4.3.1 Wavelength).

After developing auricular acupuncture Nogier used laser therapy for stimulating auricular points. Using a low, tissue-protective intensity, he experimented with different frequencies (› table 4.3-1) and, based on his observation, developed recommendations for clinical application. Further representatives of Western acupuncture using laser therapy and who have compiled their experiences include Elias, Voll, and Bahr.

4.1.2 Physical Foundation

Technical Data

- **Energy:** in Joule $(1J = 1mWs)$
- **Frequency:** frequency of the periodically repeating light pulse; in Hertz $(1/s = 1Hz)$.
- **Coherence:** A fixed phase relationship (spatial and temporal) exists among all parts of the laser radiation; therefore laser represents light with an extremely high degree of order (coherent light)
- **Power:** in Watt (W) or Milliwatt (mW).
- **Spectrum:** Laser is typically monochromatic (light of only one wavelength) in contrast to white light which contains all colours.
- **Projection:** Typically, the divergence of the laser light beam is very low (to a large extent parallel), resulting in a point-like image of the beam on the skin.
- **Wave length** (› 4.3.1): in nanometres (nm)

Penetration depth

This is the depth at which a third of the original radiation is still detectable (Monte Carlo definition).

The penetration depth is determined by the following factors:
- **Power** (› 4.3.2): decisive factor; the penetration depth is directly proportional to the power
- **Wave length** (› 4.3.1): the greater the wave length, the greater the penetration depth
- **Frequency** (› 4.3.3): has only a negligible effect on the penetration depth
- **Angle of incidence** (› 4.3.3): lowest reflection loss (20–30 %) at an impact angle of 90° ('vertical laser'). With increasing impact angle there is increasing reflection and therefore a lower penetration depth.
- **Type of tissue:** Different tissues absorb and reflect the beam differently. Penetration depth (in decreasing order): fat > skin > muscle > bone

- **Colour of skin:** the darker the skin pigmentation the greater the reflection and absorption of the laser beam
- **Body hair:** the more body hair, the more shallow the penetration. The same applies to garments. Therefore clothes should be removed before laser therapy (e.g. tights).

The penetration depth can be increased by applying pressure on the tissue with the laser. The pressure pushes the blood out of the capillaries so that there is less haemoglobin absorbing the light.

Performance

The performance is calculated as the factor of the irradiation time and the power of the laser. The weaker the power of the device the longer the point has to be irradiated in order to obtain the same dose. Although the same dose tends to have the same result a more powerful laser achieves also a higher density effect, i.e. the light effect per area unit is higher.

4.1.3 Effects of Laser Therapy

Theoretical model

Tissue reflects, absorbs, and disperses light thus expressing its effect as defined by the laws of physics. It is assumed that laser causes local changes in electrical skin conductivity and that laser beam vibrations transmit information to each individual cell. This has a positive effect on cell metabolism. In other words, the laser beam provides a stimulus which penetrates to a depth of a few millimetres and can therefore stimulate auricular acupuncture points. While the penetration depth is a limiting factor this does not play a significant role as ear points (similarly to body acupuncture points) are located more superficially.

Effects

Cellular effects
- increased ATP, DNA, and RNA synthesis (in E. coli)
- increased synthesis of collagen and protein
- increased neovascularization
- reduction of prostaglandines
- improved cellular respiration

Systemic effects
- immunostimulant
- anti-inflammatory
- analgesic
- improves circulation

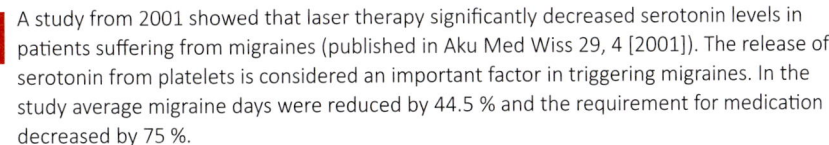

A study from 2001 showed that laser therapy significantly decreased serotonin levels in patients suffering from migraines (published in Aku Med Wiss 29, 4 [2001]). The release of serotonin from platelets is considered an important factor in triggering migraines. In the study average migraine days were reduced by 44.5 % and the requirement for medication decreased by 75 %.

Range of effects

Acupuncture points are best stimulated with devices with a low, tissue-protective perfor-mance. However, the stimulus is less intense than with acupuncture needles. While the penetration depth is limited, with more recent powerful models it can reach up to 4 cm (500 mW). Since ear points do not require a great penetration depth laser is certainly suita-ble for auricular acupuncture. As in body acupuncture, children respond particularly sensi-tively to the light stimulus. Laser therapy will therefore always be sufficient for the treatment of children but the effect in adults will be less than with needle acupuncture. In adults, laser therapy for auricular treatments should therefore be used only if fear of needling and the as-sociated pain exceed the understanding of the beneficial effects of acupuncture; especially since fear of pain increases the pain stimulus. Further indications: › 4.2.1.

> **box**
>
> The effect of laser therapy in children compares positively to acupuncture with needling in adults for the following reasons:
> - In children, acupuncture points are located more superficially and are therefore more easily accessible by the light energy of the laser beam.
> - Based on experience, the energetic system of children tends to react more strongly to therapeutic stimuli. The reason for this is believed to be that, compared to adults, the energetic system in children is still relatively unencumbered by environmental toxins, multiple diseases etc. and can therefore respond more effectively to therapeutic stim-uli.
> - The treatment is pain-free and therefore more acceptable for children.

4.1.4 Laser Classification

- **Class 1:** not suitable for therapeutic purposes. These devices have a specified, very low intensity below the threshold required for therapeutic purposes. Examples are laser videos, laser printers, laser demo pens etc. These devices must under no circumstance exceed the specified intensity.

- **Class 2:** not suitable for treatments, wavelengths between 400–710 nm (visible spec-trum), low intensity. Eye damage possible if exposure exceeds 0.25 seconds, upper limit 1 mW.

- **Class 3A:** suitable for treatments, wavelengths also within the visible spectrum (400–710 nm); medium intensity. Eye damage with exposure exceeding 0.25 seconds, upper limit 5 mW.

- **Class 3B:** suitable for therapeutic purposes, infrared wavelength range. No upper limit for eye damage, i.e. eye damage can occur with exposure of less than 0.25 seconds.

- **Class 4:** only suitable for use when triggered (i.e. rhythmic disruption of the contin-uous beam, mid laser › 4.3.3). High intensity. No upper limit for exposure of eye and skin – skin damage can therefore occur with even minimal exposure. All lasers with an intensity of an average of >0.5 W fall within this category.

4.2 Clinical Practice

4.2.1 Application

- **Advantages** of laser therapy:
  - pain-free, therefore also suitable for the treatment of children
  - no risk of infection
  - no risk of local skin irritations (inflammation)
- **Disadvantages** of laser therapy:
  - less effective than needling (applies only to adults). However, research studies (›
    chapter 11) showed that the effectiveness of the new generation of laser devices (e.g.
    LightNeedle, Reimers & Janssen) is comparable to acupuncture with needling
  - high initial cost
  - high maintenance (proper working order has to be regularly checked)
- **Indications:** children, pain-sensitive patients, patients with needlephobia, inflamed
  surface of the ear, chondritis
- **Contraindications:** skin surface hypersensitive to laser light
  - **absolute contraindications:** photo reaction (hypersensitivity to light) in atopic pa-
    tients (generally after 2–3 treatments); skin previously damaged by UV light, X-rays,
    or gamma rays
  - **relative contraindications:** certain drugs may result in hypersensitivity to laser light
    (cytostatics, immunosuppressants, arsenic-containing drugs)
- **Side effect/risks:** retinal damage due to illuminating the pupil; the head should therefore always be in a fixed position (especially in children); ask the parent or assistant to
  hold the head.
- **Limitation of usage:** insufficient effect, penetration depth to shallow for deep body acupuncture points.

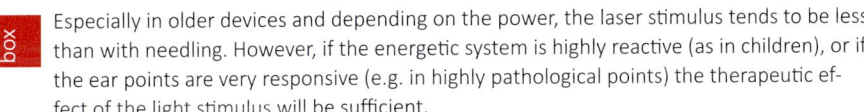

box Especially in older devices and depending on the power, the laser stimulus tends to be less
than with needling. However, if the energetic system is highly reactive (as in children), or if
the ear points are very responsive (e.g. in highly pathological points) the therapeutic effect of the light stimulus will be sufficient.

4.2.2 Method

- **Treatment room:** has to be marked with relevant warning signs. **Caution:** reflecting
  objects (mirrors, chrome etc.) have to be removed!
- Laser light must not enter the eye (**Caution:** risk of retinal injury); the patient is required to wear protective glasses; patient information is essential. **Caution:** When
  treating children their head has to be held.
- **Point selection:** Both ears are examined for pathological points which have to be
  marked. The actual treatment should begin only once all points to be treated have been
  located.

- **Marking selected points:** with a marker pen (› 2.4.4). **Caution:** coloured marks have to be removed with a disinfection agent before the laser treatment as the colour can change the light energy of the laser.
- **Settings:** Depending on the device the desired time, output and frequency (possibly also frequency cycle › 4.3.3) have to be set.
- **Positioning:** the laser is held (in the dominant hand) a few millimetres above the pathological point, or, if indicated, placed directly onto the skin (exception Twin-Laser › 4.3.1); impact angle ideally 90° to the surface of the skin.
- **Diagnosis:** Some laser devices have a diagnostic setting. This reduces the output to 1 mW (therapy: 10–500 mW). When using a device without an option for diagnosis pathological auricular points have to be selected with a 3-Volt hammer or a gold-silver hammer (RAC-palpation) and then treated by laser.
- **Irradiation:** the laser beam is activated by pressing the relevant button; many devices emit an acoustic or optical signal when the set irradiation time is over; the exposure time can also be determined by RAC-palpation. If the laser device is not equipped with a narrow, elongated outlet, an attachment for auricular acupuncture has to be used which also allows locating hidden points **Caution:** Laser treatment should be administered only by therapists with the relevant training.

 Regarding point prescription, treatment approach, and treatment course the same rules apply to both auricular laser therapy and auricular acupuncture.

4.2.3 Forms of Application

Laser monotherapy

All pathological auricular points are treated by laser stimulation only.
- **Method:** › 4.4.2
- **Time of exposure:** depends on the output of the laser device.
  - 10 mW: 25–30 seconds
  - 50 mW: 10–15 seconds
  - 150 mW: 5 seconds

Hybrid therapy

Combination of laser acupuncture and needling; after inserting the needle the insertion site is stimulated with laser light (exposure time depends on the output of the device); purpose: to increase the effect of acupuncture
- **Indication:** severe, therapy-resistant disorders
- **Method:** The pathological ear point is needled first. The needle is then stimulated with laser (frequency › 4.3.3). The laser beam should be directed at the tip of the inserted needle
- **Exposure time:** depends on the output of the device:
  - 10 mW: 5 seconds
  - 50 mW: 1–2 seconds
  - 150 mW: 1–2 seconds

LightNeedle System (Reimers & Janssen)

This device is equipped with several fibre glass probes (e.g. 12 channels, in combination with Physiolaser/Aku-Wave, manufacturer: Reimers & Janssen) allowing the simultaneous stimulation of several acupuncture points. For use in body acupuncture the laser beam can be deviated at the end of the probe by 90°. To this end the tip of the probe is fixed to the acupuncture needle for the duration of the treatment. The fibre optics used for auricular acupuncture does not deviate the beam as it is easier to use a straight beam. The devices currently on the market have an output of up to 50 mW/655 nm.

- **Indications:** for sensitive or needle-phobic patients
- **Method:** Following RAC-palpation a probe is placed on each pathological point, all points are then stimulated.
- **Exposure time:** The exposure time depends on the frequency and the therapy programme. The device calculates the correct time and switches off automatically.

Combination: Laser therapy and TCM

Laser therapy can also be combined with TCM (including Chinese herbal medicine). In children it is recommended to stimulate both ear and body points by laser.

- **Method:** The ear is examined and treated with laser first. Only then should body acupuncture points be treated. If this order is reversed it is more difficult to locate pathological auricular points by RAC-palpation due to the therapeutic effect of the body acupuncture.
- **Exposure time:** as in monotherapy (see above)

It is also possible to combine laser therapy with conventional medicine and other naturopathic therapies (as described in section › 1.2.3 with regards to auricular acupuncture).

Local therapy

Local therapy refers to the irradiation of surface areas of the body.

- **Indications:** acute sports injuries (sprains, contusions, swellings and haemtomas), skin conditions (in particular for eczema that improves in sunlight, e.g. psoriasis, neurodermatitis etc.)
- **Method:** Firstly the ear should be examined and treated with laser. Only after that is it advisable to irradiate the affected body area by moving the laser beam over it or by attaching a surface irradiation adapter.
- **Exposure time:**
  - **Musculoskeletal disorders:** preferably with Nogier frequency C (9.12 Hz); 50 mW: 80–120 seconds/cm², 150 mW: 25–40 seconds/cm²
  - **Skin disorders:** preferably with Nogier frequency A (292 Hz); 50 mW: 40–80 seconds/cm², 150 mW: 15–30 seconds/cm²
- **Treatment course:**
  - **Musculoskeletal disorders:** during the first two weeks after the trauma every 1–2 days
  - **Skin disorders:** the same treatment intervals as with acupuncture, i.e. once weekly

box
The treatment effect can be reinforced by giving acupuncture (body/ear) in addition to local laser therapy. This can significantly shorten the healing process in comparison to conservative treatments (poultices, physiotherapy).

Combination: Local therapy and auricular laser therapy

- **Indication:** acute sports injuries (sprains, contusions, swellings and haemtomas), skin conditions (in particular for eczema that improves in sunlight, e.g. psoriasis, neurodermatitis etc.)
- **Method:** first auricular acupuncture, followed by laser irradation of the affected muscle, joint, or skin area
- **Exposure time:** depends on the output of the laser device. Auricular points are treated first:
  - 10 mW: 25–30 seconds
  - 50 mW: 10–15 seconds
  - 150 mW: 5 seconds

  Affected areas on the body are treated afterwards:
  - 10 mW: 200–600 seconds/cm^2 (only limited suitability for local therapy)
  - 50 mW: 40–120 seconds/cm^2
  - 150 mW: 15–40 seconds/cm^2

4.3 Technical Variations

4.3.1 Wavelength

In auricular acupuncture two types of laser with different wavelengths are used:
- **Infrared laser:** generally a laser diode or semiconductor laser with a wavelength of approximately 780–904 nm. For orientation a visible, red light beam (directional beam) is added. *Advantage:* deeper penetration. *Disadvantage:* more expensive than red laser
- **Red laser:** Helium-neon-laser, wavelength 635 nm. *Advantage:* cheaper than infrared laser. *Disadvantage:* least penetration.

> **Twin-Laser:** A device combing both red and infrared lasers; selective or combined application possible. Special features: both beams meet approximately 5 mm after emission; the distance to the treated point has to be closely monitored! *Advantage:* reaches several tissue layers according to the penetration depths of both wavelengths. *Disadvantage:* most expensive option.

4.3.2 Output

The higher the output the deeper the penetration depth and the greater the effect on the tissue; this reduces the required exposure time. The following types of laser are commonly used:
- **Soft laser:** Output 10–1,000 mW. *Application:* Body and auricular acupuncture, also for surface irradiation in dermatology and sports medicine
- **Mid laser:** Laser with up to 10 W; moderated to the effect of a soft laser by rhythmically disrupting the continuous beam. *Application:* only for body/auricular acupuncture
- **Hard/power laser (surgical laser):** Laser with higher output (> 30 W). *Application:* surgical interventions

The following wavelengths are necessary for reaching the following output:

- 635 nm for 10 mW
- 670 nm for 20 mW
- 785 nm (infrared) for 50 mW
- 820 nm (infrared) for 150 mW
- 904 nm (infrared, impulsed laser) for 10 W

4.3.3 Frequencies

The frequency refers to the periodically repeating light impulse (in Hertz [Hz]); the individual frequencies are generated by interrupting the continuous beam for different periods of time.

- **Frequency range:** from 1–100,000 Hz. Correlating individual frequencies with particular conditions is mostly based on empirical values; variations exist between different authors (› Table 4.3-1–4.3-5, Frequencies after Nogier, Elias, Voll, Bahr and Reininger). All recommendations regarding frequencies apply to both auricular and body acupuncture. To date there have not been any detailed research studies. Experience shows that low frequencies (10–100 Hz) have a stronger analgesic effect, medium frequencies (100–500 Hz) are beneficial for the treatment of oedema, while higher frequencies (2.500–5.000 Hz) are best for treating inflammatory processes (Hode, Tuner 2002).
- **Variation: Continuous laser:** Laser with a continuous beam without frequency-generating disruption; preferred by some authors to the use of frequencies
- **Variation: Frequency cycle:** Device with a programmable frequency sequence within a defined period of time; the combination of different frequencies with a similar effect enhances the treatment effect.

Tab. 4.3-1 Nogier frequencies in potentiated and non-potentiated (in brackets) form

	Frequency	Indication (selection)
Frequency A	292 (2.28) Hz	Acute disorders, 'frequency of non-organisation' (e.g. tumours, rheumatism, allergies, scars, inflammation)
Frequency B	584 (4.56) Hz	Chronic disorders, intoxication, metabolic disorders (e.g. arthritis, ulcers)
Frequency C	1,168 (9.12) Hz	Musculoskeletal disorders and restrictions
Frequency D	2,336 (18.24) Hz	Psychological disorders, exhaustion ('running on empty')
Frequency E	4,672 (36.48) Hz	Disorders affecting nerve pathways (e.g. herpes zoster, trigeminal neuralgia)
Frequency F	9,344 (72) Hz	Emotional disorders (e.g. depression, disorientation, lack of concentration)
Frequency G	18,688 (144) Hz	Personality disorders (e.g. intellectual disorders, identity problems)
Frequency U	1.14 Hz	Universal frequency; scars, interference fields
Frequency A″	37,376.00 Hz	Double potentiated frequency A

Tab. 4.3-2 Frequencies after Elias

	Frequency	Indications (selection)
Frequency 1	F 25 Hz	Difficulty concentrating (especially in children), stress
Frequency 2	F 50 Hz	Anti-inflammatory, immuno-stimulating; circulation, connective tissue
Frequency 3	F 160 Hz	Emotionally balancing, psychologically stabilising
Frequency 4	F 350 Hz	Strengthens the musculo-skeletal system
Frequency 5	F 475 Hz	Laterality disorders
Frequency 6	F 2,800 Hz	Regulates the peripheral nervous system (pareses, neuralgias)
Frequency 7	F 6,500 Hz	Psychosomatic disorders
Frequency 8	F 8,000 Hz	Pain frequency

Tab. 4.3-3 Frequencies after Voll

Frequency	Indications	Frequency	Indications
1.2 Hz	Tachycardia	6.0 Hz	Flaccid paralysis
1.7 Hz	Abscesses, acne, furuncles	6.3 Hz	Headaches, irritability
2.2 Hz	Fatigue	6.6 Hz	Flaccid paralysis
2.45 Hz	Sinusitis, insomnia, contusions	7.7 Hz	Cerebral palsy
2.65 Hz	Gallbladder disorders	8.25 Hz	Flaccid paralysis
2.9 Hz	Rhinitis	9.2 Hz	Hypertension, renal insufficiency
3.3 Hz	Arteriosclerosis		
3.5 Hz	Lithiasis, tremors	9.35 Hz	Flaccid paralysis
3,8 Hz	Spasms, burning tongue	9.4 Hz	Stomach, joint, bladder, prostate
3.9 Hz	Neuralgias	9.45 Hz	Angina pectoris, gonadal dysfunction
4.0 Hz	Endocrine disorders		
4.9 Hz	Dysmenorrhoea, stiff neck	9.5 Hz	Hypertension, migraines
5.55 Hz	Paraesthesias	9.6 Hz	Arthritis, chronic polyarthritis
5.8 Hz	Anxiety, headaches	9.7 Hz	Sciatica, chronic polyarthritis
5.9 Hz	Cerebral palsy	10 Hz	Varicose veins, phlebitis, venous ulcers

Tab. 4.3-4 Frequencies after Bahr

	Frequency	Indications (selection)
Frequency 1	599.50 Hz	Deep tissue layers
Frequency 2	1,199.00 Hz	Middle tissue layers
Frequency 3	2,398.00 Hz	Superficial layer (dominant ear)
Frequency 4	4,796.00 Hz	Superficial layer (non-dominant ear)
Frequency 5	9,592.00 Hz	Frequency of 'order', anti-oscillation, cardinal points
Frequency 6	19,184.00 Hz	Masked psychological interference fields
Frequency 7	38,368.00 Hz	Contained interference fields (e.g. teeth)

Tab. 4.3-5 New frequencies after Bahr

	Frequency
Allergies	1,927.00 Hz
Appetite suppressant	4,070.00 Hz
Anti-Aging	4,141.00 Hz
Detoxification	969.00 Hz
Hysteria	1,131.00 Hz
Insulin (Dr. Wirz)	3,323.00 Hz
Om	136.10 Hz
Parkinson's disease (Dr. Wirz)	9,617.00 Hz
Qi-movement	7,695.00 Hz
Pain/Thalamus	963.50 Hz
Pain/Prostaglandin E1	1,152.00 Hz
Self-healing	4,625.00 Hz
Serotonin	9,637.00 Hz
Simillimum	7,708.00 Hz
Detoxification	969.00 Hz
Addiction	1,719.00 Hz
Tinnitus	641.00 Hz
Order	9,592.00 Hz
'Non-order'/interference field	292.00 Hz
Masked/'hidden' interference fields	299.75 Hz

Tab. 4.3-6 New frequencies after Bahr: Musculoskeletal system

	Frequency
Hip	873.00 Hz
Knee	893.00 Hz
Ankle	913.00 Hz
Shoulder	931.00 Hz
Elbow	952.00 Hz
Wrist	955.00 Hz
Atlas	1,039.00 Hz
C7	1,050.00 Hz
L1	1,073.00 Hz
L4	1,091.00 Hz
L5	1,093.00 Hz

Tab. 4.3-7 Frequencies after Reininger

	Frequency	Indications
Frequency RI 1	132 Hz	Constitution
Frequency RI 2	264 Hz	Adrenal stimulant
Frequency RI 3	528 Hz	Constitutional weakness
Frequency RI 4	1,056 Hz	Causative interference field point / Laterality
Frequency RI 5	2,112 Hz	Causative interference field point 1
Frequency RI 6	4,224 Hz	Vitamin absorption support
Frequency RI 7	8,448 Hz	Nosode for hereditary diseases
Frequency RII 1	113 Hz	Left reunion zone, gold
Frequency RII 2	226 Hz	Right reunion zone, gold
Frequency RII 3	452 Hz	Left reunion zone, silver
Frequency RII 4	904 Hz	Right reunion zone, silver
Frequency RII 5	1,808 Hz	Personal master point 1, VIP 1 (very important point)
Frequency RII 6	3,616 Hz	Personal master point 2, VIP 2 (very important point)
Frequency RII 7	7,232 Hz	Point for underlying causes
Frequency RIII 1	114 Hz	Simillimum
Frequency RIII 2	228 Hz	Psychological blockages point
Frequency RIII 3	456 Hz	Frequency of points on the Governing Vessel
Frequency RIII 4	912 Hz	Frequency of points on the Conception Vessel
Frequency RIII 5	1,824 Hz	Bach Flower frequency
Frequency RIII 6	3,648 Hz	Allergy frequency
Frequency RIII 7	7,296 Hz	Master point of Order

Tab. 4.3-8 Meridian frequencies after Reininger

Frequency	Indication
442 Hz	Liver
471 Hz	Stomach
497 Hz	Heart
530 Hz	Cardiovascular system/sexuality
553 Hz	Colon
583 Hz	Gallbladder
611 Hz	Kidney
667 Hz	Bladder
702 Hz	Spleen/pancreas
732 Hz	Triple Warmer
791 Hz	Small intestine
824 Hz	Lung

Tab. 4.3-9 New frequencies after Reininger: Anti-frequencies

	Frequency
Psyche	129.00 Hz
Anti-psyche	4,221.00 Hz
Autonomic Nervous System	112.00 Hz
Anti-ANS	3,665.00 Hz
Addiction	101.00 Hz
Anti-addiction	3,305.00 Hz
Carcinoma	108.00 Hz
Anti-carcinoma	3,534.00 Hz
Pain	119.00 Hz
Anti-pain	3,894.00 Hz
Inflammation	128.00 Hz
Anti-inflammation	4,189.00 Hz
Allergy	104.00 Hz
Anti-allergy	3,416.00 Hz
Tinnitus	125.00 Hz
Anti-tinnitus	4,090.00 Hz
Immunity	102.00 Hz
Anti-immunity	3,351.00 Hz
General	384.00 Hz

5 Diagnostic and Therapeutic Principles

5.1 Medical History

Procedure

The medical history has to be taken before locating any points. This helps to speed up the selection process for the point prescription by limiting the number of points to be tested.

- **Limiting the number of points to be tested:** RAC-palpation is considered an objective method which allows the experienced practitioner to select relevant pathological points, but it would be extremely difficult and time-consuming to test all 250 known ear points in each and every patient.

The medical history further provides the following information:

- **Severity of symptoms:** Pathological points provide information only about the type but not the severity of a disorder. *Example:* If the point 'Resentment' tests RAC-positive, it will do so regardless if the resentment is caused by failing to find a parking space, or by anger and desperation about a malignant disease.

- **Causes of the disorder:** Pathological points do not indicate the causes of symptoms. *Example:* An interference field due to nephritic scarring will trigger a RAC identical to one caused by nephrolithiasis.

- **Pathological processes** initially not verifiable by RAC-palpation: severely pathological points can 'mask' other points (in particular adjacent ones) so that it can be extremely difficult to find them. 'Masked' points often become more obvious after treating the more overtly pathological points. It can therefore happen that, as the treatment course progresses, there are more pathological points than in the beginning despite an improvement in the patient's condition.

Medical History: check list

- **Current signs and symptoms:** Ear points related to known disorders can be targeted directly for RAC-diagnosis and treatment (› 3.1.4).

- **Handedness (chirality):** Certain points are located only on the dominant or non-dominant ear (› 5.4). In right-handed people the right ear is dominant, in left-handed people the left ear.

- **Duration of existing disorders:** The duration of the disorder as well as knowing about acute or chronic diseases provides information about the duration of the treatment. Acute symptoms generally respond more quickly than long-standing, chronic complaints.

- **Psychological problems:** Psychological points should be checked (› 6.8).

- **Pre-existing disorders:** These may provide information about general weaknesses. *Example:* chronic physical weakness during childhood following recurrent infections treated with antibiotics. When compiling the point prescription energetically stabilising points should be considered for quicker treatment results.

- **Surgeries:** Even if scars do not cause any symptoms they can have the effect of an interference field (› 5.7.1). If the affected area tests RAC-positive it has to be treated.

- **Current medication:** Both effects and side-effects need to be considered as they can mask symptoms (*Example:* no knee pain due to antirheumatic drugs but RAC for the knee is pathological!); or new symptoms can appear (*Example:* ringing in the ears due to antihypertensive drugs but RAC for the ear is not pathological!). Antibiotics, cortisone as well as other immunosuppressants (› 5.9.1 Adjunctive medication) are considered as having an interfering effect on auricular acupuncture treatments.

5.2 Physcial Examination

5.2.1 General Examination

The general examination is carried out according to the principles of conventional medicine. Based on the patient's complaint or diagnosis (according to Western medicine) the patient should be checked for the following to prevent any medical emergencies:

- **General physical condition:** if this is impaired in any way the patient should be referred to a physician.
- **Blood pressure:** to exclude hyper/hypotension (**Caution:** risk of needle collapse!)
- **Pulse:** provides information about arrhythmias; important for interpreting the RAC (› 3.1.4)
- **Signs of inflammation/infection:** fever, reddening, swelling, enlarged lymph glands; if indicated, refer to a physician
- **Signs of malignancies:** e.g. cachexia, visible tumours, non-movable lymph glands; if indicated, refer to a physician
- **Scars:** may represent interference fields (› 5.7.1); particular attention should be paid to the following scars: tonsillectomy, appendectomy, cholecystectomy, surgical drains, hysterectomy, episiotomy, umbilical laparoscopy
- **Amalgam fillings:** may present interference fields (› 5.7.5)
- **Other foreign bodies:** e.g. total endoprostheses, breast implants, and coils may also present an obstacle to treatment (› 5.9)

5.2.2 Examination of the Ear

Before the actual auricular acupuncture treatment the ear should be carefully examined with particular attention to the following features:

- **Form of the ear:** There is practically no other part of the human body with such variable anatomical features as the ear. The location of auricular points has therefore to be adapted accordingly but can generally be determined by the relationship of the anatomical landmarks to each other (› fig. 5.5-1 to fig. 5.5-4). The determining factor for the location of a particular point is always RAC-palpation.
- **Ear wax:** This should be removed with cotton wool from relevant areas before starting the treatment (risk of infection).
- **Ear rings/Ear piercing:** These can act as interference fields (› 5.9.3 Ear rings, › 5.9.4 Piercing); ear rings should always be removed before the treatment (piercing jewellery generally require pliers for removal).
- **Injuries/infections:** These need to be documented for forensic reasons; they can act as

interference fields; treatment of the affected ear is contraindicated due to forensic reasons.

- **Tumours** (e.g. basal cell carcinoma)/**'brown spots'**: These should always be documented; treatment of the affected ear is contraindicated and the patient should be referred for further investigation.

5.3 Patient Position

- **Treatment couch:** width approximately 80 cm, height approximately 60 cm, ideally with an adjustable headrest; knee bolsters are helpful in providing spinal support.
- **Patient position:** supine, head turned to the side with the ear to be treated on top. After needling, the head can be returned to a central position.
- **Practitioner position:** seated at the top of the couch, behind the patient's head

Lying down generally has a relaxing effect and helps to prevent needle collapse.

5.4 Which Side to Treat

The following theoretical considerations are intended to make locating pathological points easier. The principles listed below should be observed:

- Unpaired organs are always represented on the same side as that organ; e.g. spleen on the left ear, liver on the right ear.
- Superordinate points (points which cannot be assigned a specific side [e.g. psychological points, analgesic points]) that require tonification or stimulation are **generally** found on the side corresponding to the patient's handedness (= dominant side, e.g. in right-handed persons on the right-hand side).
- Superordinate points (points which cannot be assigned a specific side [e.g. psychological points, analgesic points]) that require sedation or calming are **generally** found on the side opposite to the patient's handedness (= non-dominant side, e.g. in right-handed persons on the left-hand side).
- The effect of a small number of points depends on whether the dominant or non-dominant ear is treated: e.g. Anxiety on the dominant ear, Worry on the non-dominant ear (› 5.4.1 Dominant Side). This will always be pointed out in the text.

5.4.1 Dominant Side

The patient's handedness determines which ear is dominant. In right-handed people the right ear is dominant, in left-handed people the left ear.

- Some points are found only on the dominant ear:
  - **Joy** (› 6.13.2)
  - **Anxiety** (› 6.8.5)

- **Caffeine** (› 6.7.1)
- **PGE**₁ (in combination with the point **Thymus** (› 6.7.6)
- Some points are found only on the non-dominant ear:
  - **Sorrow** (› 6.13.2)
  - **Worry** (› 6.8.5)
  - **Barbiturate** (› 6.7.1)
  - **Thymus** (in combination with **PGE**₁ (› 6.11.4)

It is therefore important to establish the patient's handedness before the treatment

In left-handed persons who have been trained to write with their right hand (› 5.8 Unstable Laterality) the natural dominance will continue to persist, even if the person predominantly uses their right hand in their adult life.

5.4.2 Organ Representation

Unpaired Organs

According to the French School, unpaired organs are always represented on the side where they are located anatomically. Therefore some acupuncture points are located only on one side, irrespective of the person's handedness ('laterality').

- The following points are located on the right ear only:
  - **Liver** (› 6.4.1)
  - **Gallbladder** (› 6.4.1)
- The following points are located on the left ear only:
  - **Spleen** (› 6.4.1)
  - **Tail of Pancreas** (› 6.4.1)

Paired Organs

If in a paired organ only one side is affected by a disorder, **generally** only the point on the affected side will be pathological, e.g. in right-sided pneumonia the corresponding pathological point will be on the right ear. However, if both points (on the left and the right ear) trigger a RAC-response, both points must be needled.

5.5 Point Variations

Although the anatomical structures of the ear are well defined, they vary significantly from person to person (› Fig. 5.5-1 to Fig. 5.5-15):

- **C7** (› 6.1.1)
- **Elbow** (› 6.2.1)
- **Hip** (› 6.2.3)
- **Testes/Ovaries** (› 6.5.2)
- **Anxiety** (› 6.8.4)
- **Maxillary Sinus** (› 6.8.3)

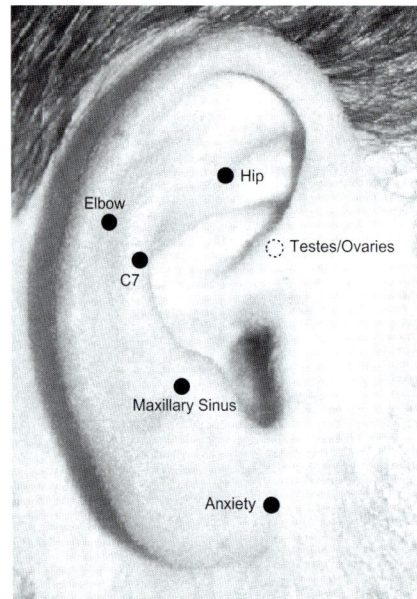

Abb. 5.5-1

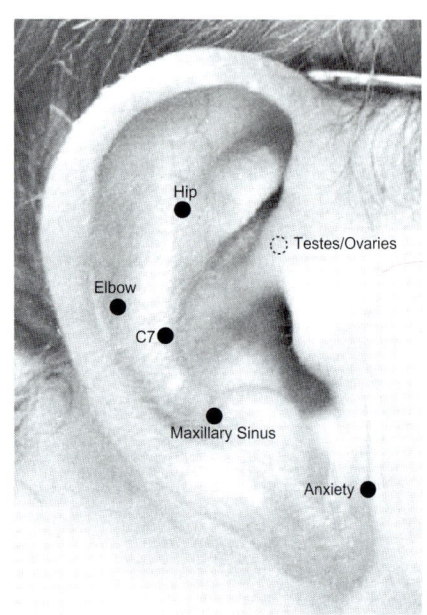

Abb. 5.5-2

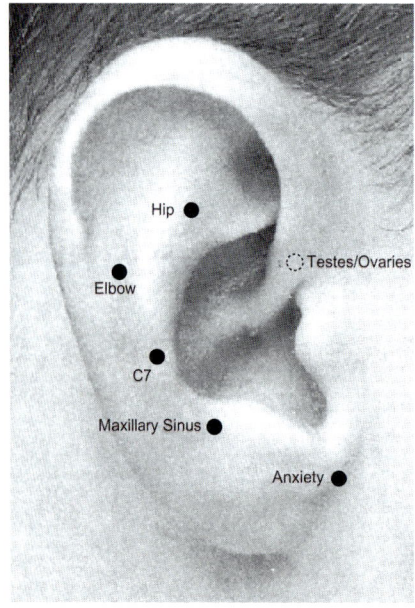

Abb. 5.5-3

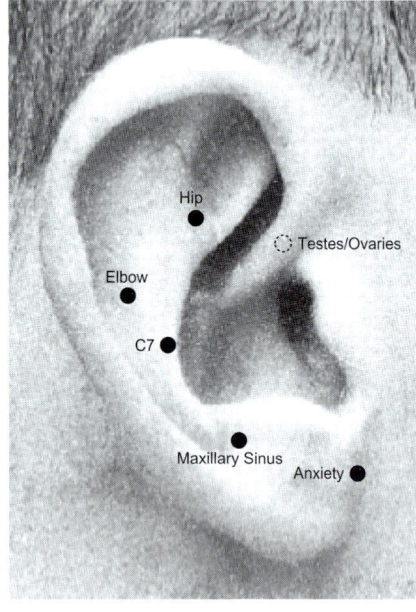

Abb. 5.5-4

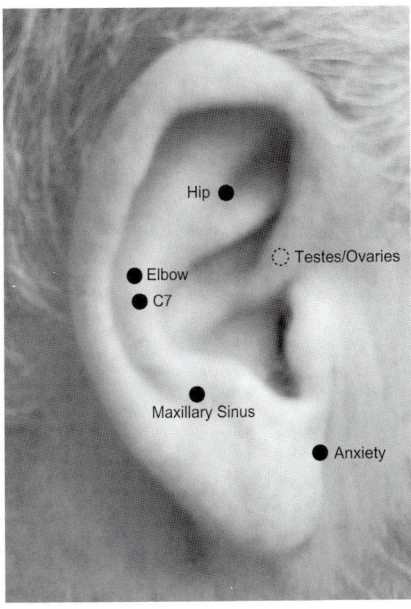

Abb. 5.5-5

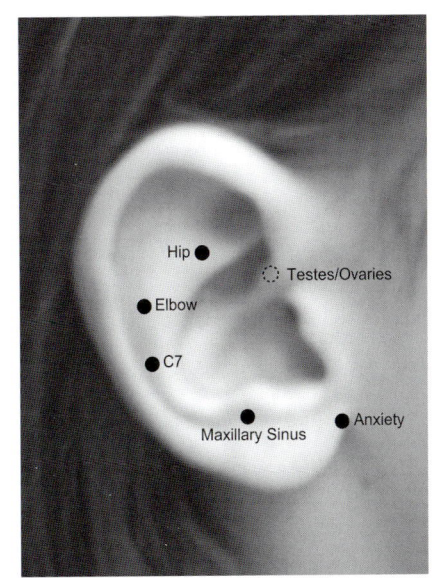

Abb. 5.5-6

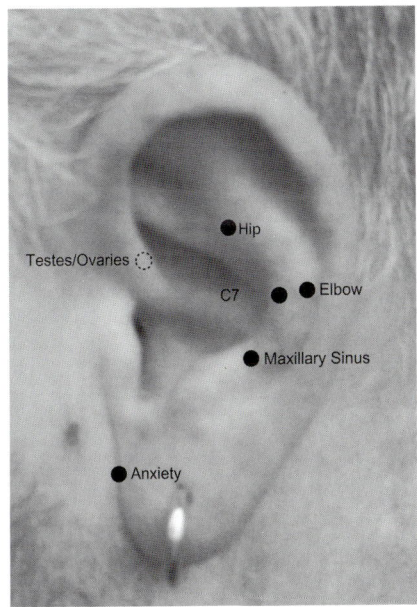

Abb. 5.5-7

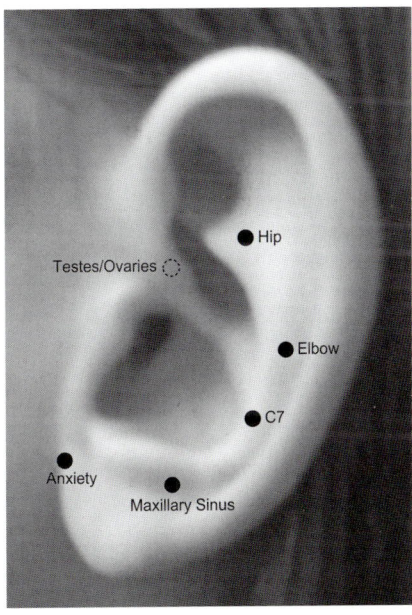

Abb. 5.5-8

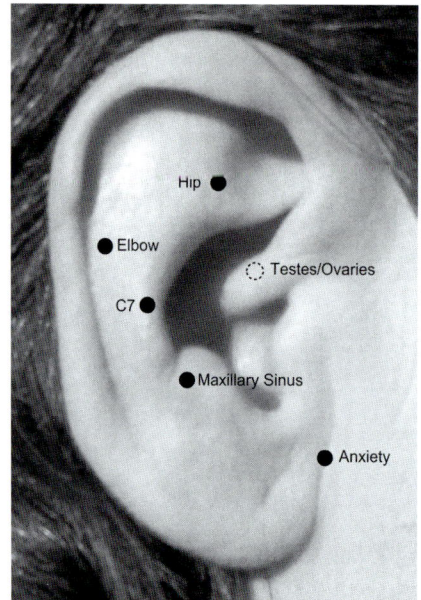

Abb. 5.5-9

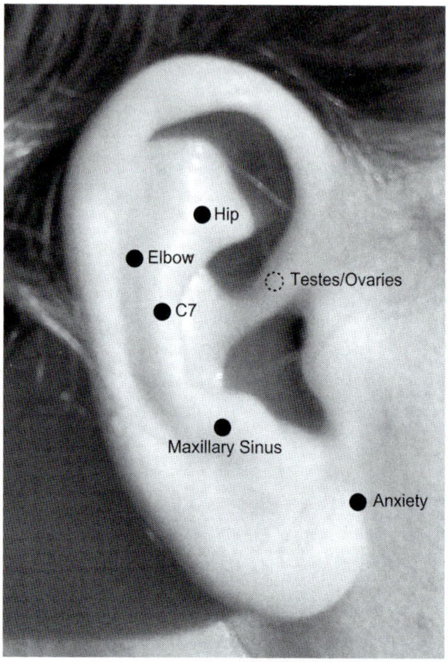

Abb. 5.5-10

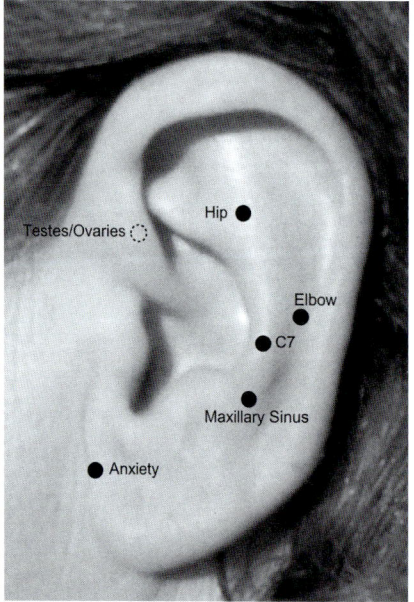

Abb. 5.5-11

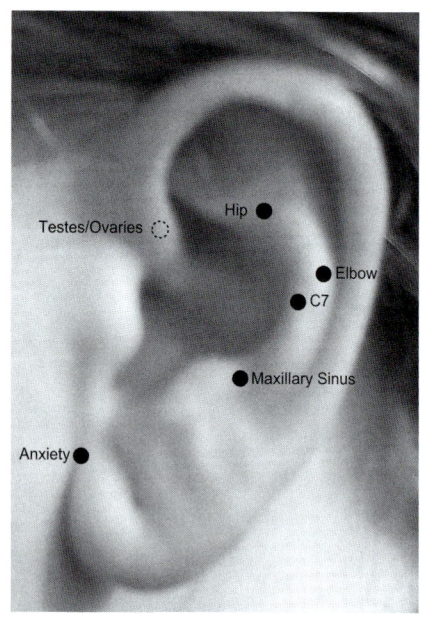

Abb. 5.5-12

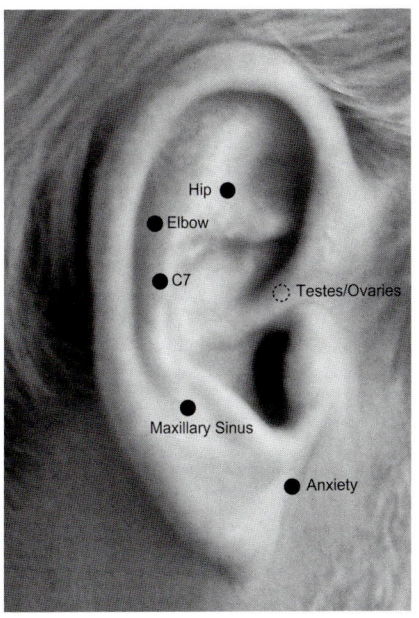

Abb. 5.5-13

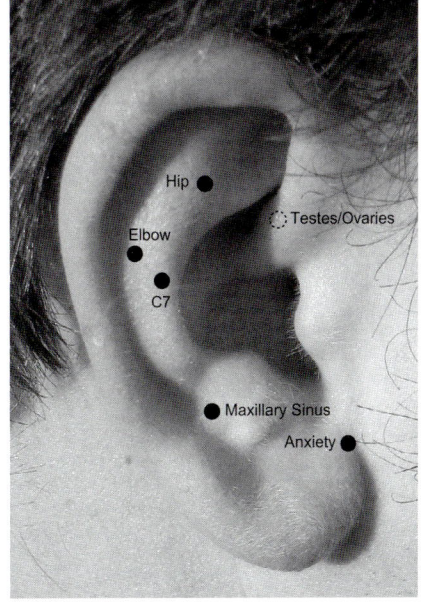

Abb. 5.5-14

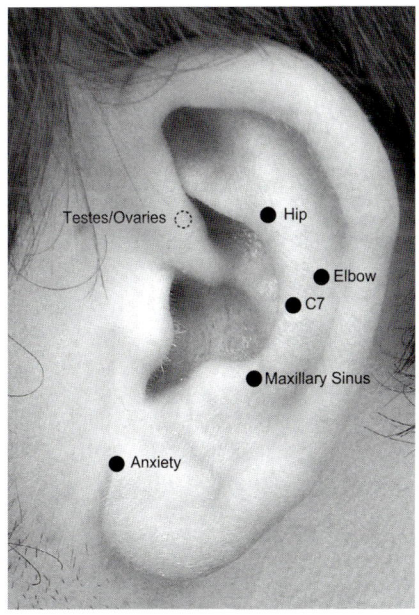

Abb. 5.5-15

5.6 Time Considerations

5.6.1 Duration of an Acupuncture Treatment

- **Introductory talk at the first appointment:** about 20 minutes
- **Medical history and examination:** before every treatment, approximately 10–15 minutes for experienced practitioners, 40–60 minutes for beginners
- **Locating pathological points:** RAC-palpation on both ears, approximately 5–10 minutes for experienced practitioners, 30–40 minutes for beginners
- **Needling of pathological points:** approximately 5 minutes for experienced practitioners, 30–40 minutes for beginners.
- **Needle retention:** at least 20 minutes

> **box** The duration of a treatment session depends very much on the practitioner's experience.

5.6.2 Treatment Intervals

Treatment intervals vary from case to case. The following list is therefore for guidance only. Suggestions are provided in chapters 7 and 8 so that average treatment intervals for a particular disorder can be estimated.

Acute disorders

Acute disorders (< 1 week)

Initially daily or **2–3 times weekly**:
- Cervical myalgia (› 7.1.1)
- Lower back pain (› 7.1.2)
- Sciatica (› 7.1.3)
- Epicondylitis (› 7.1.6)
- Carpal tunnel syndrome (› 7.1.7)
- Hip pain (› 7.1.9)
- Ankle sprain (› 7.1.13)
- Vascular headaches (› 7.3.4)
- Angina (› 8.1.3)
- Bronchial asthma (› 8.2.1)
- Bronchopulmonary infection (› 8.2.3)
- Nephrolithiasis (› 8.4.4).

Acute disorders (duration: > 1 week)

1–2 times weekly until symptoms have disappeared, e.g.
- Intercostal neuralgia (› 7.2.4).

Chronic disorders

Chronic disorders (symptoms occurring daily to weekly)

Initially one treatment per week; when symptoms improve one treatment every other week until symptoms have completely disappeared, e.g. complex regional pain syndrome (› 7.2.2)

- Arthritis (› 7.2.3)
- Urinary retention (› 8.4.3)
- Anorexia (› 8.13.4).
- Phantom pain (› 7.2.5)
- Incontinence (› 8.4.2)
- Benign prostatic hyperplasia (› 8.4.5)
- Neurodermatitis (› 8.5.1)
- Insomnia (› 8.12.1).

Chronic disorders (symptoms > once weekly)

Treat **every other week**, e.g.
- Head aches (› 7.3)
- Hormonal migraines (› 7.4.2)
- Premenstrual syndrome (› 8.10.1).

Disorders with danger to self

Daily treatments until the patient is stable, e.g. depression (› 8.13.1).

5.6.3 Treatment Course

The treatment course for a particular disorder varies for each individual case. The information provided in chapters 7 and 8 (treatment protocols) are for guidance only.

The following basic rules apply:
- The more recent the onset of the disorder, the shorter the treatment course required.
- The longer standing the disorder, the longer the treatment course.
- If the disorder is at the level of the energetic system only and has not yet developed into a physical condition (impaired well-being) the treatment course will be shorter.
- 'Deep-seated' disorders presenting with physical symptoms require a longer treatment course. Less 'deep-seated' (acute) disorders tend to resolve first, other concurrent disorders later, generally in the order in which they first occurred.
- The higher the number of concurrent disorders the longer will be the treatment course.
- The more weakened the patient is on an energetic level (e.g. following severe previous illnesses, many births, old age), the longer will be the treatment course.
- The presence of interference fields (› 5.7) will extend the duration of the treatment course.

Tab. 5.6-1 Duration of treatment courses for specific disorders (for guidance only)

Disorder	Treatment period
Acute sciatica	A few hours to several days
Bronchopulmonary infection	Several hours to a few days
Ankle sprain	A few days to 4 weeks
Acute lower back pain	A few days to 4 weeks
Herpes zoster	Several weeks to 3 months
Palpitations	Several weeks to 3 months
Arthritis	Several weeks to months
Intercostal neuralgia	Several weeks to 6 months
Trigeminal neuralgia	Several weeks to 6 months
Complex regional pain syndrome	6 months
Chronic headaches	6 months to 1 year
Migraines	6 months to 2 years
Psoriasis	Several months to 2 years
Chronic polyarthritis	1–2 years
Atopic dermatitis	1–2 years and longer
Bronchial asthma	2 years and longer

5.7 Interference Fields

Interference fields represent a physical and/or energetic taxation by continuously draining the body's energy and its powers of self-healing. In this respect they further weaken the patient, which, in turn, inevitably exacerbates the patient's overall signs and symptoms.

- **Common interference fields:** scars (› 5.7.1), chronic sinusitis (› 5.7.2), chronic tonsillitis (› 5.7.3), focal tooth infection (5.7.4), amalgam fillings (› 5.7.5), psychosomatic intestinal disorders (› 5.7.6), restricted joint movements (› 5.7.7)

- **General symptoms:** Interference fields can manifest with clinical symptoms and present as a physical disorder; or they can be asymptomatic but still weaken the body's energetic system. Typical symptoms include:
  - exacerbation of the underlying disorder
  - impaired wellbeing, e.g. fatigue, lack of motivation, psychological disorders

- **Diagnosis:** considering common interference fields when taking the medical history; RAC-palpation of the ear for possible 'interference field points'

- **Treatment:** continuous treatment of the 'interference field point' in tandem with treating the primary disorder. *Example:* If a tonsillectomy scar (even if asymptomatic) triggers a RAC at the tonsil point, this point must always be treated in addition to other pathological points. Sometimes disorders previously not responding to treatment can be resolved by treating an interference field discovered by RAC-palpation (and which the patient was not aware of).

– **Technique:** In case of a pathological RAC the relevant 'interference field point' is treated with a semi-permanent needle retained for approximately one week (or shorter in case the needle spontaneously falls out), followed by a break of 3–4 days. *Alternative:* needling of the 'interference field point' at every session.
– **Selecting the side:** If a RAC-response is found on only one side, only that side is treated; if there is a RAC-response on both sides both ears are treated.
– **Treatment course:** Treatments are necessary until the interference field has disappeared (interference field: chronic, reversible disorder e.g. sinusitis) or until the primary disorder has been resolved (interference field: irreversible defect e.g. a scar).

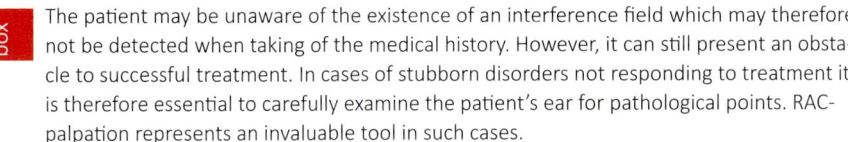

The patient may be unaware of the existence of an interference field which may therefore not be detected when taking of the medical history. However, it can still present an obstacle to successful treatment. In cases of stubborn disorders not responding to treatment it is therefore essential to carefully examine the patient's ear for pathological points. RAC-palpation represents an invaluable tool in such cases.

Some common interference fields are described below.

5.7.1 Scars

Scars are the most common causes of interference fields.

- **Possible explanation:** Scar tissue impedes or even blocks the energy flow in the affected channels. The resulting stagnation on one side of the blockage and/or the lack of energy on the other side can lead to physical symptoms or weaken the patient's energetic system.

- **Character of the scar:** The size of the scar provides no information about the nature of its interference field. However, a scar crossing several meridians is considered a particular obstacle to treatment. More important than the size is the orientation of the scar. Generally, scars perpendicular to the body's alignment or the course of the meridians result in more severe blockages than scars with a parallel alignment. For locating 'interference field points' see table 5.7-1.

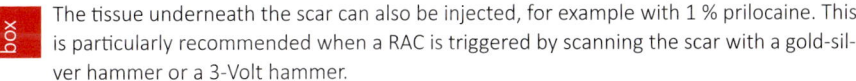

The tissue underneath the scar can also be injected, for example with 1 % prilocaine. This is particularly recommended when a RAC is triggered by scanning the scar with a gold-silver hammer or a 3-Volt hammer.

5.7.2 Chronic Sinusitis

- **Mechanism:** Exacerbation of the primary disorder due to a weakening of the immune system.
- **Special feature:** Typical symptoms of chronic sinusitis include nasal obstruction which often exists since childhood, as well as a permanent or recurrent runny nose in form of a chronic cold. These complaints often persist for many years so that the patient doesn't register them anymore and, unless specifically asked, will not mention them as part of the medical history. For locating 'interference field points' › table 5.7-2.

Tab. 5.7-1 Surgical scars causing interference fields: location of common auricular 'interference field points'

Scar following	Auricular 'interference field point'	Possible side (based on RAC)
Tonsillectomy	**Tonsils:** directly inferior to the point **TMJ** (at the inferior end of the **Vegetative Groove**)	On both sides
Appendectomy	**Appendix IV (90):** in the superior concha, adjacent to the helix root, in the area of **Cecum**	Generally on the right-hand side
Cholecystectomy	**Gallbladder:** a zone in the superior concha, on the lower border of the antihelix, superior to the helix root	Always on the right-hand side
Surgical drain	Depends on the location of the drain	On both sides
Hysterectomy	**Uterus:** on the inside of the helix brim, superior to the intersection point between helix and antihelix	On both sides
Episiotomy	**Haemorrhoids:** in the upper medial corner of the concha, medial to the intersection of the helix and antihelix	On both sides
Umbilical laparoscopy	**Point Zero:** 0.5 cm superior to the helix root, palpable as a distinct notch	On both sides

Tab. 5.7-2 Chronic sinusitis: 'Interference field points' on the ear in decreasing order of frequency (combinations possible)

Affected sinus	'Interference field points' and their location
Maxillary sinus	**Maxillary sinus:** inferior to the point **Atlanto-occipital Joint** (at the end of the **Vegetative Groove**)
Frontal sinus	**Frontal Sinus:** at the tip of the antitragus
Ethmoid sinus	**Ethmoid Sinus:** lateral and slightly superior to the point **Frontal Sinus**, just inferior to the antitragus
Sphenoid sinus	**Sphenoid Sinus:** lateral and superior to the point **Ethmoid Sinus**, just inferior to the antitragus

5.7.3 Chronic Recurrent Tonsillitis

- **Mechanism:** exacerbation of the primary disorder due to a weakening of the immune system. *Vicious circle:* Frequent antibiotics contribute to chronic recurrent tonsillitis since each course of antibiotics weakens the immune system. For this reason antibiotics should be used only as a last resort (**Caution:** Throat culture!). Especially during the early stages of tonsillitis treatment with auricular acupuncture and TCM is often sufficient.

- **Special features:** Even during symptom-free intervals chronic recurrent tonsillitis can often be detected by RAC. Since an interference field weakens the body, it becomes more susceptible to other illnesses. It is therefore beneficial to treat during symptom-free intervals, as this will considerably reduce the number of future tonsil infections. For locating 'interference field points' › table 5.7-3.

Tab. 5.7-3 Chronic recurrent tonsillitis: 'Interference field points' on the ear in decreasing order of frequency (combinations possible)

Auricular 'interference field points'	Location
Tonsils (most common finding)	Directly inferior to the point **TMJ**
Tonsil I (73)	At the apex of the helix
Tonsil II (74)	On the helix rim, slightly inferior to **Point Zero**
Tonsil III (75)	On the helix tail, approximately at the same level as the tip of the antitragus
Tonsil IV (10)	Approximately in the centre of zone VIII

5.7.4 Focal Tooth Infections

- **Causative mechanism:** Purulent roots and devitalised teeth present a burden to the energetic system and therefore have the potential to exacerbate any primary disorder.
- **Special feature:** The affected tooth can be located by scanning both the upper and lower jaw (not on the ear!) – possibly directly in the oral cavity – with a 3-Volt hammer or a gold-silver hammer. The affected tooth should be treated and possibly extracted. For locating 'interference field points' › table 5.7-4.

Tab. 5.7-4 Focal tooth infections: Location of 'interference field points' on the ear

Auricular 'interference field points'	Location
Upper Jaw	On an imaginary line between the point **TMJ** and the insertion of the ear lobe, slightly medial to the point **TMJ**
Upper Jaw (5)	In the centre of zone III, lateral and inferior to the point **Tonsils**
Lower Jaw	At a right angle to **Upper Jaw** and the gradually terminating helix
Lower Jaw (6)	Slightly superior to the point **TMJ**, at the end of the **Vegetative Grove**
Tooth (1)	In zone I, approximately 1 cm lateral to the insertion of the ear lobe
Tooth (7)	Approximately in the centre of zone IV

5.7.5 Amalgam Load

- **Causative mechanism:** By releasing mercury amalgam-fillings present a strain on the body which is already taxed by an increasing number of environmental toxins. Defective fillings significantly increase the amalgam load. Having fillings made of different materials is also problematic since gold fillings, due to their electric conductivity, dissolve mercury in amalgam fillings (galvanisation)
- **Special features:** Every person reacts differently to amalgam fillings. Even if a patient has several amalgam fillings they may not necessarily act as an interference field. Psychological aspects (fear of environmental toxins) should be considered.

- Amalgam-indicative point: the Ω_1-**Point** often indicates an amalgam-related distur-bance ('interference field point').

> - The Ω_1-Point (› 6.8.1) is also of psycho-emotional importance (depression, tension).
> - The medical history should allow to make a decision whether a RAC at the Ω_1-Point is caused by an amalgam load or related to a psycho-emotional disorder. If the point is found by RAC-palpation it should always be needled.
> - If there is an amalgam load and the primary disorder improves as a result of the treat-ments it is advisable to replace the fillings with a more compatible material (e.g. palla-dium-free gold) as well as draining the mercury (including by treating the amalgam-in-dicative point).

5.7.6 Psychosomatic Intestinal Disorders

- **Causative mechanism:** Pathological intestinal colonisation (e.g. with candida albicans) or chronic intestinal disorders (e.g. Crohn's disease, ulcerative colitis) weaken the im-mune system and impair the absorption of nutrients, thus exacerbating the primary disorder.
- **Special features:** Since the intestinal mucosa have a huge surface area the associated interference field can be equally extensive. Therapeutic intervention therefore often re-quires the combination of auricular acupuncture with other naturopathic therapies such as body acupuncture and Chinese herbal medicine. For locating 'interference field points' › table 5.7-5.

Tab. 5.7-5 Psychosomatic intestinal disorders: location of auricular 'interference field points'

Auricular 'interference field points'	Location
Duodenum (88)	In the superior concha, superior to the ascending helix root
Small Intestine (89)	Superior to the helix root, adjacent to the point **Duodenum (88)**;
Cecum	In the superior concha, at the junction of the lower and mid-dle third of the ascending helix root
Colon (91)	In the superior concha, level with the middle to upper third of the helix root
Rectum	The area extending from **Colon (91)** to the transition of the concha to the helix, medial and inferior to the intersection between the antihelix and helix
Point Zero	0.5 cm superior to the helix root, clearly palpable as a notch

5.7.7 Restricted Joint Movement

- **Causative mechanism:** Restricted movement in a joint can strain the body without necessarily causing pain. However, it weakens the body which in turn can lead to other disorders. Any joint that triggers a RAC should therefore be treated with auricular acu-puncture, even if it is free of pain.
- **Special features:** In general, joint problems are not considered as interference fields. However, any asymptomatic joint that triggers a RAC should be considered as suspi-cious.

Craniosacral therapy is the therapy of choice for supporting the treatment of restricted joints.

Tab. 5.7-6 Commonly restricted joints: location of auricular 'interference field points'

Affected joint	Auricular 'interference field points' and their location
Temporo-mandibular joint	At the intersection of an imaginary line through **Point Zero** and **Atlanto-occipital Joint**, at the lower end of the **Vegetative Groove**
Sacroiliac joint	**Buttocks (53):** at the edge of the antihelix, superior to **L2**
Sternocostal joint (1st rib)	**Thoracic Spine (39):** on the antihelix, level with **C7**

5.8 Imbalances between the Cerebral Hemispheres

Generally, one hemisphere is always dominant, or certain functions are carried out preferentially by the relevant dominant or non-dominant hemisphere. If this assignation is no longer clearly defined this is referred to as unstable laterality.

Theoretical background: If a patient is energetically imbalanced he/she will constantly consume energy to regulate his/her balance which will result in a continuous weakening of the body. Unstable laterality is an expression of such an energetic imbalance and is comparable to an interference field (› 5.7) as it exacerbates the underlying disorder and weakens the immune system. The body will find it more difficult to fight off external disorders (e.g. infections) which, as a result, will occur more frequently.

Indicators of unstable laterality

- Pathological RAC on the **Laterality Point** (› 6.8.6), possibly also on **Point Zero** (› 6.10.3).
- Further indicators of ambiguous handedness: right-handed persons leading with the left foot (normally right-handed persons lead with the right foot and vice versa). The 'clapping test' is also helpful in cases of unclear handedness: in right-handed persons the right hand will lie on top, in left-handed persons it will be the bottom hand.

Causes

- **Long-standing chronic disorders:** These deplete the body's energy reserves causing an energetic imbalance. Typical examples: chronic polyarthritis, bronchial asthma, multiple sclerosis, addictions (› 5.7). Certain long-term medication (e.g. tricyclic antidepressants or cortisone) can further contribute to unstable laterality.
- **Re-education of left-handed persons:** A person's handedness is determined by the dominant cerebral hemisphere. If this innate dominance is not respected and left-handed children are re-educated the energetic system is continuously challenged. The brain requires energy to re-programme innate responses (e.g. writing).
- **Psychological stress:** Psychological stress consumes energy, particularly if the stress-causing situation is not changed. The longer-standing the stress, the greater the imbalance. In addition, acute, profound psychological strain can cause instability, e.g. death of a life partner, severe trauma, anxiety syndromes (› 8.1.2).

Typical disorders with unstable laterality

- Atopic dermatitis, psoriasis, eczema in general
- Hay fever
- Bronchial asthma
- Difficulty concentrating, depressive moods, insomnia
- Chronic polyarthritis
- Multiple sclerosis
- Childhood development disorders, bedwetting, dyslexia

These disorders are usually multifactorial and unstable laterality should not be regarded as the sole cause. This has to be considered especially with regards to the treatment.

Treatment

The following approach applies to all forms of unstable laterality:

- **Treatment principle:** If at all possible the cause of the unstable laterality should be treated or eliminated; this is a requirement for restoring energetic balance. For this reason it is difficult to achieve a sustained stabilisation in long-term re-educated left-handed persons.
- **Procedure:** If the Laterality Point (› 6.8.6) can be found by RAC, it should be needled. When using semi-permanent needles, there should be a 3-day break between removing a needle and inserting a new one to avoid the body becoming accustomed to the stimulation.
- **Selecting the side to be treated:** The side with a pathological RAC is treated.
- **Duration of treatment:** Treatments with auricular acupuncture should continue until the Laterality Point does not show a RAC-response any longer or until the underlying disorder has been resolved.

5.9 Further Obstacles to Treatment

5.9.1 Medication

Conventional medication can, and sometimes has to, continue alongside auricular acupuncture and TCM. Medication is always necessary for severe acute disorders (emergency medical treatment) or if there are pre-existing disorders which cannot be resolved by treating the body energetically (e.g. insulin-dependent diabetes mellitus). Combining auricular acupuncture with conventional therapy generally does not compromise one or the other. However, with certain kinds of medication interactions with acupuncture have to be taken into consideration.

Cortisone preparations and other immunosuppressants

Auricular acupuncture in combination with drugs containing cortisone or immunosuppressants can often result in an exacerbation of symptoms. This is particularly the case when treating ear points that stimulate the immune system, e.g. **ACTH** (› 6.6.6), **Adrenal Cortex** (› 6.6.1) or **Immune Axis**(› 6.12.3).

Explanatory model: Cortisone suppresses the immune system resulting in a weakening of many functions in the body. This is a desired effect to inhibit inflammatory reactions, although often accompanied by considerable side effects. Auricular acupuncture, in contrast, supports the body energetically and promotes self-healing. This calms the immune system by strengthening it while possibly impeding the effects of cortisone. When treating patients who are taking cortisone the risk of an initial worsening of symptoms has to be taken into account.

Antibiotics

Bacterial infections will generally subside quickly if treated correctly with antibiotics. However, with repeated courses of antibiotics one can often observe an increased susceptibility to infections.

Explanatory models:

- Repeated courses of antibiotics result in the immune system not being sufficiently challenged. It thus becomes more susceptible to further infections.
- Due to the nature of antibiotics some energetic information regarding the infection remains in the body. The more such information accumulates (through repeated courses of antibiotics) the more the body is energetically challenged. This could result in a persistent weakening and therefore an increased susceptibility to infection.

 Auricular acupuncture has the potential to arrest the progression of infections (especially when given at an early stage), and thus accelerate the healing process. A pre-existing susceptibility to infections will often decrease.

5.9.2 Energetic Disturbances

Auricular acupuncture influences the body's energetic system. It regulates and harmonises, drains blockages, supplements energy in deficient areas (mainly by redistribution), and resolves stagnation. This, in turn, influences the physical and physiological aspects of the disorder, enabling the body to reverse the dysregulation so that affected organ systems can regenerate and heal. This process has its limits only when the disease has already caused irreversible physical damage (e.g. amputations, cirrhosis of the liver, etc.).

The rate of recovery depends on how quickly and how strongly the therapeutic information provided by auricular acupuncture can be integrated by the patient's energetic system.

Energetic disturbances can either store energy or cause its loss so that it is not available for therapeutic purposes. Energetic disturbances can thus slow down or impair the healing process.

Examples of energetic disturbances:

- **Longstanding, severe diseases**
- **Multiple disorders affecting different areas of the body,** e.g. migraines, scars and sinusitis all at the same time; this situation can result in a kind of 'fragmentation' of the therapeutically available energy.
- **Interference fields** binding energy so that it is therapeutically unavailable (› 5.7)
- **Continuous strain** on the energetic system by toxins, radiation (e.g. high-voltage power lines, transmission towers), or stress

- **'Deep-seated' blockages** of the energetic system due to chronic disorders; the longer-standing the disorder, the more it becomes engrained in the energetic system, blocking the flow of energy
- **Old age:** with increasing age, the life essence is used up. **Caution:** Age itself is no indication if a disorder can be treated or not since the innate life essence varies considerably.

5.9.3 Earrings

- **Historical background:** It was already common in the Middle Ages for sailors to wear an earring in one ear. This was supposed to improve eyesight. Carpenters and farmers, too, made use of this method. The area where the ear lobe was pierced corresponds to the French and Chinese **Eye**-point. While auricular acupuncture was not known in Western culture at that time similar observations led to the same conclusion: that visual acuity can be influenced by piercing a point on the earlobe.
- **Acute effect:** If an earring is located on a pathological, irritated ear point there will be a short-lived therapeutic effect. However, this effect is diminished by the ear being pierced front and back as this represents an energetic short circuit (› 3.2.2). If non-pathological points are pierced there will be no reaction.
- **Long-term effect:** After a few weeks the effect of a permanent stimulus such as an earring (cf. semi-permanent needle › 2.5.3) will subside. The body adapts to the stimulus, comparable to the adaptation to odours which happens within minutes.

> box
> - Usually, piercing the ear for attaching an earring does not cause any pathological symptoms.
> - If the hole does not close up after removing the earring that point is lost for auricular acupuncture. The more holes were pierced the more limited are the therapeutic options.

5.9.4 Ear Piercing

Ear piercing (and in particular ear tunnels) causes a loss of substance because of the generally larger diameter. This can lead to systemic physical symptoms, especially if the piercing affects the auricular cartilage. In contrast to earrings, piercing jewellery can trigger physical symptoms associated with the pierced points. Example: piercing the antihelix (projection area of the spine) can cause back pain. Piercing jewellery on other parts of the body can act as interference fields (› 5.7.1). In particular navel rings can weaken the energetic system (similar to laparoscopy scars).

5.10 Emergencies

5.10.1 Needle Stick

- **Procedure:** large-scale disinfection, e.g. with 70 % alcohol; bathe affected area in beta-dine solution; possibly send the needle for microbiological investigation; if hepatitis or HIV is suspected blood should be taken from both the injured person and the patient for testing; surgical care for the injury.
- **Documentation:** Every injury has to be recorded in a permanent format (e.g. accident book) including a description of the incident, date and time as well as emergency measures carried out.
- **Accident reporting procedure:** if an employee is injured this has to be reported to the relevant authority without delay.

5.10.2 Needle Collapse

- **Occurrence:** in patients with orthostatic dysregulation or when treating a seated or standing patient.
- **Action:** If the patient is not lying down already, move her/him into shock position (legs up), keep the patient warm and responsive, set pain stimuli (pinching the cheek), check blood pressure and pulse; for suspected underlying cardiovascular disease call emergency services.
- **Emergency points** (body acupuncture) for needle collapse: **GV-26** (between the upper and middle third of the philtrum, at the inferior end of the nasal septum), **PC-6** (2 cun superior to the midpoint of the palmar wrist fold, where a wrist watch is worn) and **Ex-UE-11** (tips of the ten fingers).

5.10.3 Emergency Equipment

Emergency equipment (First-Aid kit etc.) as required by the relevant authority and/or professional organisation must be kept at a well-accessible place in the clinic.

6 Point Locations

6.1 Spine

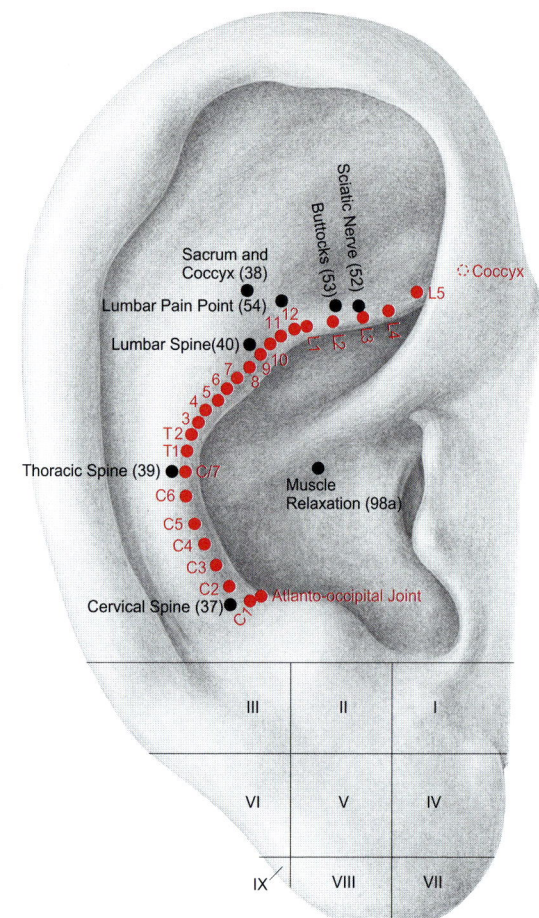

Sciatic Nerve (52)
Buttocks (53)

Sacrum and
Coccyx (38)

Lumbar Pain Point (54)

Lumbar Spine(40)

◌ Coccyx

L5

11 12

Thoracic Spine (39)

T2
T1

C/7

C6

C5

C4

C3

C2

Cervical Spine (37)

C1

Atlanto-occipital Joint

Muscle
Relaxation (98a)

III   II   I

VI   V   IV

IX   VIII   VII

Fig. 6.1-1

6.1.1 Antihelix (› Fig. 6.1-1)

The antihelix can be divided into three sections by palpating with a stirrup probe for notches in the auricular cartilage (› 2.2.1):

- 1st notch: at the junction of the antitragus and the antihelix where **Atlanto-occipital Joint** is located
- 2nd notch: at the junction of **C7** and **T1**, where the relief of the concha wall widens
- 3rd notch: in the area where the antihelix divides into superior and inferior crus; at the junction of **T12** and **L1** where the relief of the concha wall narrows

The three sections are divided according to the number of vertebrae:

- **C1–C7:** 7 sections between the 1st and 2nd notch; indication: pain therapy
- **T1–T12:** 12 sections between the 2nd and 3rd notch; indication: pain therapy
- **L1–L5:** 5 sections between the 3rd notch and the point of intersection between helix and antihelix; indication: pain therapy

Further points on the antihelix:

- **Cervical Spine (37):** at the inferior end of the antihelix, between **C1** and **C2**; indication: pain therapy
- **Thoracic Spine (39):** corresponds to the sternocostal joint; on the antihelix at the level of **C7**; indication: pain therapy, restricted movement of the sternocostal joint (interference field)
- **Lumbar Spine (40):** on the antihelix, at the level of **T10**; indication: pain therapy
- **Coccyx:** adjacent to the points **L1–L5**, at the junction of antihelix and helix, covered by the helix brim; indication: pain therapy
- **Sacrum and Coccyx (38):** at the point where the antihelix bifurcates, at the beginning of the superior crus; indication: pain therapy
- **Sciatic Nerve (52):** slightly lateral to the antihelix inferior crus, superior to **L3**; indication: pain therapy
- **Buttocks (53):** corresponds to the sacroiliac joint; at the edge of the antihelix, superior to **L2**; indication: pain therapy, blockages of the sacroiliac joint
- **Lumbar Pain Point (54):** in the area where the antihelix begins to divide; indication: pain therapy

> box
> The width of the helix brim varies. The lumbar section up to L4 can therefore be covered. Sometimes, however, even the point **Sacrum** can be visible.

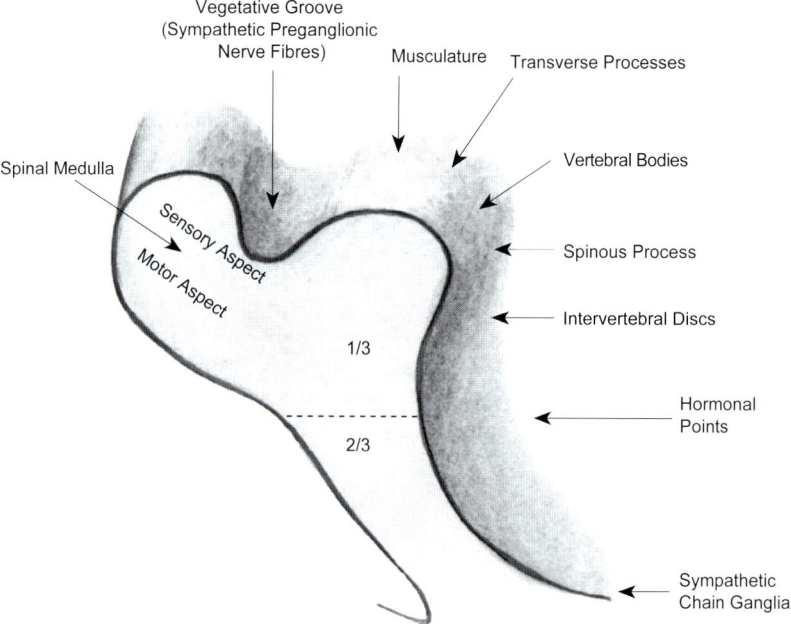

Fig. 6.1-2

6.1.2 Antihelix Cross Section (› Fig. 6.1-2)

- **Musculature:** 2mm lateral to the antihelix edge; indication: pain therapy
- **Transverse Processes:** 1mm lateral to the antihelix edge; indication: fractures
- **Vertebral Body:** directly on the antihelix edge, needle insertion at a 90° angle; indication: fractures
- **Spinous Processes:** 1mm inferior to the antihelix edge; indication: fractures
- **Intervertebral Discs:** when dividing the concha wall into three sections, superior to the junction between the 1st and 2nd third; indication: disc protrusion/prolapsed disc

6.1.3 Concha (› Fig. 6.1-1)

- **Muscle Relaxation (98a):** in the inferior concha, slightly inferior to the helix root; indication: pain therapy

6.2 Musculoskeletal System

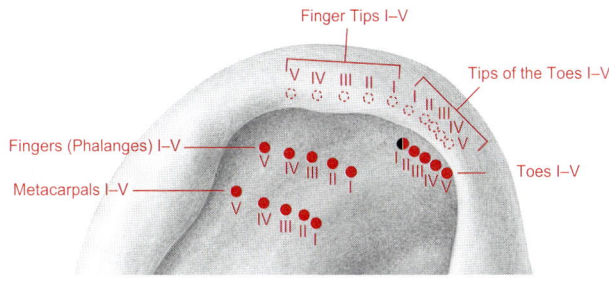

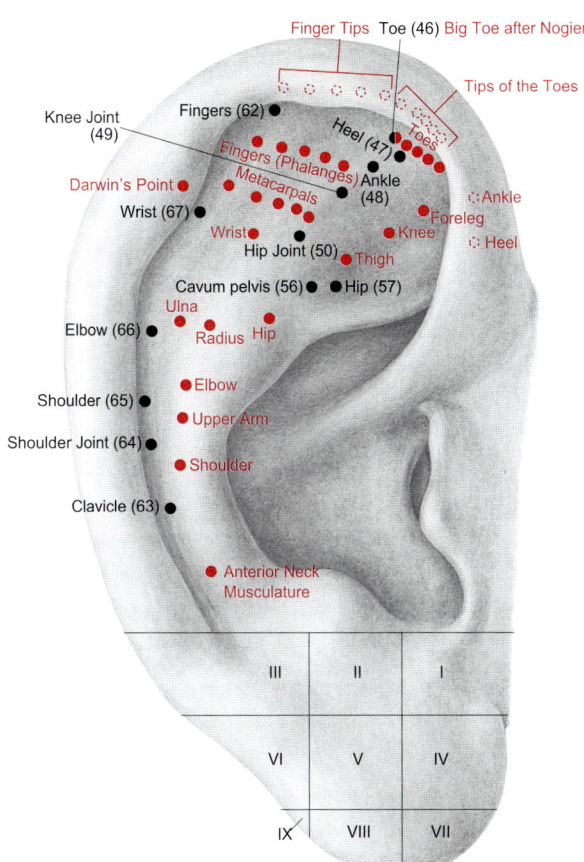

Fig. 6.2-1

6.2.1 Scapha (› Fig. 6.2-1)

- **Anterior Neck Muscles:** approximately at the level of **C2**, between the **Vegetative Groove** (› 6.9.1) and the occipital musculature, just lateral to the antihelix (› 6.1.2); indication: pain therapy

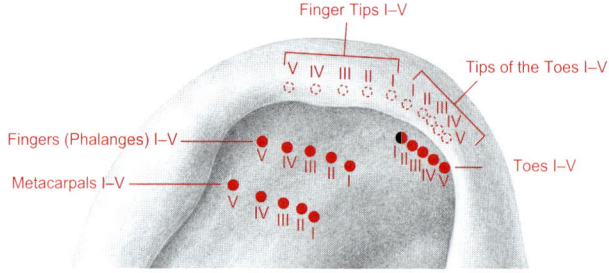

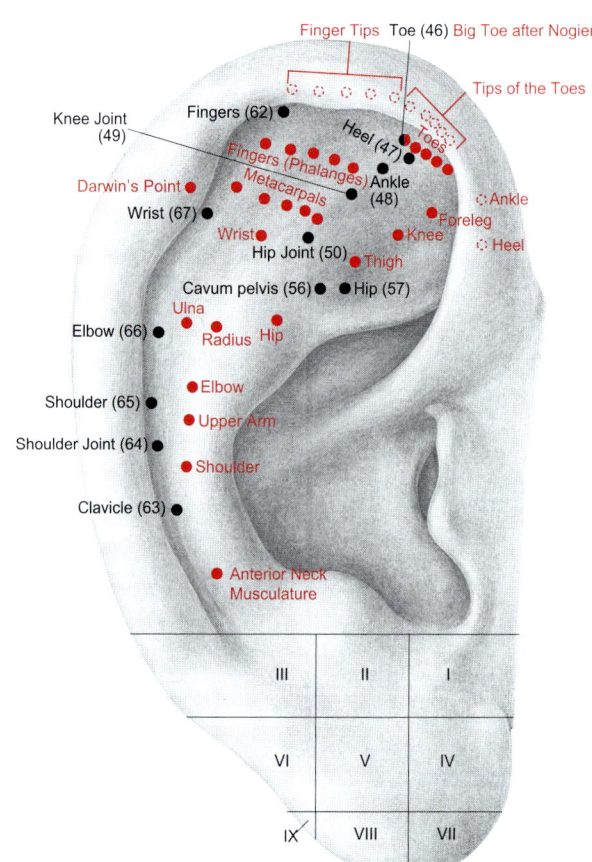

Fig. 6.2-1

Upper Extremity

- **Clavicle (63):** just medial to the **Vegetative Groove,** level with **C5**; indication: pain therapy
- **Shoulder:** between **C7** and the **Vegetative Groove**; indication: pain therapy
- **Shoulder (65):** slightly medial to the **Vegetative Groove,** level with **T4**; indication: pain therapy
- **Shoulder joint (64):** slightly medial to the **Vegetative Groove,** level with **T1**; indication: pain therapy
- **Upper arm:** between **Shoulder** and **Elbow,** level with **T2/3**; indication: pain therapy
- **Elbow** (after Nogier): in the extension of the lumbar spine area of the antihelix and medial to the **Vegetative Groove**; indication: pain therapy
- **Elbow (66):** slightly medial to the **Vegetative Groove** and inferior to the lower border of Darwin's tubercle; indication: pain therapy
- **Ulna:** lateral to the midpoint of an imaginary line between **Elbow** and **Wrist**; indication: pain therapy
- **Radius:** between **Elbow** and **Wrist,** but more medial to this line; indication: pain therapy
- **Wrist** (after Nogier): on a horizontal line extending laterally from **Knee**, medial to the **Vegetative Groove**; indication: pain therapy
- **Wrist (67):** in the scapha, level with Darwin's tubercle; indication: pain therapy
- **Metatarsals I–V:** in the superior part of the scapha, medial to Darwin's tubercle; indication: pain therapy
- **Fingers (Phalanges) I–V:** in the superior part of the scapha, inferior to the helix brim; indication: pain therapy
- **Fingers (62):** in the scapha, just before the helix brim, somewhat superior and lateral to Darwin's tubercle; indication: pain therapy
- **Finger tips I–V:** in the superior part of the scapha, covered by the helix brim, below the **Vegetative Groove**; indication: pain therapy

Lower Extremity

- **Toes I–V, Toe I = Toe (46):** in the upper section of the superior crus of the antihelix, slightly anterior to the helix brim; **Toes** form a mirror image to **Fingers (Phalanges),** i.e. **Toe I** (big toe) is adjacent to **Finger I** (thumb); indication: pain therapy
- **Tips of the Toes I–V:** superior to **Toes,** covered by the helix brim; indication: pain therapy
- **Toe (46):** lateral to the superior crus of the antihelix, slightly inferior to the helix brim; indication: pain therapy

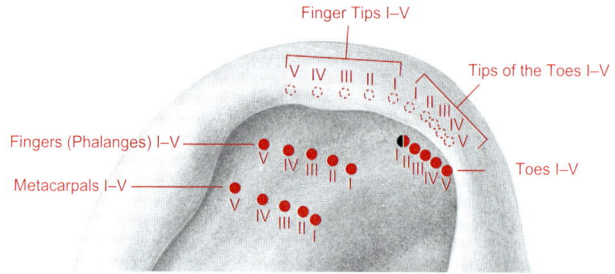

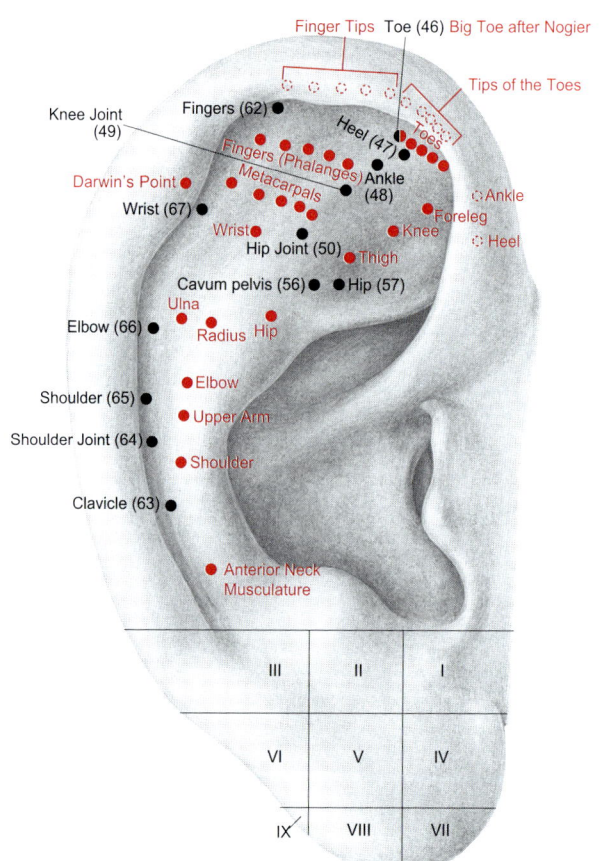

Fig. 6.2-2

6.2.2 Antihelix (› Fig. 6.2-2)

- **Hip (57):** at the apex of the triangular fossa; indication: pain therapy
- **Hip Joint (50):** on the superior crus of the antihelix, opposite the deepest point of the triangular fossa (**Knee** after Nogier); indication: pain therapy
- **Knee Joint (49):** on the superior crus of the antihelix, superior and medial to **Hip Joint (50)**; indication: pain therapy
- **Ankle (48):** on the superior crus of the antihelix, superior to **Knee Joint (49)**; indication: pain therapy
- **Heel (47):** on the superior crus of the antihelix, slightly inferior to the helix brim; indication: pain therapy

6.2.3 Triangular Fossa (› Fig. 6.2-2)

Lower Extremity

- **Hip** (after Nogier): at the apex of the intersection point of the inferior and superior crus of the antihelix; this point can sometimes be raised; indication: pain therapy
- **Pelvic Cavity (56):** at the intersection where the inferior and superior crus divide; indication: pain therapy
- **Thigh:** between **Hip** and **Knee**; indication: pain therapy
- **Knee:** at the deepest point of the triangular fossa; indication: pain therapy
- **Lower Leg:** between **Knee** and **Ankle**; indication: pain therapy
- **Ankle:** on the extension of a line connecting **Hip** and **Knee**, at the transition into the helix; indication: pain therapy
- **Heel:** 2mm superior to the intersection between antihelix and helix, covered by the helix brim; indication: pain therapy

6.2.4 Helix (› Fig. 6.2-2)

- **Darwin's Tubercle:** a cartilaginous protrusion on the lateral aspect of the helix; in evolutionary terms it represents the tip of the ear in mammals; indication: pain therapy, especially of the lower extremities

6.3 Skull

6.3.1 Helix (› Fig. 6.3-1)

- **Tonsil I (73):** on the top of the superior helix brim; indication: tonsillitis, tonsillectomy scar representing an interference field (› 5.7.1)

- **Tonsil II (74):** on the edge of the helix tail, somewhat inferior to the level of **Point Zero**; indication: tonsillitis, tonsillectomy scar representing an interference field (› 5.7.1)

- **Tonsil III (75):** on the helix tail, approximately level with the apex of the antitragus; indication: tonsillitis, tonsillectomy scar representing an interference field (› 5.7.1)

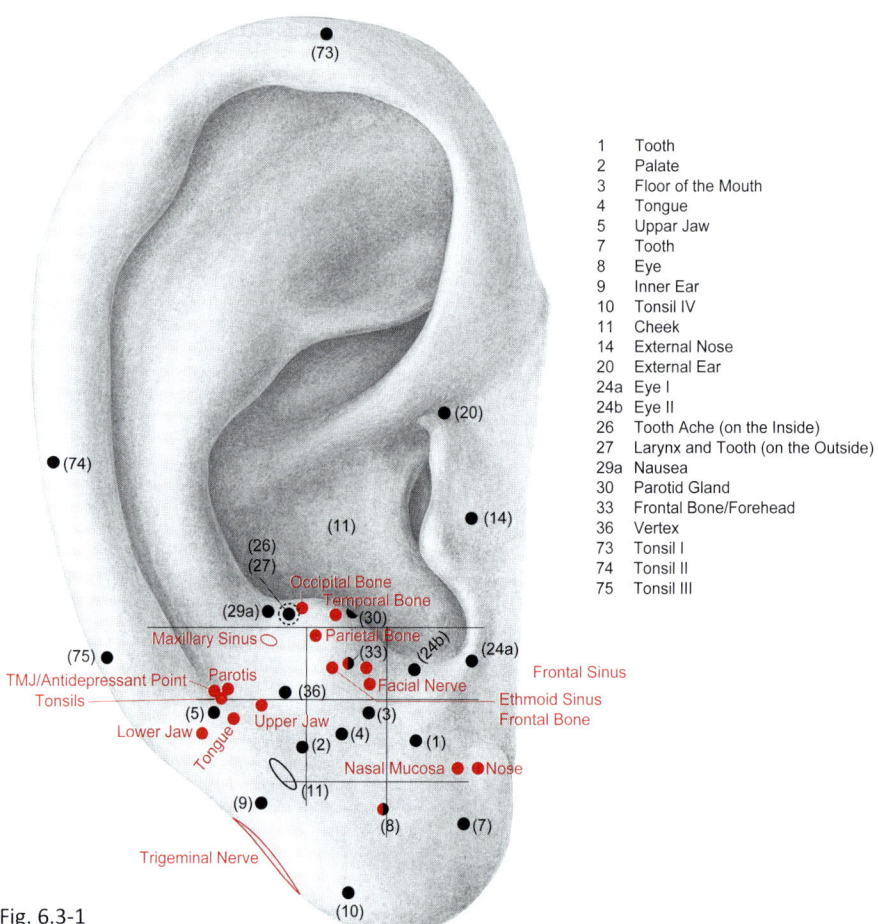

1	Tooth
2	Palate
3	Floor of the Mouth
4	Tongue
5	Uppar Jaw
7	Tooth
8	Eye
9	Inner Ear
10	Tonsil IV
11	Cheek
14	External Nose
20	External Ear
24a	Eye I
24b	Eye II
26	Tooth Ache (on the Inside)
27	Larynx and Tooth (on the Outside)
29a	Nausea
30	Parotid Gland
33	Frontal Bone/Forehead
36	Vertex
73	Tonsil I
74	Tonsil II
75	Tonsil III

Fig. 6.3-1

6.3.2 Tragus (› Fig. 6.3-1)

- **External Nose (14):** in a groove at the inferior tragus protrusion; indication: infections (cold, flu), allergic rhinitis
- **Inner Nose (16):** in the lower third of the inside of the tragus; indication: infections (cold, flu), allergic rhinitis
- **External Ear (20):** in the corner between helix root and tragus; indication: ear injury

6.3.3 Antitragus (› Fig. 6.3-1)

- **Frontal Bone/Forehead (33):** close to the antitragus protrusion; indication: pain therapy
- **Parietal Bone:** at the midpoint of the inferior edge of the antitragus; indication: pain therapy
- **Temporal Bone:** at the midpoint of the superior edge of the antitragus; indication: pain therapy
- **Occipital Bone:** on the antitragus, at the end adjacent to the base of the antihelix; indication: pain therapy
- **Frontal Sinus:** on the antitragus protrusion, more medial than **Frontal Bone**; indication: sinusitis
- **Ethmoid Sinus:** lateral and generally somewhat superior to **Frontal Sinus**, slightly inferior to the antitragus; indication: sinusitis, interference field
- **Sphenoid Sinus:** lateral and superior to **Ethmoid Sinus**, slightly inferior to the antitragus; indication: sinusitis, interference field
- **Maxillary Sinus:** inferior to the point **Atlanto-occipital Joint**, slightly inferior to the antitragus; indication: sinusitis, interference field
- **Nasal Mucosa:** slightly lateral to **Nose**; indication: infections (cold, flu), allergic rhinitis
- **Eye (8):** in the centreof the lobe; indication: all eye disorders
- **Tooth Ache (26):** on the inside of the antitragus, at its lateral end; indication: pain therapy
- **Larynx and Tooth (27):** on the outside of the tragus, opposite the point **Tooth Ache (26)** located on the inside; indication: sore throat
- **Parotid Gland (30):** at the midpoint of the antitragus ridge; indication: parotitis
- **Vertex (36):** medial to the inferior end of the **Vegetative Groove (TMJ)**, on the intersection of a vertical line through **Atlanto-occipital Joint**; indication: pain therapy
- **Nausea (29a):** just slightly inferior to the point **Atlanto-occipital Joint**, on a line perpendicular to a second line extending laterally to the points **Point de Jérome (29b)** (› 6.8.2), **Occiput (29)** (› 6.7.4) and **Desire (29c)** (› 6.8.3)

> **box**
> There are five different Chinese points for the tonsils and the teeth. For the eye there are three points; Eye (8) is indicated for any eye disorder, Eye I (24a) for non-inflammatory eye disorders and Eye II (24b) for inflammations of the eye. RAC-palpation is essential for selecting the appropriate point (› 3.1.4).

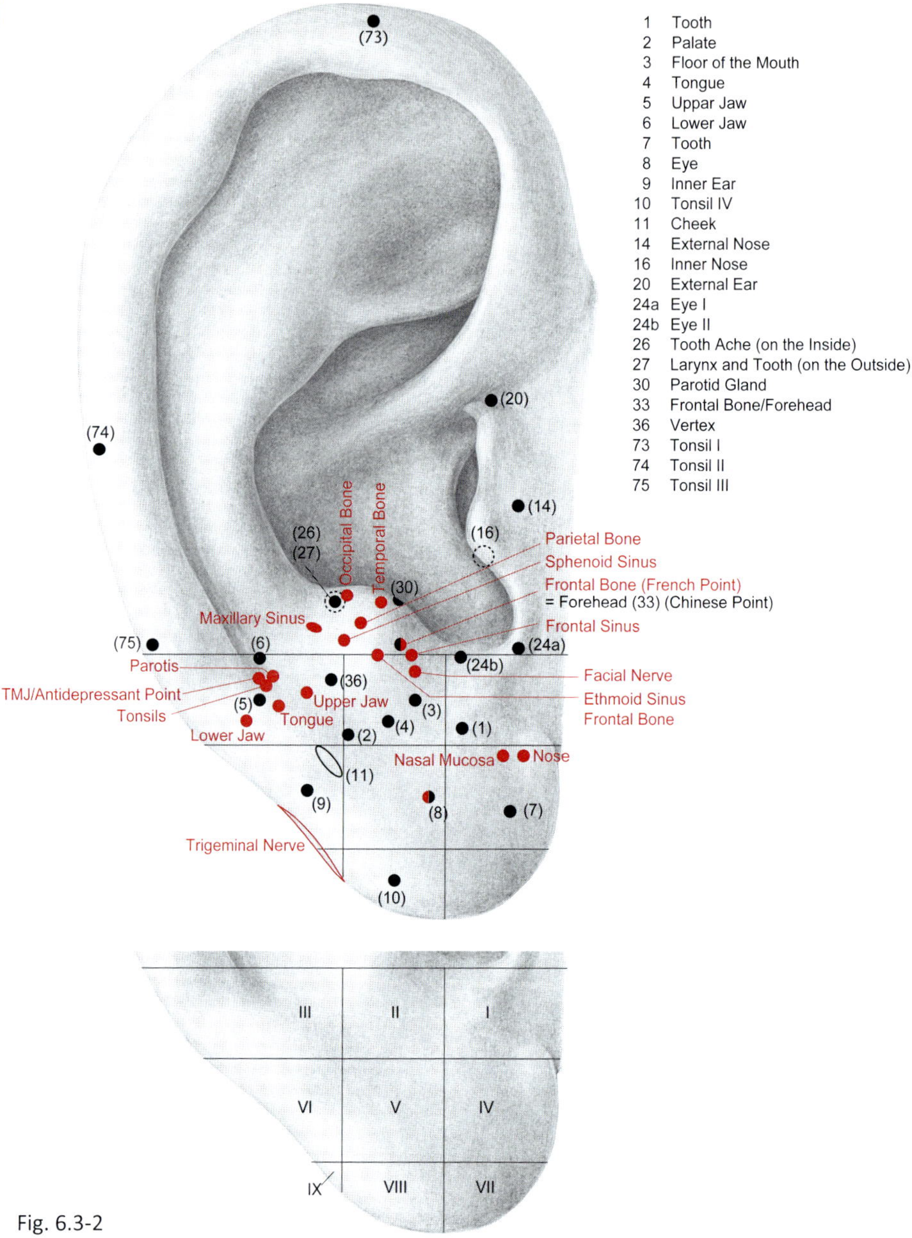

(73)

1   Tooth
2   Palate
3   Floor of the Mouth
4   Tongue
5   Uppar Jaw
6   Lower Jaw
7   Tooth
8   Eye
9   Inner Ear
10 Tonsil IV
11 Cheek
14 External Nose
16 Inner Nose
20 External Ear
24a Eye I
24b Eye II
26 Tooth Ache (on the Inside)
27 Larynx and Tooth (on the Outside)
30 Parotid Gland
33 Frontal Bone/Forehead
36 Vertex
73 Tonsil I
74 Tonsil II
75 Tonsil III

(74)

(20)

(14)

Occipital Bone
Temporal Bone
(26)
(27)
(16)
Parietal Bone
Sphenoid Sinus
Frontal Bone (French Point)
= Forehead (33) (Chinese Point)
(30)
Maxillary Sinus
Frontal Sinus
(75)
(6)
(24a)
Parotis
(36)
(24b)
Facial Nerve
TMJ/Antidepressant Point
(5)
Upper Jaw
(3)
Ethmoid Sinus
Tonsils
Tongue
(4)
(1)
Frontal Bone
Lower Jaw
(2)
Nasal Mucosa
Nose
(11)
(9)
(8)
(7)
Trigeminal Nerve
(10)

III   II   I

VI   V   IV

IX   VIII   VII

Fig. 6.3-2

6.3.4 Lobe (› Fig. 6.3-2)

The lobe is divided in to nine zones to facilitate point location.

- **TMJ/Antidepressant Point:** at the lower end of the **Vegetative Groove**, at the intersection of an imaginary line through **Point Zero** and **Atlanto-occipital Joint**; indication: pain therapy, blockages
- **Upper Jaw:** on an imaginary line connecting the point **TMJ** and the lobular insertion, slightly medial to the point **TMJ**; indication: pain therapy, tooth problems
- **Upper Jaw (5):** in the centre of zone III, lateral and inferior to **Tonsil**; indication: pain therapy, tooth problems
- **Lower Jaw:** at the transition between the end of the helix and the lobe; indication: pain therapy, tooth problems
- **Lower Jaw (6):** slightly superior to the point **TMJ**, at the lower end of the **Vegetative Groove**; indication: pain therapy, tooth problems
- **Teeth (1):** in zone I, approximately 1cm lateral to the attachment of the lobe; indication: pain therapy, tooth problems
- **Teeth (7):** approximately in the centre of zone IV; indication: pain therapy, tooth problems
- **Tonsil:** directly inferior to the point **TMJ**; indication: tonsillitis, tonsillectomy scar representing an interference field (› 5.7.1)
- **Tonsil IV (10):** approximately in the centre of zone VIII; indication: tonsillitis, tonsillectomy scar representing an interference field (› 5.7.1)
- **Palate (2):** in the lateral, inferior corner of zone II, on a line extending from the **Vegetative Groove**; indication: laryngitis, for example in conjunction with flu
- **Floor of the Mouth (3):** in zone II, slightly inferior to the medial end of the antitragus; indication: infections
- **Cheek (11):** at the intersection of zones II, III, V and VI, in the extension of the **Vegetative Groove**; indication: infections
- **Tongue:** between the points **Upper** and **Lower Jaw**; indication: speech impediments
- **Tongue (4):** between **Palate (2)** and **Floor of the Mouth (3)**; indication: speech impediments
- **Parotid Gland:** medial to the point **TMJ**; indication: parotitis
- **Nose:** slightly lateral to the insertion of the lobe; indication: infections, allergic rhinitis
- **Eye I (24a):** medial to the intertragic notch; indication: non-inflammatory eye disorders
- **Eye II (24b):** lateral to the intertragic notch; indication: inflammatory eye disorders
- **Trigeminal Nerve:** on the lateral border of the ear, on the extension of an imaginary line connecting **Point Zero** and the antitragus; indication: pain therapy
- **Facial Nerve:** slightly inferior to **Frontal Sinus**; indication: pareses
- **Inner Ear (9):** at the transition of the helix tail to the lobe; indication: tinnitus, vertigo

6.4 Inner Organs

6.4.1 Concha (› Fig. 6.4-1a+b)

- **Mouth (84):** slightly superior to the ear canal; indication: infections
- **Gullet Point:** on the upper border of the ear canal; indication: addiction, difficulty swallowing

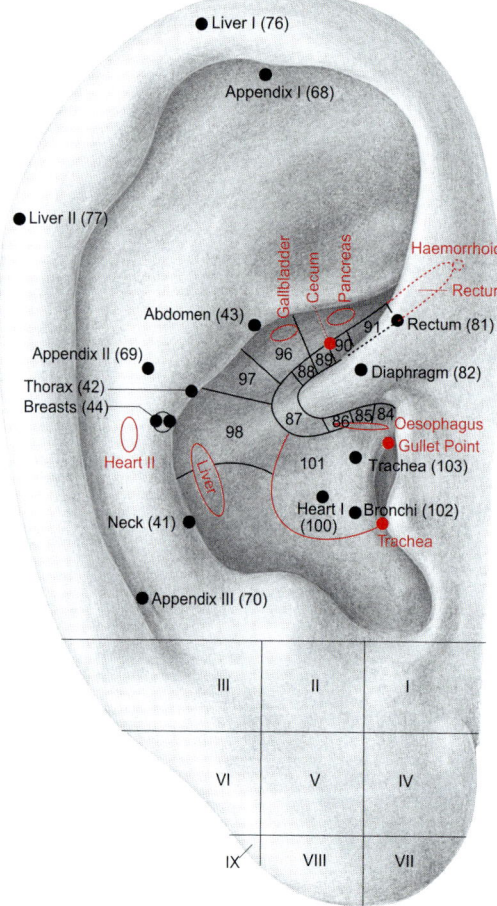

84 Mouth
85 Oesophagus
86 Cardia
87 Stomach
88 Duodenum
89 Small Intestine
90 Appendix IV
91 Colon
96 Pancreas/Gallbladder
97 Liver
98 Spleen
101 Lungs

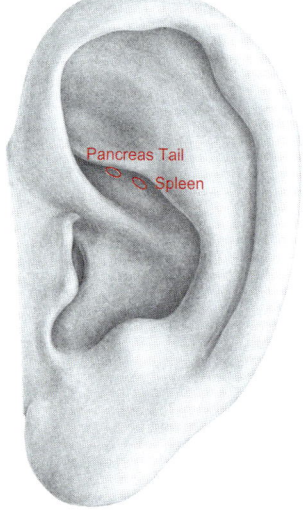

Fig. 6.4-1a+b

- **Oesophagus:** using the point **Gullet Point** as reference, slightly inferior to the ascending helix; indication: oesophagitis, reflux
- **Oesophagus (85):** at the midpoint of the inferior border of the helix root; indication: oesophagitis, reflux
- **Cardia (86):** lateral to **Oesophagus (85)**; indication: gastritis, ulcers
- **Stomach (87):** in the concha, curving around the helix root; indication: gastritis, ulcers
- **Duodenum (88):** in the superior concha, superior to the ascending helix root; indication: duodenitis
- **Small intestine (89):** superior to the helix root, adjacent to **Duodenum (88)**; indication: enteritis, Crohn's disease
- **Appendix IV (90):** in the superior concha, adjacent to the helix root, in the area of **Cecum**; indication: appendicitis
- **Cecum:** at the junction of the lower and middle third of the ascending helix root, in the superior concha; indication: appendicitis, enteritis, Crohn's disease
- **Colon (91):** in the superior concha, level with the middle to upper third of the helix root; indication: colitis, bowel irregularities
- **Rectum:** the area reaching from **Colon (91)** to the transition of the concha to the helix, medial and inferior to the intersection between the antihelix and helix; indication: enteritis, bowel irregularities
- **Haemorrhoids:** medial and inferior to the intersection between antihelix and helix; indication: haemorrhoids
- **Trachea:** on the lower border of the ear canal; indication: pulmonary infections, tracheitis
- **Trachea (103):** in the concha, lateral to the upper part of the ear canal; indication: tracheopulmonary infections, tracheitis
- **Bronchi (102):** in the concha, lateral to the lower part of the ear canal; indication: bronchopulmonary infections
- **Lung (101):** in the lower half of the inferior concha, surrounds the point **Heart I (100)** in the shape of a leaf; indication: pulmonary infection
- **Heart I (100):** approximately 1cm lateral to the ear canal, approximately on the midline of the ear; indication: heart disorders
- **Pancreas** (right ear: **Pancreas Head**): superior and medial to **Gallbladder**; indication: pancreatitis
- **Pancreas** (left ear: **Pancreas Tail**): superior and medial to **Spleen**; indication: pancreatitis, diabetes mellitus
- **Pancreas/Gallbladder (96):** a zone in the superior concha, approximately level with **T9–L1**; indication: pancreatitis, cholecystitis, cholecystolithiasis
- **Liver** (right ear only): a zone in the upper half of the inferior concha, parallel to the antihelix; indication: hepatitis
- **Liver (97):** in the superior concha, approximately level with **T5–9**; indication: hepatitis
- **Gallbladder** (right ear only): a zone in the superior concha, on the lower border of the antihelix, superior to the helix root; indication: cholecystitis, cholecystolithiasis

- **Spleen** (left ear only): same location as **Gallbladder** but in the left ear; indication: disorders of the haemopoietic system, fear
- **Spleen (98):** a zone in the medial concha, lateral to the helix root; indication: disorders of the haemopoietic system, fear

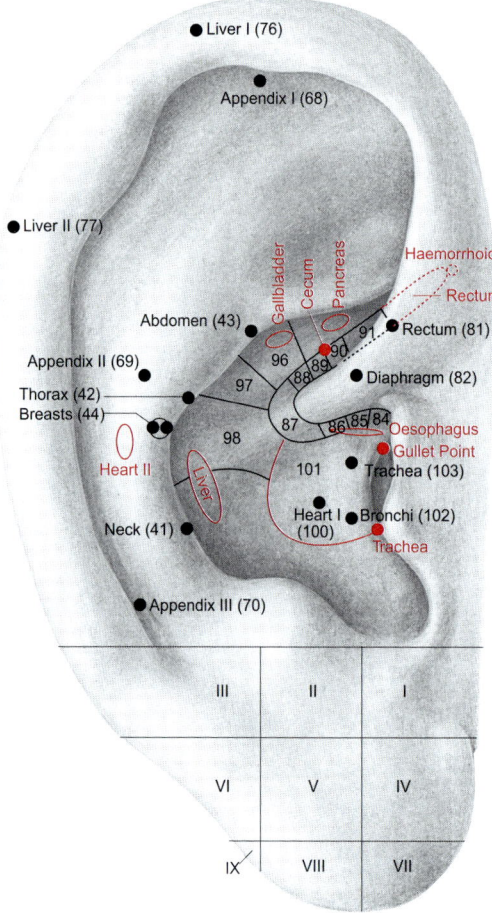

84 Mouth
85 Oesophagus
86 Cardia
87 Stomach
88 Duodenum
89 Small Intestine
90 Appendix IV
91 Colon
96 Pancreas/Gallbladder
97 Liver
98 Spleen
101 Lungs

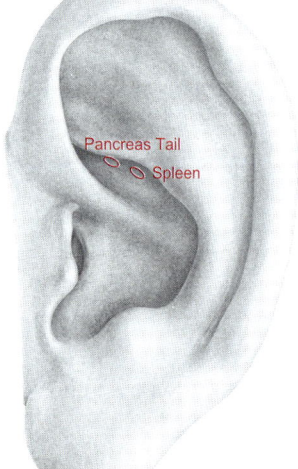

Fig. 6.4-2a+b

The variability of the abdominal location of the appendix is mirrored in the ear. Appendix IV can be found at the helix root but also more superiorly by up to one transverse process. In contrast, the locations of the points Appendix I, II, and III respectively hardly vary at all.

6.4.2 Scapha (› Fig. 6.4-2a)

- **Appendix I (68):** in the scapha, anterior to the edge of the helix brim, near **Finger Digit IV**; indication: appendicitis, interference field following appendectomy
- **Appendix II (69):** between helix and antihelix, level with the points for the lower thoracic spine; indication: appendicitis, interference field following appendectomy
- **Appendix III (70):** at the inferior end of the **Vegetative Groove**; indication: appendicitis, interference field following appendectomy
- **Heart II:** the area lateral to the antihelix, approximately level with **C7–T1**; indication: heart disorders

6.4.3 Helix (› Fig. 6.4-2a)

- **Diaphragm (82):** on the ascending helix, slightly superior to **Point Zero**; indication: supports the Middle
- **Liver I (76):** on the helix, at the superior end of Darwin's tubercle; indication: hepatitis
- **Liver II (77):** on the helix, at the inferior end of Darwin's tubercle; indication: hepatitis
- **Rectum (81):** on the helix, superior to the French point **Rectum** located in the concha; indication: enteritis, bowel irregularities
- **Anus:** on the lateral border of the ascending helix, level with the intersecting point of antihelix and helix; indication: anal fissures, haemorrhoids

6.4.4 Antihelix (› Fig. 6.4-2a)

- **Gullet Point (41):** on the edge of the antihelix, level with **C4**; indication: sore throat, colds, viral infections
- **Thorax (42):** on the antihelix, opposite the helix root near **T4/5**; indication: pulmonary infections
- **Mammary Glands (44):** divided into two points, one on the antihelix level with **T1**, the other slightly lateral to the first point; indication: mastitis, lumps, interference field following mastectomy
- **Abdomen (43):** on the edge of the antihelix, level with **T11**; indication: diffuse abdominal disorders

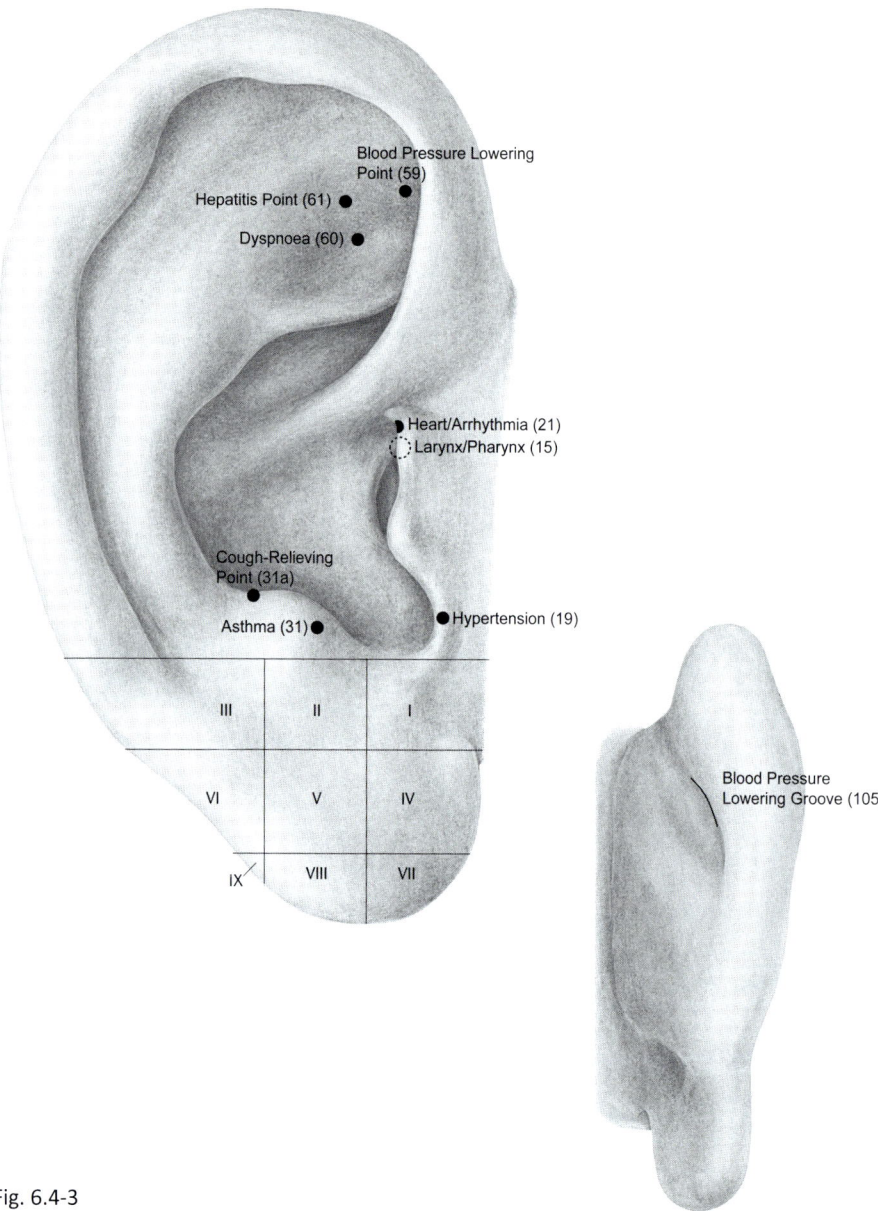

Blood Pressure Lowering
Point (59)

Hepatitis Point (61)

Dyspnoea (60)

Heart/Arrhythmia (21)
Larynx/Pharynx (15)

Cough-Relieving
Point (31a)

Asthma (31)

Hypertension (19)

III   II   I

VI   V   IV

IX   VIII   VII

Blood Pressure
Lowering Groove (105)

Fig. 6.4-3

6.4.5 Tragus (› Fig. 6.4-3)

- **Heart/Arrhythmia (21):** on the edge of the tragus, at its superior end, slightly inferior to the helix; indication: cardiac arrhythmia
- **Larynx/Pharynx (15):** on the lateral inner edge of the tragus, level with the superior edge of the ear canal; indication: inflammation, difficulty swallowing
- **Hypertension (19):** on the inferior end of the tragus; indication: hypertension

6.4.6 Antitragus (› Fig. 6.4-3)

- **Asthma (31):** on the medial inferior third of the antitragus protrusion; indication: asthma, allergies, dyspnoea
- **Cough-Relieving Point (31a):** at the lateral superior end of the antitragus; indication: chronic urge to cough, chronic irritation of the throat

6.4.7 Triangular Fossa (› Fig. 6.4-3)

- **Blood Pressure Lowering Point (59):** slightly inferior to the end of the superior crus of the antihelix, not covered by the helix brim; indication: hypertension
- compare with **Blood Pressure Lowering Groove (105)** on the posterior ear (› 6.11.3)
- **Hepatitis Point (61):** in the triangular fossa, inferior to the midpoint of the superior crus of the antihelix; indication: hepatitis
- **Dyspnoea (60):** in the centre the triangular fossa, near the point **Knee** (› 6.2.3); indication: dyspnoea

box
- The point Glans Penis/Clitoris corresponds to the Frustration Point, while the point Testes/Ovaries corresponds to the point Testosterone/Oestrogen.
- The urogenital points on the helix brim (Uterus, Ovaries/Oestrogen/Testes/Testosterone, Prostate) are needled from below.

6.5 Urogenital System

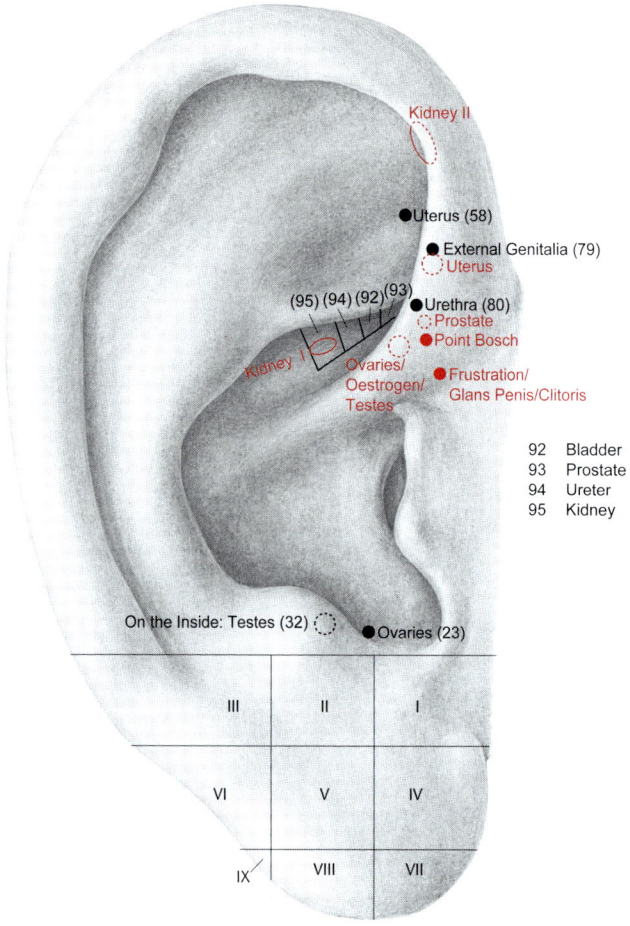

Fig. 6.5-1

6.5.1 Concha (› Fig. 6.5-1)

- **Kidney I:** in the 'cave' of the superior concha, inferior to **L2** (after Nogier); indication: nephrolithiasis, nephritis
- **Kidney (95):** in the 'cave' of the superior concha, inferior to **L2** (after Nogier); indication: nephrolithiasis, nephritis
- **Ureter (94):** between **Kidney (95)** and **Bladder (92)**; indication: ureterolithiasis, urinary tract infection
- **Bladder (92)**(= **sensitive bladder**): in the 'cave' of the superior concha, slightly lateral to the intersection between antihelix and helix, slightly inferior to **L4**; indication: urinary tract infection; compare to **Bladder /Motor Function** (muscular aspect) on the posterior ear (› 6.11.3)

- **Prostate (93):** in the 'cave' of the superior concha, lateral to the intersection between helix and antihelix; indication: prostate hypertrophy, prostatitis
- **Ovaries (23):** in the inferior concha, lateral to the intertragic notch; indication: ovarian cysts, adnexitis; considered equivalent to gonadotropin (› 6.6.7) by some schools
- **Point Bosch** (genital region after Nogier): on the lateral edge of the helix brim, inferior to the intersection between helix and antihelix; indication: impotence
- **Prostate:** on the inside of the edge of the helix brim, inferior to the intersection between helix and antihelix; indication: prostate hypertrophy, prostatitis
- **External Genitalia (79):** on the helix, slightly superior to the intersection between helix and antihelix; indication: impotence
- **Frustration/Glans Penis/Clitoris:** on the medial upper edge of the ear, slightly inferior to the ascending helix; indication: impotence, frustration
- **Urethra (80):** on the helix brim, slightly inferior to the intersection between helix and antihelix; indication: urinary tract infection

6.5.2 Helix (› Fig. 6.5-1)

- **Uterus:** on the inside of the helix brim, superior to the intersection point between helix and antihelix; indication: fibroids, dysmenorrhoea
- **Ovaries/Oestrogen/Testes/Testosterone:** on the inside of the helix brim, there is often a cartilaginous protrusion, approximately 1 transverse process inferior to the intersection between helix and antihelix; indication: ovarian cysts, adnexitis, impotence, hydrocoele
- **Point Bosch** (genital region after Nogier): on the lateral edge of the helix brim, inferior to the intersection between helix and antihelix; indication: impotence
- **Prostate:** on the edge of the inside of the helix brim, inferior to the intersection between helix and antihelix; indication: prostate hypertrophy, prostatitis
- **External Genitalia (79):** on the helix, slightly superior to the intersection between helix and antihelix; indication: impotence
- **Frustration/Glans Penis/Clitoris:** on the medial upper edge of the ear, slightly inferior to the ascending helix; indication: impotence, frustration
- **Urethra (80):** on the helix brim, slightly inferior to the intersection between helix and antihelix; indication: urinary tract infection

6.5.3 Antitragus (› Fig. 6.5-1)

- **Testes (32):** on the inside of the antitragus, opposite **Asthma (31)** (› 6.4.6), which is located on its external surface; indication: impotence, hydrocoele

6.5.4 Triangular Fossa (› Fig. 6.5-1)

- **Kidney II:** at the gradually terminating end of the superior crus of the antihelix, partially covered by the helix brim; indication: nephrolithiasis, nephritis
- **Uterus (58):** at the superior end of the triangular fossa, slightly lateral to the helix brim; indication: fibroids, dysmenorrhoea

6.6 Hormonal Points

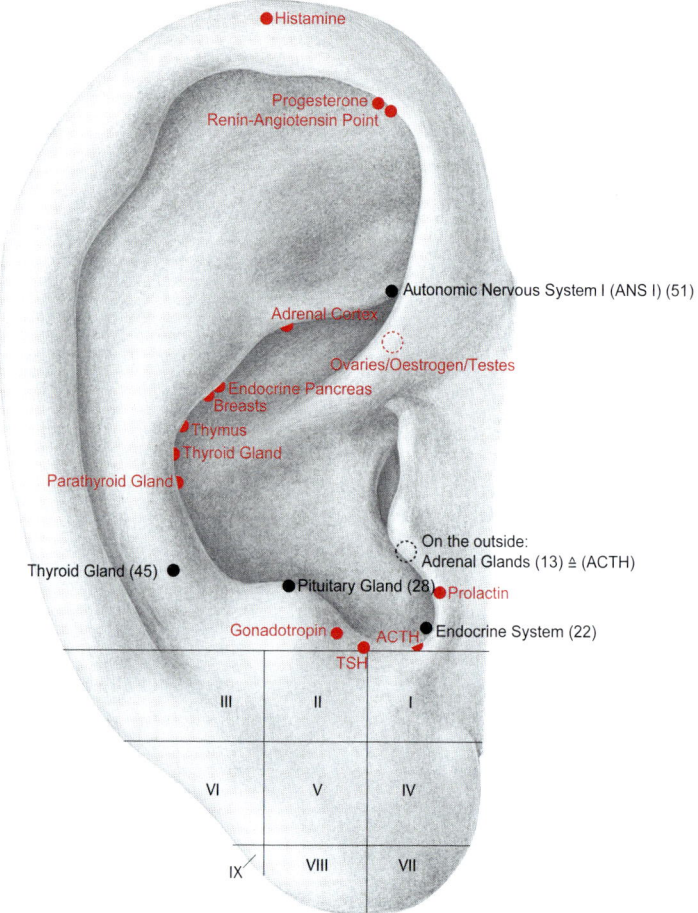

Histamine

Progesterone
Renin-Angiotensin Point

Autonomic Nervous System I (ANS I) (51)

Adrenal Cortex

Ovaries/Oestrogen/Testes

Endocrine Pancreas
Breasts

Thymus

Thyroid Gland

Parathyroid Gland

On the outside:
Adrenal Glands (13) ≙ (ACTH)

Thyroid Gland (45)

Pituitary Gland (28)   Prolactin

Gonadotropin   ACTH   Endocrine System (22)

TSH

III   II   I

VI   V   IV

IX   VIII   VII

Fig. 6.6-1

6.6.1 Hormonal Line on the Antihelix Wall (› Fig. 6.6-1)

The points of the Hormonal Line can be found on an imaginary line, which is located ⅓ from the upper edge and ⅔ from the base of the antihelix wall (› Fig. 6.1-2)

- **Parathyroid Gland:** inferior to **C6**; indication: calcium metabolism disorders
- **Thyroid Gland:** inferior to **C7**; indication: hypo/hyperthyroidism
- **Thymus Gland:** inferior to **T2/3**; indication: resistance against infections, exposure to radiation, interference fields
- **Breast:** inferior to **T5**; indication: mastitis, lumps
- **Endocrine Pancreas:** inferior to **T6**; indication: diabetes mellitus
- **Adrenal Cortex:** inferior to **L1**; indication: weak immune system, auto-immune disorders, allergies

6.6.2 Concha (› Fig. 6.6-1)

- **Endocrine System (22):** at the deepest point of the intertragic notch; indication: stabilisation of the immune system, auto-immune disorders

6.6.3 Scapha (› Fig. 6.6-1)

- **Renin-Angiotensin Point:** at the end of the superior crus of the antihelix, just at the edge of the helix brim, lateral and superior to the area of **Kidney II**; indication: hypertension
- **Progesterone:** lateral and superior to the **Renin-Angiotensin Point**; indication: dysmenorrhoea, premenstrual syndrome, migraines

6.6.4 Helix (› Fig. 6.6-1)

- **Histamine:** on the highest point of the helix, at the tip of the ear, which is formed by folding the ear forward; indication: allergies, interference fields
- **Oestrogen** (in men **Testosterone**, corresponds to the points **Ovaries/Testes**): on the inside of the helix brim, approximately 1 transverse process inferior to the intersection between helix and antihelix; indication: dysmenorrhoea, premenstrual syndrome, migraine

6.6.5 Antihelix (› Fig. 6.6-1)

- **Thyroid (45):** slightly lateral to the antihelix wall, approximately level with **C2**; indication: hypo/hyperthyroidism
- **Autonomic Nervous System I (ANS I) (51):** on the inferior crus of the antihelix, on the intersecting point with the helix; indication: cardiovascular dysregulation, dizziness, dystonia

6.6.6 Tragus (› Fig. 6.6-1)

- **ACTH:** 2mm inferior to the intertragic notch; indication: weak immune system, auto-immune disorders, allergies
- **Prolactin:** medial and superior to the intertragic notch; indication: lactation disorders
- **Adrenal Glands:** slightly inferior to the inferior tragus protrusion; indication: weak immunity, auto-immune disorders, allergies

6.6.7 Antitragus (› Fig. 6.6-1)

- **Pituitary Gland (28):** on the ridge of the antitragus, at the junction of its upper and medial third; indication: stabilises the immune system
- **TSH:** slightly lateral to the intertragic notch; indication: goitre
- **Gonadotropin:** at the medial end of the antitragus; indication: dysmenorrhoea, premenstrual syndrome, migraines; according to some schools this point corresponds to the point **Ovaries (23)**

6.7 Analgesic and Medication-analogous Points

6.7.1 Scapha (› Fig. 6.7-1a+b)

- **Barbiturate/Caffeine:** level with **C7,** slightly medial to the **Vegetative Groove**; indication: pain therapy, anxiety. Barbiturate: located only on the non-dominant ear, caffeine: located only on the dominant ear; indication of Caffeine: influences sleep rhythm
- β-**Receptor:** level with **T3,** slightly medial to the **Vegetative Groove**; indication: tachycardia, palpitations

> **box**
> The point Barbiturate/Caffeine has a sedating effect similar to barbiturates on the non-dominant ear only; on the dominant ear it has a stimulating effect similar to caffeine. On the dominant ear, the point β-Receptor has a rather sympathomimetic effect, while on the non-dominant ear its effect is rather sympatholytic.

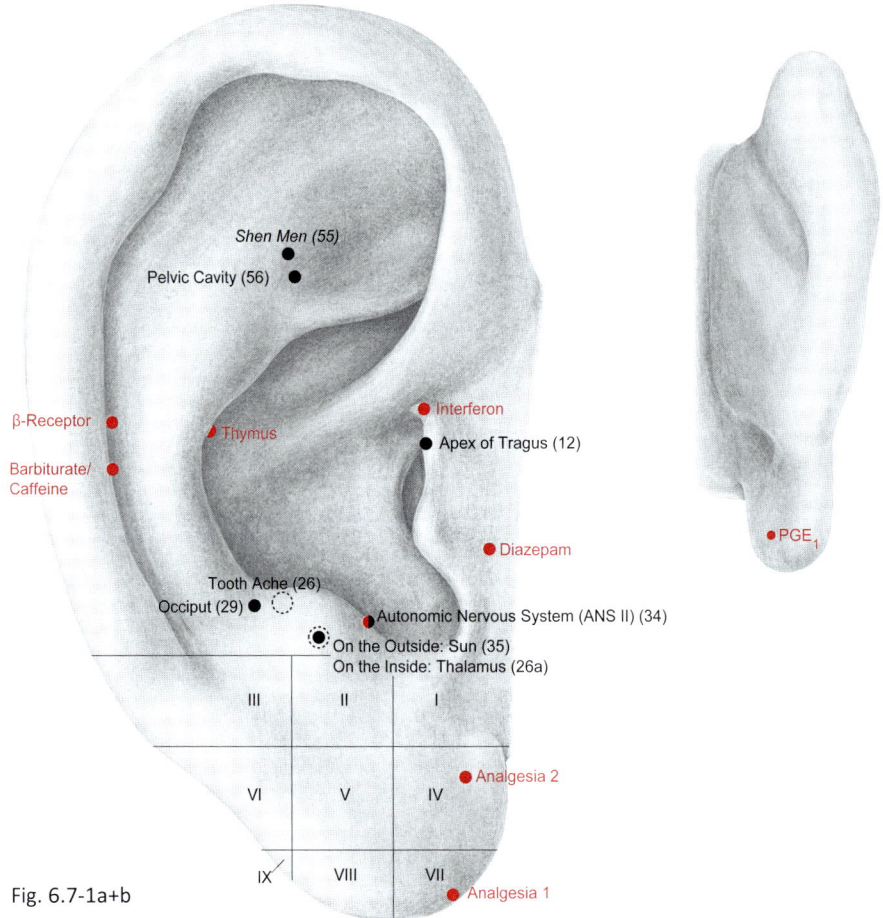

Shen Men (55)
Pelvic Cavity (56)
β-Receptor
Thymus
Barbiturate/Caffeine
Interferon
Apex of Tragus (12)
Diazepam
PGE₁
Tooth Ache (26)
Occiput (29)
Autonomic Nervous System (ANS II) (34)
On the Outside: Sun (35)
On the Inside: Thalamus (26a)
III   II   I
VI   V   IV
Analgesia 2
IX   VIII   VII
Analgesia 1

Fig. 6.7-1a+b

6.7.2 Antihelix (› Fig. 6.7-1a+b)

- **_Shen Men_ (55):** in the triangular fossa, slightly superior to where the superior crus of the antihelix begins; indication: pain therapy
- **Pelvic Cavity (56):** precisely in the corner where the superior and inferior crus divide; indication: pain therapy in the pelvic and hip area

6.7.3 Tragus (› Fig. 6.7-1a+b)

- **Diazepam:** in a groove medial to the tragus protrusion, slightly inferior to the tip of the tragus; indication: pain therapy for myalgia, relaxation, anxiety
- **Interferon:** on the superior end of the tragus, in the angle which is formed by the ascending helix; indication: infections, allergies
- **Apex of Tragus (12):** on the lateral, superior edge of the tragus, level with the upper border of the ear canal; indication: pain therapy, inflammations

6.7.4 Antitragus (› Fig. 6.7-1a+b)

- **Thalamus (26a)/Thalamus:** at the tip of a triangle which forms when folding the antitragus outward, actually located in the concha; indication: pain therapy
- **Occiput (29):** on the lateral, superior end of the antitragus; indication: pain therapy
- **Sun (35):** on the outside of the antitragus, opposite the point **Thalamus (26a)**; indication: pain therapy
- **Tooth Ache (26):** on the inside of the antitragus, at its lateral end; indication: pain therapy
- **Autonomic Nervous System II (ANS II) (34)/Grey Matter/Subcortex:** on the inside of the antitragus ridge, towards its medial end; indication: pain therapy, inflammations

6.7.5 Lobulus (› Fig. 6.7-1a+b)

- **Analgesia 1:** on the inferior medial edge of the lobe, in zone VII; indication: pain therapy
- **Analgesia 2:** slightly lateral to the insertion of the lobe; indication: pain therapy

6.7.6 Combinations (› Fig. 6.7-1a+b)

- **Diclofenac:** combination of **PGE$_1$** (› 6.11.4) on the dominant side and **Thymus** (› 6.6.1) on the non-dominant side; indication: pain therapy
- **Valoron:** combination of **Analgesia 2** and **Thalamus (26a)**; indication: pain therapy

> Occiput (29), Sun (35), Shen Men (55), and Thalamus (26a) are primary analgesic points, particularly suitable for headaches and migraine. Apex of Tragus (12) and ANS II (34) have an analgesic as well as an anti-inflammatory effect.

6.8 Psycho-emotional Points

6.8.1 Concha (› Fig. 6.8-1)

- **Neural Liver Point/Resentment:** in the sympathetic groove (› Fig. 6.9-1a) level with **T 5/6** (› 6.1.1); indication: resentment, aggression
- Ω_1-**Point:** in the superior concha, slightly lateral to the intersection between antihelix and helix, but located more closely to the antihelix; indication: depression, tension

> If the Ω_1-Point is found by RAC-palpation, this can be an indication of amalgam contamination. Treating this point will promote its drainage. The Ω_1-Point corresponds to the hypogastric plexus and the inferior mesenteric ganglion after Bourdiol.

6.8.2 Scapha (› Fig. 6.8-1)

- **Point de Jérome (29b):** between **Atlanto-occipital Joint** and **TMJ** (at the end of the **Vegetative Groove**), in the inferior part of the scapha; indication: insomnia, diffuse anxiety

6.8.3 Helix (› Fig. 6.8-1)

- Ω_2-**Point:** on the helix, on a vertical line above the intersecting point between the helix and antihelix; indication: depression, tension
- **Frustration(Glans Penis/Clitoris)** (› 6.5.2): on the medial edge of the ear, slightly below the ascending helix; indication: frustration, depression, tension
- **Weather Change:** on the ascending helix, on the extension of the lateral edge of the tragus; indication: pain therapy
- **Desire (29c):** at the inferior end of the helix, where it gradually terminates; indication: addiction therapy

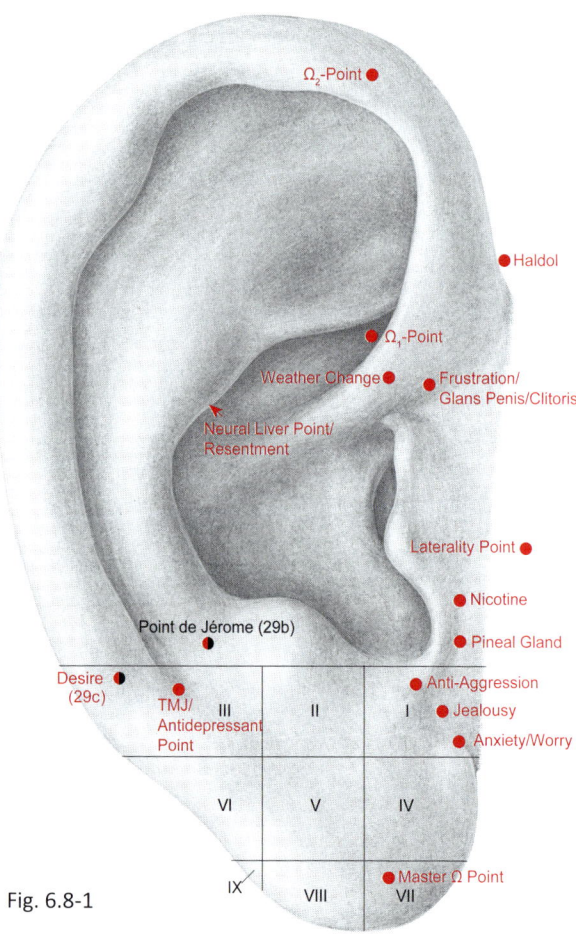

Ω_2-Point

Haldol

Ω_1-Point

Weather Change

Frustration/
Glans Penis/Clitoris

Neural Liver Point/
Resentment

Laterality Point

Nicotine

Point de Jérome (29b)

Pineal Gland

Desire
(29c)

Anti-Aggression

TMJ/
Antidepressant
Point

III   II   I

Jealousy

Anxiety/Worry

VI   V   IV

IX   VIII   VII

Master Ω Point

Fig. 6.8-1

6.8.4 Tragus (› Fig. 6.8-1)

- **Nicotine:** in the tragus fold at the insertion of the ear, level with the midpoint of a line connecting the tip of the tragus with the intertragic notch; indication: addiction therapy
- **Pineal Gland:** in the tragus fold, towards the insertion of the ear, slightly superior to the level of the intertragic notch; indication: disturbed sleep

6.8.5 Lobe (› Fig. 6.8-2)

- **Antidepressant Point/TMJ (PT 3)** (› 6.3.4, 6.13.2): at the end of the **Vegetative Groove**, on a line through the points **Atlanto-occipital Joint** and **Point Zero**; indication: depression, tension
- **Master Ω Point:** in zone VII, on a vertical line below the intersecting point of helix and antihelix; indication: depression, tension
- **Anti-Aggression (PT 1)** (› 6.13.2): a few millimetres inferior to the intertragic notch; indication: aggression, addiction therapy
- **Jealousy:** on the medial border of the ear, slightly superior to the insertion of the lobe; indication: jealousy
- **Anxiety (PT 2)** (› 6.13.2): on the anterior aspect of the ear, at the insertion of the lobe; located only on the dominant ear (**Worry** on the non-dominant ear); indication: anxiety
- **Worry (PT 2):** (› 6.13.2): on the anterior aspect of the ear, at the insertion of the lobe; only on the non-dominant ear (**Anxiety** on the dominant ear); indication: anxiety

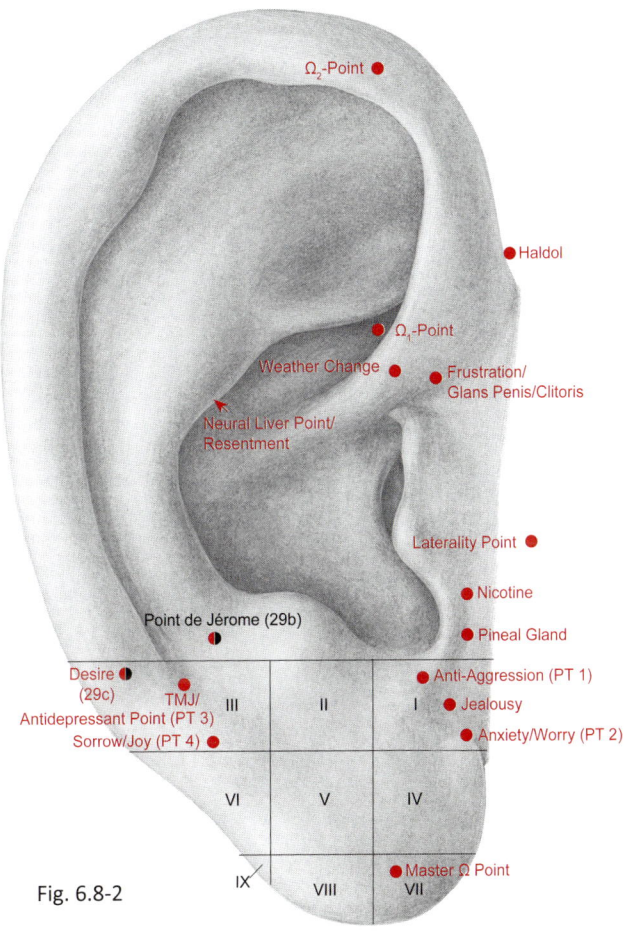

Ω_2-Point

Haldol

Ω_1-Point

Weather Change

Frustration/
Glans Penis/Clitoris

Neural Liver Point/
Resentment

Laterality Point

Nicotine

Point de Jérome (29b)

Pineal Gland

Desire (29c)

Anti-Aggression (PT 1)

TMJ/
Antidepressant Point (PT 3)

III

II

I

Jealousy

Sorrow/Joy (PT 4)

Anxiety/Worry (PT 2)

VI

V

IV

IX

VIII

Master Ω Point

VII

Fig. 6.8-2

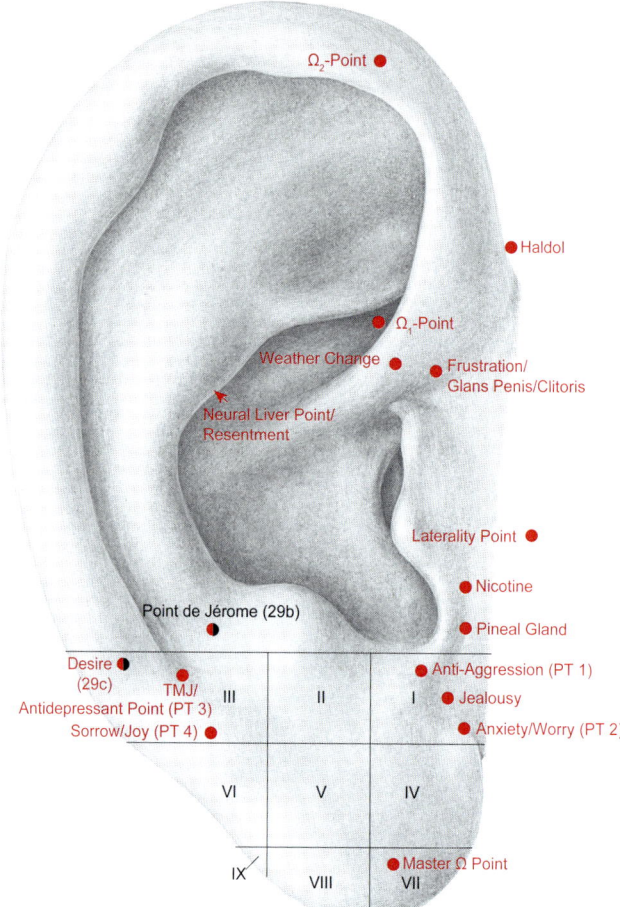

Ω_2-Point

Haldol

Ω_1-Point

Weather Change

Frustration/
Glans Penis/Clitoris

Neural Liver Point/
Resentment

Laterality Point

Nicotine

Point de Jérome (29b)

Pineal Gland

Desire
(29c)

Anti-Aggression (PT 1)

TMJ/
Antidepressant Point (PT 3)

Jealousy

Sorrow/Joy (PT 4)

Anxiety/Worry (PT 2)

III

II

I

VI

V

IV

Master Ω Point

IX

VIII

VII

Fig. 6.8-2

- **Sorrow/joy (PT 4):** (› 6.13.2): on an imaginary extension of the **Vegetative Groove**, on a horizontal line connecting with the point pair **Anxiety/Worry**, level with the insertion of the lobe; **Joy** on the dominant ear, **Sorrow** on the non-dominant ear; indication: lethargy, lack of vitality

6.8.6 Facial Area (› Fig. 6.8-2)

- **Laterality Master Point:** on the face, on a horizontal line level with the midpoint of the inferior tragus protrusion, approximately 3cm from the tip; indication: depression, tension, stabilises handedness, allergies
- **Haldol (Bourdiol):** on the face, on an imaginary extension of the antihelix, slightly medial to the helix; indication: depression, tension, restlessness

6.9 Vegetative and Sympathetic Groove

6.9.1 Vegetative Groove (› Fig. 6.9-1a+b)

The Vegetative Groove is located in the transitional area between the scapha and the helix. It extends from the groove below the lateral end of the antitragus to the inferior crus of the antihelix. The Vegetative Groove corresponds to the sympathetic trunk (› Fig. 6.1-2).

- The auricular points located along this groove correspond to the spinal segments; they can be found by 'drawing' a line through **Point Zero** and the relevant spinal segment (**C1–L 5**) and then extending this line to the Vegetative Groove.

- Indication: pain therapy for disorders of the spine (according to the corresponding spinal points on the antihelix). Needling the corresponding points in the **Vegetative Groove** can increase the effect of needling the individual spinal segments.

box Often points in the Vegetative Groove have a stronger RAC-response than the corresponding muscular points of the affected spinal segments (C1–L5). Both points should be needled for best therapeutic results!

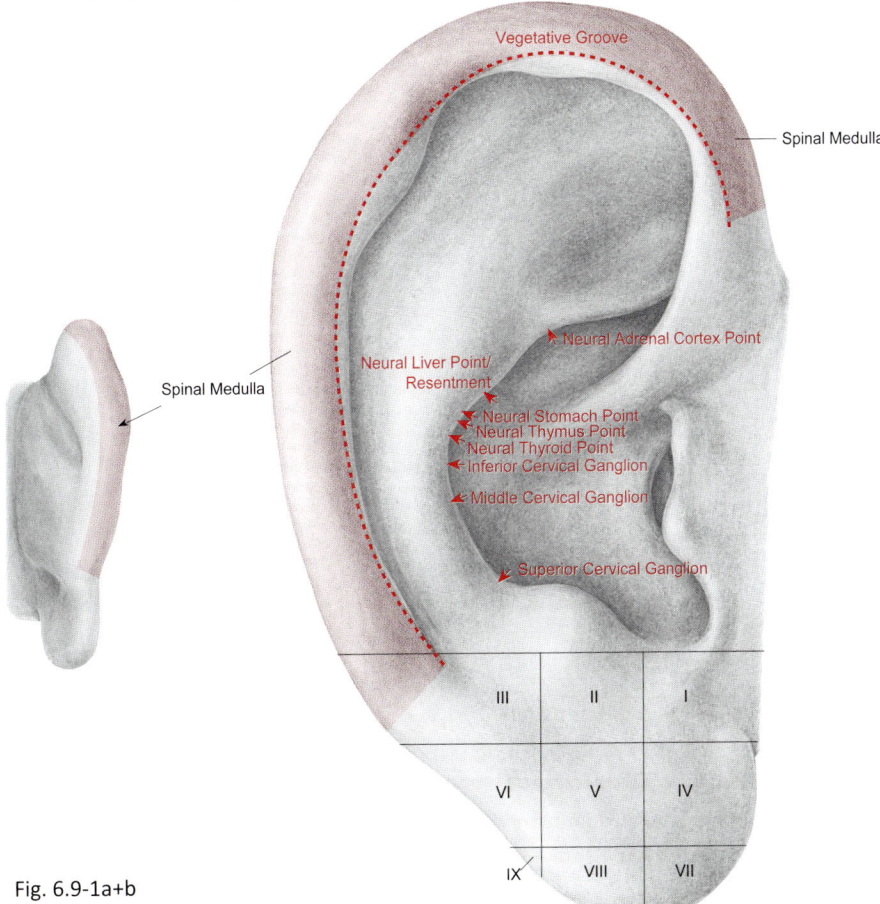

Fig. 6.9-1a+b

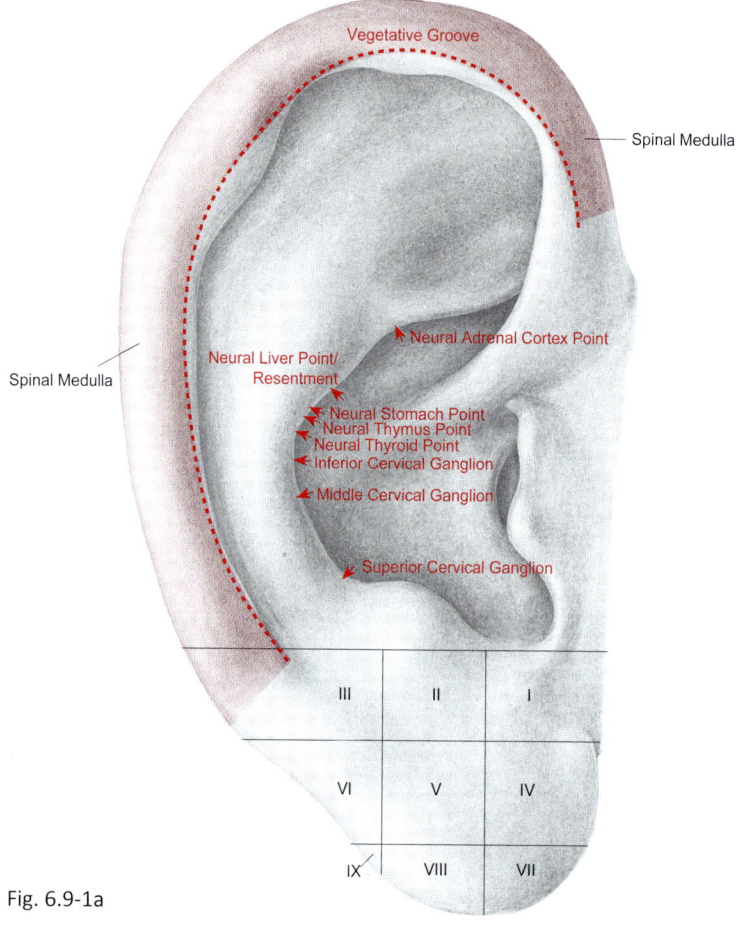

Fig. 6.9-1a

6.9.2 Sympathetic Groove (› Fig. 6.9-1a+b)

Located at the junction of the concha and the antihelix wall (› 6.1.2).

- **Superior Cervical Ganglion:** level with **C1/2**; indication: sympathetic dysregulation, glaucoma
- **Middle Cervical Ganglion:** level with **C5/6**; indication: blood pressure dysregulation
- **Inferior Cervical Ganglion /Stellate Ganglion:** level with **C7**; indication: pain therapy of the cervical spine, migraines, hyperemesis gravidarum (morning sickness)
- **Neural Thyroid Point:** level with **T2**; indication: hypo/hyperthyroidism
- **Neural Thymus Point:** level with **T2/3**; indication: stimulates the immune system
- **Neural Stomach Point:** level with **T3/4**; indication: ulcers, gastritis
- **Neural Liver Point /Resentment:** level with **T5/6**; indication: resentment
- **Neural Adrenal Cortex Point:** level with **T12**; indication: blood pressure dysregulation

6.9.3 Spinal Cord (› Fig. 6.9-1a+b)

- On the helix, beginning at the intersection of the ascending helix with the antihelix and extending to the transitional area between the helix root and the lobe
- The sensory nerve fibres are represented on the anterior aspect of the helix (› Fig. 6.9-1a)
- The motor nerve fibres are represented on the posterior aspect of the helix (› Fig. 6.9-1b+c)

Indication: regeneration following ischaemic damage (e.g. tumours of the spinal cord, post-operative, post-stroke rehabilitation, cerebral palsy)

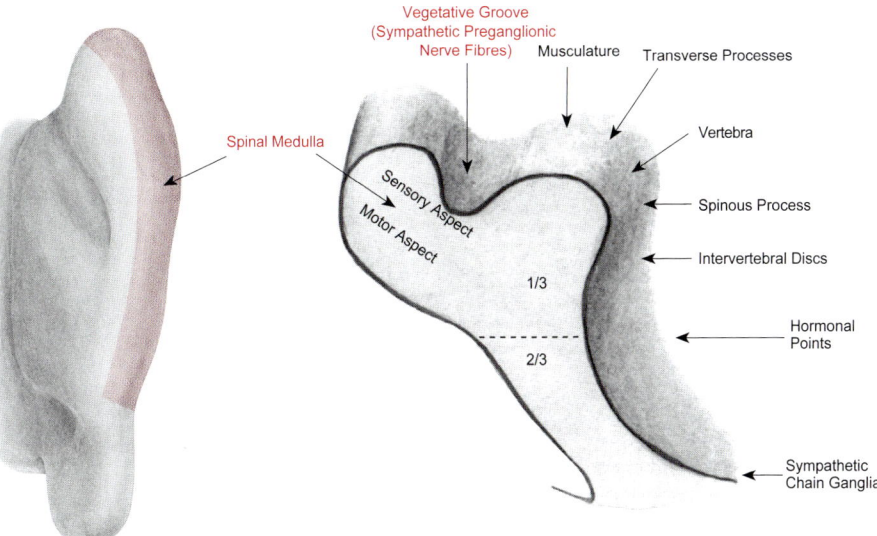

Fig. 6.9-1b+c

6.10 Extra Points

6.10.1 Concha (› Fig. 6.10-1)

- **Cardiac Plexus**: in the lateral inferior concha, level with **C4/5** between the **Sympathetic groove** (› 6.9.2) and the **Liver** area (› 6.4.1); indication: cardiac disorders
- **Bronchopulmonary Plexus:** in the inferior concha, slightly inferior to the helix root; indication: stabilising effect for lung disorders, depression
- **Branching Point (83):** in the superior concha close to the helix root, indication: enuresis, exam nerves
- **Ascites (99):** in the superior concha, at the intersection of the zones of **Duodenum (88)**, **Small Intestine (89)**, **Pancreas/Gallbladder (96)** and **Kidney (95)**; indication: ascites
- *San Jiao* **(Triple Warmer) (104):** area in the most medial and inferior corner of the inferior concha, inferior to the ear canal; indication: chronic constipation, oedema, moves the qi, meteorism

6.10.2 Scapha (› Fig. 6.10-1)

- **Urticaria (71):** zone in the lateral scapha close to Darwin's tubercle; indication: urticaria, allergies

6.10.3 Helix (› Fig. 6.10-1)

- **Apex of Ear (78):** at the apex of the helix; indication: anxiety, pain therapy
- **Point Zero** (Centre Point): 0.5 cm superior to the helix root, a clear notch is palpable; indication: stabilising point

6.10.4 Antihelix (› Fig. 6.10-1)

- **Brainstem (25):** at the edge of the antihelix, approximately level with **C2**; indication: disturbed consciousness, meningitis, cerebral ischaemia

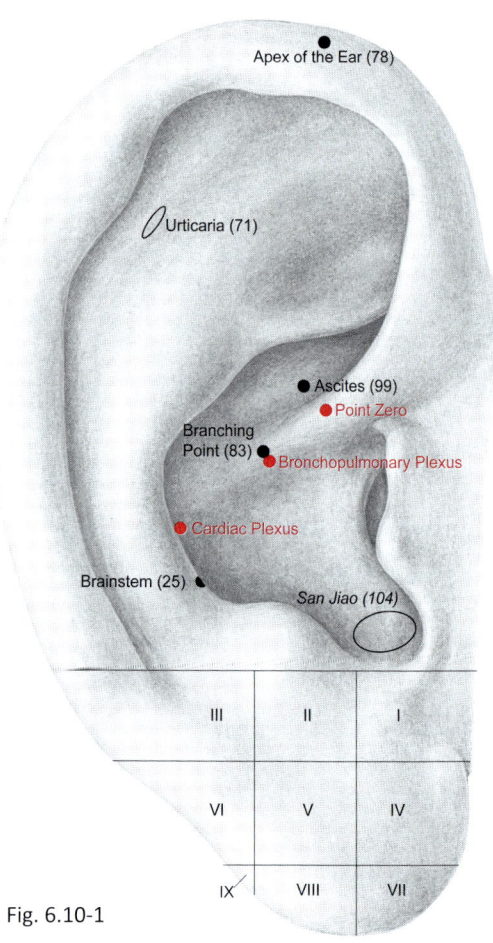

Fig. 6.10-1

6.10.5 Tragus (› Fig. 6.10-2)

- **Statoacoustic Nerve:** at the midpoint of the inferior tragus protrusion; indication: deafness, acute hearing loss
- **Thirst (17):** superior to the midpoint of the tragus, medial towards the face; indication: exsiccosis
- **Hunger (18):** inferior to the midpoint of the tragus, lateral to **Diazepam** (› 6.7.3) and **Nicotine** (› 6.8.4); indication: addiction, obesity, eating disorders

6.10.6 Antitragus (› Fig. 6.10-2)

- **Sensory Line:** a line in the antitragal groove, approximately 1cm long; the Sensory Line was originally defined by Nogier and connects the points **Occiput (29)** (› 6.7.4), **Sun (35)** (› 6.7.4), and **Forehead (33)** (› 6.3.3); indication: deafness, acute hearing loss, headaches
- **Vertigo Line** (after Drs Steinburg 1981): connects the points **Occiput (29)** (› 6.7.4), **Point de Jérome** (› 6.8.2) and **Antidepressant Point** (› 6.8.5) with the point **Atlanto-occipital Joint** (› 6.1.1), extending at a right angle to the inside of the antitragus; indication: dizziness, vertigo, acute hearing loss

6.10.7 Meatus (› Fig. 6.10-2)

- **Vagus Nerve:** a zone on the edge of the ear canal; indication: dysregulation of the cardiovascular system

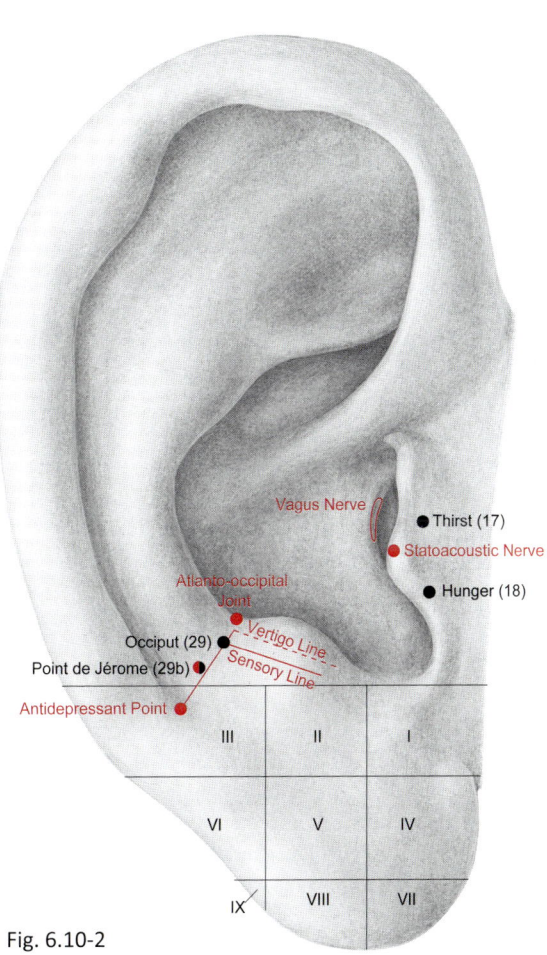

Fig. 6.10-2

6.11 Points on the Posterior Ear

The motor aspects of the organs are projected primarily on the posterior ear while the sensory aspects are found on the anterior ear. The posterior ear should therefore be included when treating the spine and the musculoskeletal system in order to increase the treatment effect. However, since the points on the posterior ear are arranged less clearly than on the anterior ear precise point location can be more difficult. Treatment of the posterior ear is therefore recommended mainly in addition to the anterior ear, especially for beginners. Stimulating the sensory aspects of the organs on the anterior ear will also have a therapeutic effect on the motor aspects (e.g. by relaxing the musculature of the spine › 6.1.2, › 6.1.3).

6.11.1 Spine (› Fig. 6.11-1)

When the ear is folded over the anatomy of its posterior aspect can be somewhat confusing. The following descriptions of the point locations should therefore be considered as a rough guide only. The precise locations should always be determined by RAC-palpation (› 3.1.4).

- **Cervical Spine:** a zone on the inferior part of the antihelix groove; indication: pain therapy
- **Thoracic Spine:** a zone in the medial part of the antihelix groove; indication: pain therapy
- **Lumbar Spine:** a zone in the groove of the inferior crus of the antihelix; indication: pain therapy
- **Cervical Spine (107):** a few millimetres medial to the midpoint of the inferior third of the antihelix groove; indication: pain therapy
- **Thoracic Spine (108):** a few millimetres medial to the midpoint of the antihelix groove; indication: pain therapy
- **Lumbar Spine (106):** a few millimetres medial to the midpoint of the superior third of the antihelix groove; indication: pain therapy

The motor aspects of the spinal cord are represented on the posterior aspect of the helix brim (in contrast to its sensory aspects on the anterior ear › 9.3). Following RAC-palpation, pain therapy should only be carried out in cases of known irreversible damage to the spinal cord. If the spinal cord is intact, as in a prolapsed disc with motor defi-

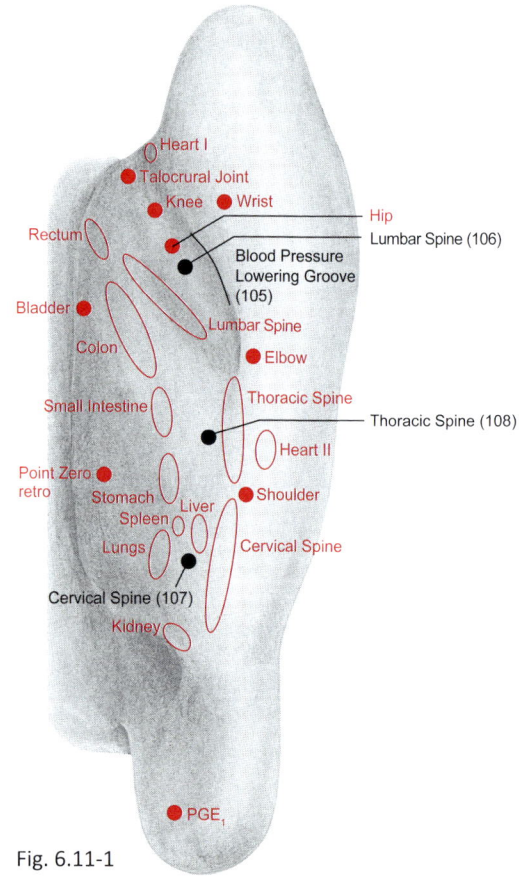

Fig. 6.11-1

cits, there is the risk of damage to the spinal cord by masking the prolapse through pain reduction which may result in delaying necessary surgical intervention.

6.11.2 Musculoskeletal System (› Fig. 6.11-1)

- **Wrist:** on the posterior aspect of the helix, lateral to the superior crus of the posterior groove, level with the point **Knee**; indication: tendovaginitis
- **Elbow:** on the medial aspect of the posterior helix, superior to **Thoracic Spine**; corresponds to the location of the anterior point **Elbow**; by piercing the ear from the anterior one would arrive precisely at the point's posterior location; indication: pain therapy
- **Shoulder:** on the medial aspect of the posterior helix, at the junction of the zone **Cervical Spine** and **Thoracic Spine**; by piercing the ear from anterior one would arrive precisely at the point's posterior location; indication: pain therapy
- **Talocrural Joint:** slightly medial to the superior end of the antihelix groove; indication: pain therapy
- **Knee:** slightly inferior to **Talocrural Joint**; indication: pain therapy
- **Hip:** slightly inferior to **Knee**, lateral to the inferior crus of the antihelix groove; indication: pain therapy

6.11.3 Internal Organs (› Fig. 6.11-2)

Regarding the internal organs the posterior ear is of only minor importance as motor deficits of these organs (e.g. cardiac infarction or pulmonary embolism) generally lead to irreversible damage that cannot be treated by acupuncture. In individual cases it may be beneficial to consider the motor aspects of the internal organs on the posterior ear, e.g. for urinary incontinence (› 8.4.2) or nausea (› 8.3.1).

- **Blood Pressure Lowering Groove/ RR↓ (105)** lateral to **Lumbar Spine**, in the superior part of the antihelix groove; indication: hypertension
- **Lungs:** a zone medial to **Cervical Spine**; indication: bronchial asthma

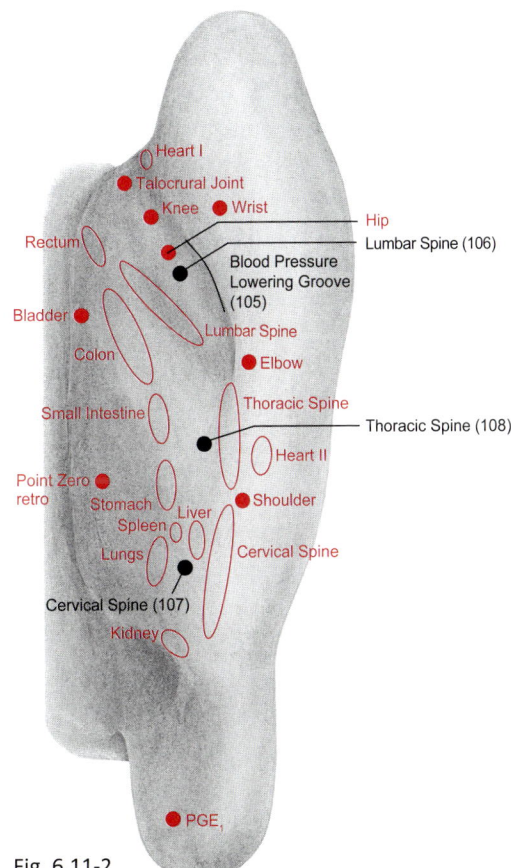

Fig. 6.11-2

- **Heart II:** lateral to the inferior part of **Thoracic Spine**, on the medial aspect of the posterior helix; indication: angina pectoris
- **Heart I:** on the upper border of the superior crus of the antihelix groove; indication: cardiac insufficiency
- **Stomach:** medial to the junction of **Cervical Spine** and **Thoracic Spine**; indication: nausea, vomiting, fullness sensation
- **Spleen:** in the area of the posterior concha, between the antihelix groove and **Stomach** area; indication: meteorism
- **Liver:** medial to the **Stomach** area, on the posterior concha, and lateral to the posterior **Point Zero**; indication: cholestasis, lumbago
- **Small Intestine:** medial to **Thoracic Spine**, approximately in the centre of the posterior ear; indication: meteorism
- **Colon:** medial to **Lumbar Spine**; indication: pain therapy, constipation
- **Rectum:** medial to the superior end of the groove corresponding to the inferior helix, extending to the insertion of the ear; indication: constipation
- **Kidneys:** on the lower border of the eminence of the concha, at the junction with the lobe; indication: nephrolithiasis
- **Bladder (Motor Aspect):** inferior to **Rectum**; indication: urinary retention, incontinence

> **box** Often it is easier to find the points **Elbow** and **Shoulder** as well as the area **Cervical Spine** and **Thoracic Spine** by piercing a rubber ear model (› 2.4.5) from anterior to posterior with a needle.

6.11.4 Miscellaneous (› Fig. 6.11-2)

- **PGE₁** (Prostaglandin E₁): on the posterior lobe, on the medial part of its lower border; indication: pain therapy
- **Point Zero (posterior):** a few millimetres lateral to the insertion of the ear; opposite **Point Zero** on the anterior ear; indication: meteorism, releases spasms

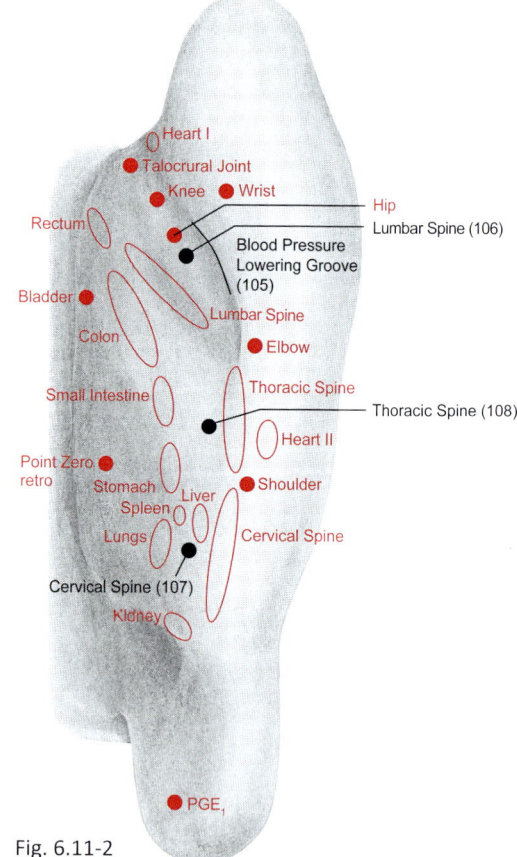

Fig. 6.11-2

6.12 Point Axes

6.12.1 Omega Axis (› Fig. 6.12-1)

- **Master Ω Point:** on the inferior part of the lobe, in zone VII, on a vertical line inferior to the intersection between helix and antihelix
- **Ω_1- Point:** in the superior concha, approximately on the intersecting point of antihelix and helix
- **Ω_2- Point:** on the helix, on a vertical line superior to the intersecting point of helix and antihelix

Indication: releasing tension, depression, anxiety, addiction

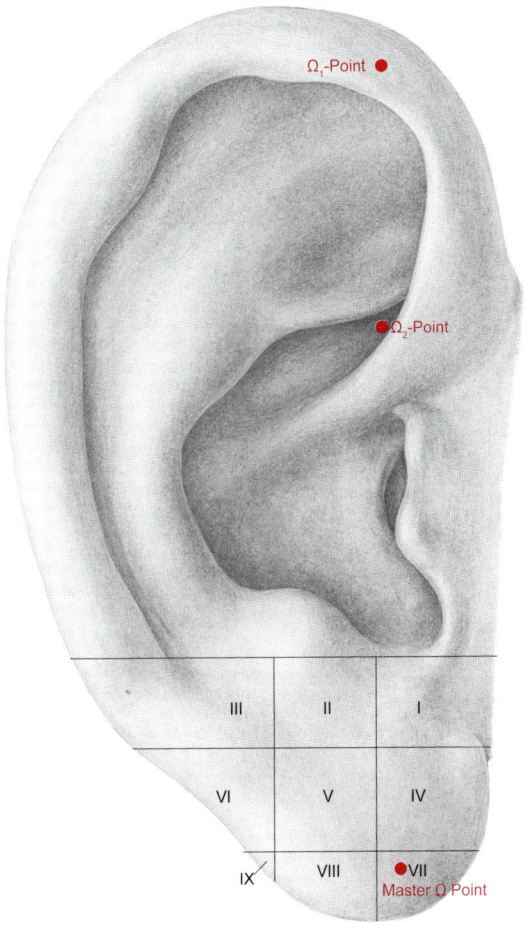

Ω_1-Point

Ω_2-Point

III II I

VI V IV

IX VIII VII
Master Ω Point

Fig. 6.12-1

6.12.2 Addiction Axis (› Fig. 6.12-2)

The Addiction Axis corresponds to the omega axis with the addition of the following points:

- **Anti-Aggression:** a few millimetres inferior to the intertragic notch
- **Bridging Point**: between **Anti-Aggression** and the **Master Ω Point;** indication: supports addiction therapy by relaxing and calming as well as by strengthening the anti-addiction component of the treatment

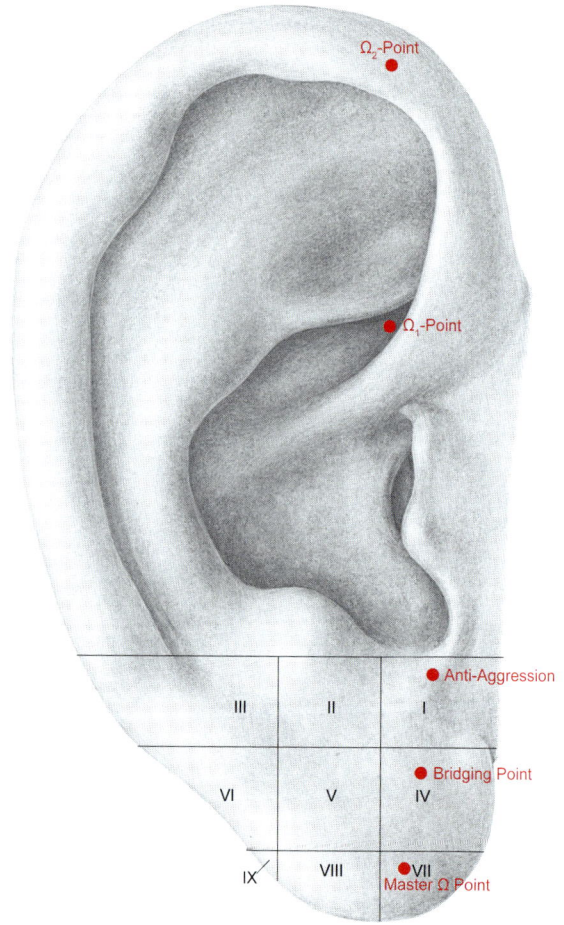

Ω_2-Point

Ω_1-Point

Anti-Aggression

Bridging Point

VII
Master Ω Point

Fig. 6.12-2

6.12.3 Immune Axis (› Fig. 6.12-3)

The Immune Axis – also called Allergy Axis – comprises the following points:

- **Histamine:** at the highest point of the helix, at the tip of the folded-over ear
- **Adrenal Cortex:** on the Hormonal Line on the antihelix wall, inferior to **L1,** (› Fig. 6.1-2)
- **ACTH:** 2mm below the intertragic notch
- **Mirror Point (imm):** on the face, slightly inferior to the insertion of the lobe

Indication: allergies, autoimmune disorders

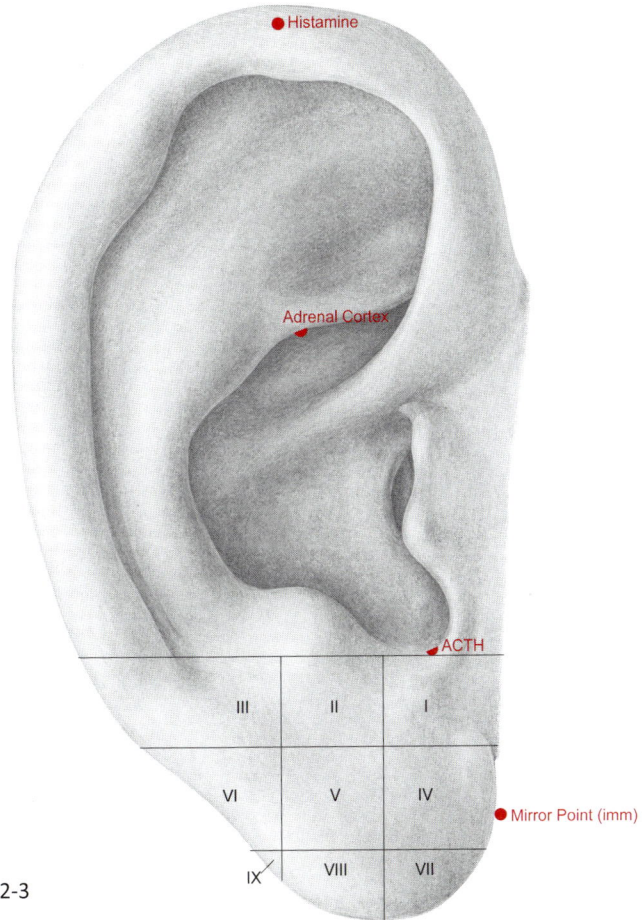

Fig. 6.12-3

6.12.4 Infection Axis (› Fig. 6.12-4, 6.13-1b)

The Infection Axis – sometimes also referred to as Immune Axis – comprises the following points:

- **Helix Brim Point (inf):** on the helix, approximately level with **C7–T2** (› 6.1.1)
- **Thymus:** level with **T2/3,** on the antihelix wall, on the Hormonal Line (› Fig. 6.1-2)
- **Interferon:** at the cranial end of the tragus, at the intersection point of the ascending helix and the tragus
- **Mirror Point (inf):** on the face, level with the cranial end of the tragus

Indication: flu-like, gastrointestinal, viral, and bacterial infections; also as adjunctive therapy during medication with antibiotics

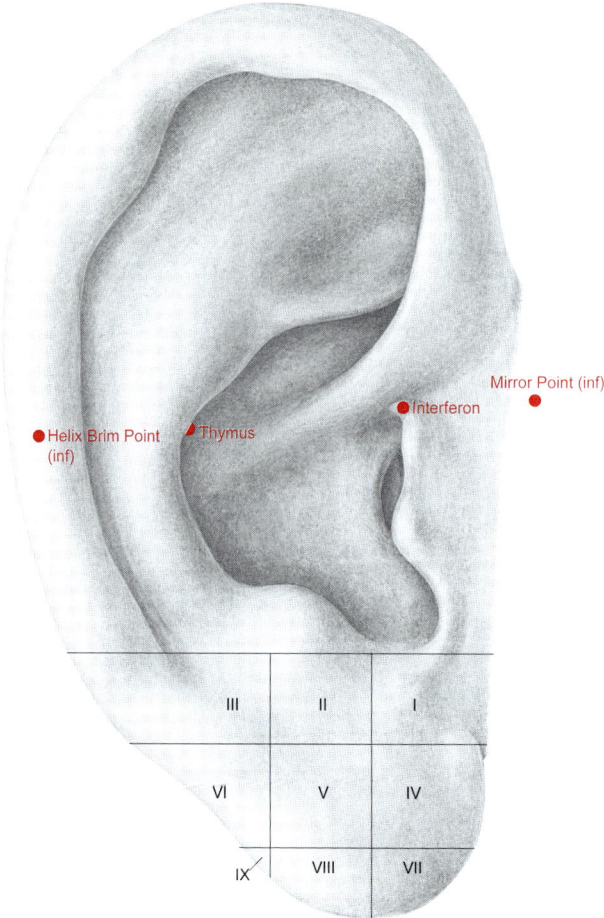

Fig. 6.12-4

6.12.5 Gynaecological Axis (› Fig. 6.12-5, 6.13-1b)

The Gynaecological Axis – also referred to as Hormonal Axis – comprises the following points:

- **Progesterone:** lateral and superior to the **Renin-Angiotensin-Point**
- **Oestrogen:** on the inside of the helix brim, approximately 1 transverse process inferior to the intersecting point between helix and antihelix
- **Gonadotropin:** at the medial end of the antitragus
- **Mirror Point (gyn):** at the lateral lower border of the lobe, in zone VIII

Indication: dysmenorrhoea, premenstrual syndrome, migraines

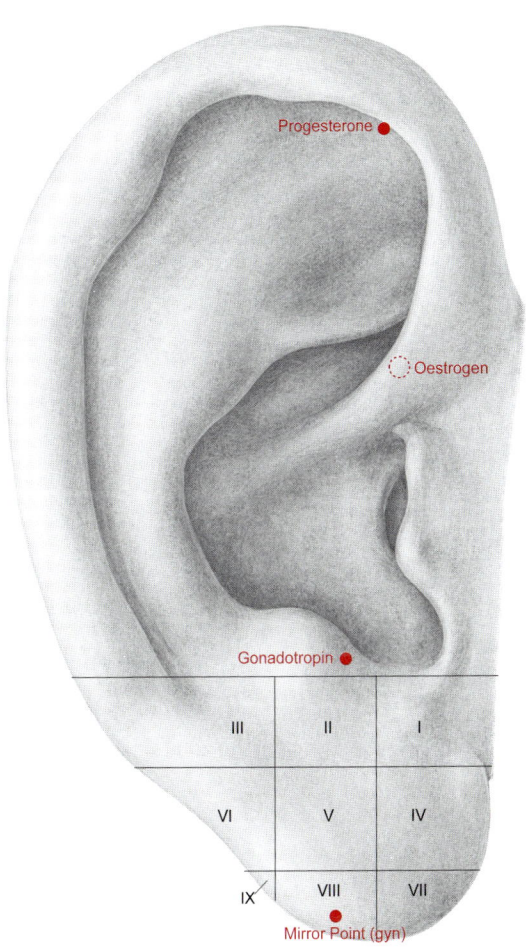

Fig. 6.12-5

6.12.6 Antidepressant Axis (› Fig. 6.12-6, 6.13-1b)

The Antidepressant Axis – also referred to as Depression Axis – comprises the following points:

- **Antidepressant Point:** at the end of the **Vegetative Groove**, on the extension of an imaginary line between the points **Atlanto-occipital Joint** and **Point Zero**
- **Bronchopulmonary Plexus:** in the concha, slightly inferior to the helix root
- **Haldol:** on the face, slightly medial to the helix, on an imaginary extension of the antihelix
- **Mirror Point (ant):** within the hairline, on an imaginary extension of the antihelix;

Indication: depression, anxiety

> box
>
> Depending on the shape of the ear, the axis points are located more or less on a straight line. All lines pass through Point Zero. When needling points on a particular axis one should not feel compelled to achieve a straight line but rather be guided by RAC-palpation. Point Zero is generally not needled.

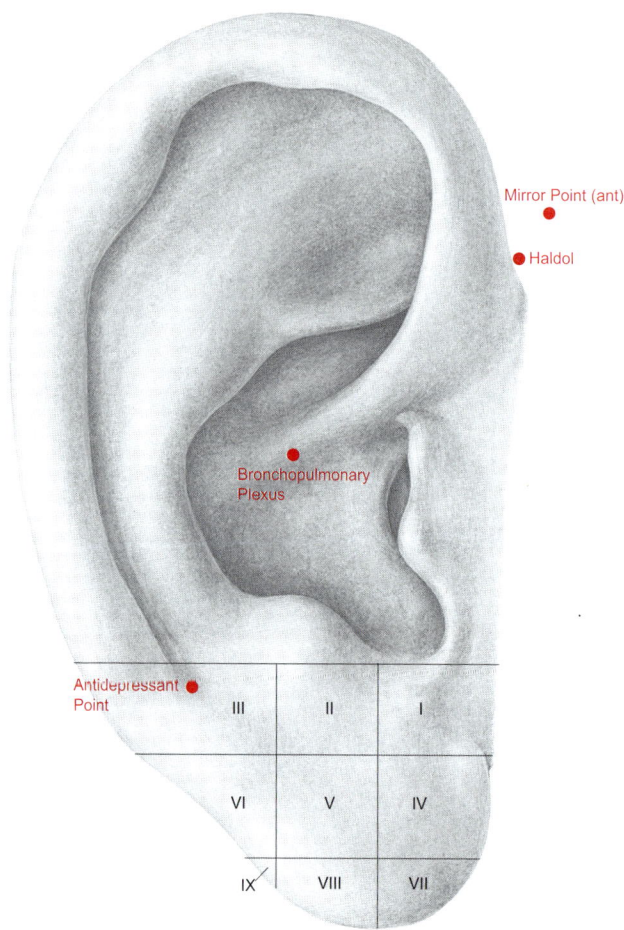

Fig. 6.12-6

6.12.7 Anxiety Axis (› Fig. 6.12-7, 6.13-1b)

The Anxiety Axis – also referred to as Vegetative Axis – comprises the following points:

- **Diazepam** (› 6.7.3): in a groove medial to the tragus, slightly inferior to the tragus tip
- **Spleen** (› 6.4.1): a zone in the superior concha, slightly superior to the level of the anti-helix root, somewhat lateral towards the concha wall
- **Helix Brim Point (anx):** level with Darwin's tubercle
- **Mirror Point (anx):** located at the same distance to the border of the ear as the Laterality Master Point (approximately 3 cm medial towards the face), level with the insertion of the lobe

Indication: relaxation, anxiety syndromes, anxiety treatment, depression

> **box** This Axis is needled on the left side only, since, per definition by the French school, the Spleen is represented only on the left side; however, often both Spleen and Anxiety are found by RAC-palpation on the dominant side and are then also treated there.

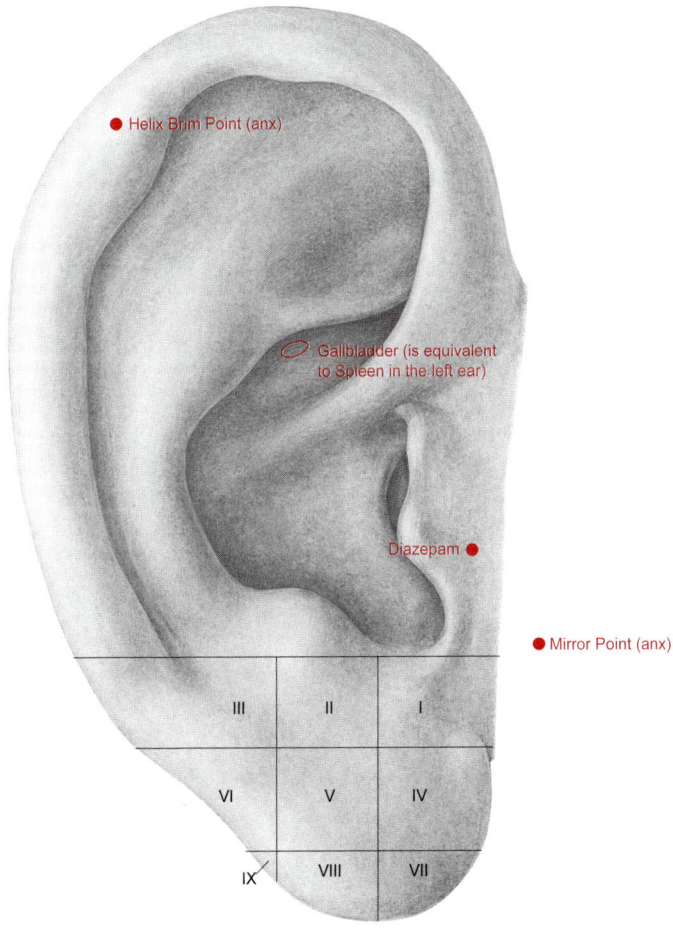

Fig. 6.12-7

6.13 New Point Locations on the Ear

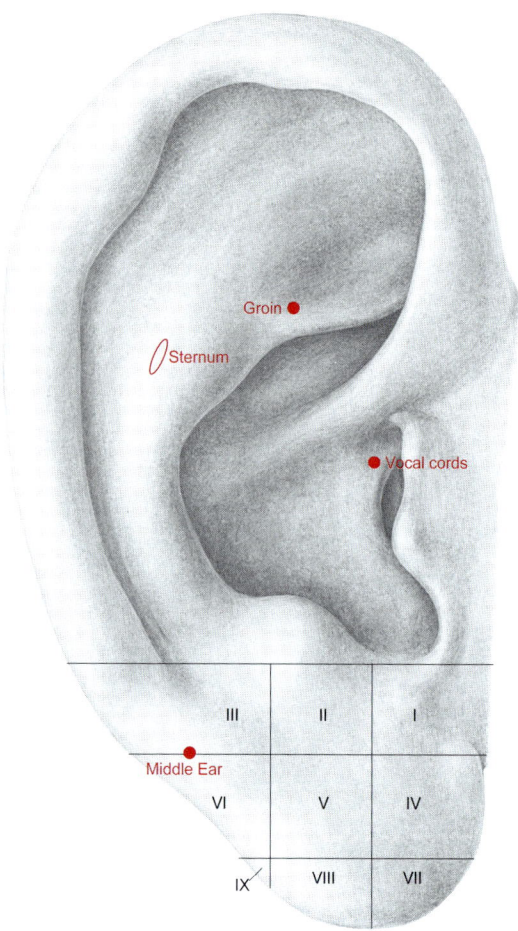

Groin

Sternum

Vocal cords

III   II   I

Middle Ear

VI   V   IV

IX   VIII   VII

Fig. 6.13-1a

6.13.1 New Point Locations after Angermaier (› Fig. 6.13-1a)

During my nearly 15 years of clinical experience in private practice with TCM and auricular acupuncture time and again the question would arise about points not covered by known point locations. In such cases experienced practitioners can correlate the patient's symptoms with individual RAC-reactions on the ear. This procedure was also used by Paul Nogier to develop his first auricular map. If the same auricular location is found in different patients with similar symptoms, a certain regularity can be assumed.

Correlation of point locations and symptoms

In my treatments it was possible to repeatedly correlate the following point locations with the same **symptoms**:

- **Vocal Cords:** lateral to the point **Gullet Point** at the upper border of the ear canal; indication: dysphonia, laryngitis
- **Groin:** in the triangular fossa, superior to L1/2 and lateral and superior to the point buttocks (53)/SI joint; indication: sports hernia, postoperative inguinal hernia pain, groin strain
- **Middle Ear:** at the junction of the helix and the lobe, between the points **Desire** (29c) and **Inner Ear** (9); indication: otitis media
- **Sternum:** an area lateral to the ribs, parallel to the thoracic spine, at the transition to the scapha; indication: complications following sternotomy: postoperative pain, poor wound healing, and posttraumatic pseudoarthritis

6.13.1 New Point Locations after Angermaier *(ctd.)* (› Fig. 6.13-1b)

Detailed terminology of the helix brim points and mirror points

- Mirror point (imm): Mirror point of the Immune Axis
- Mirror point (inf): Mirror point of the Infection Axis
- Mirror point (gyn): Mirror point of the Gynaecological Axis
- Mirror point (ant): Mirror point of the Antidepressant Axis
- Mirror point (anx): Mirror point of the Anxiety Axis
- Helix brim point (inf): Helix brim point of the Infection Axis
- Helix brim point (anx): Helix brim point of the Anxiety Axis

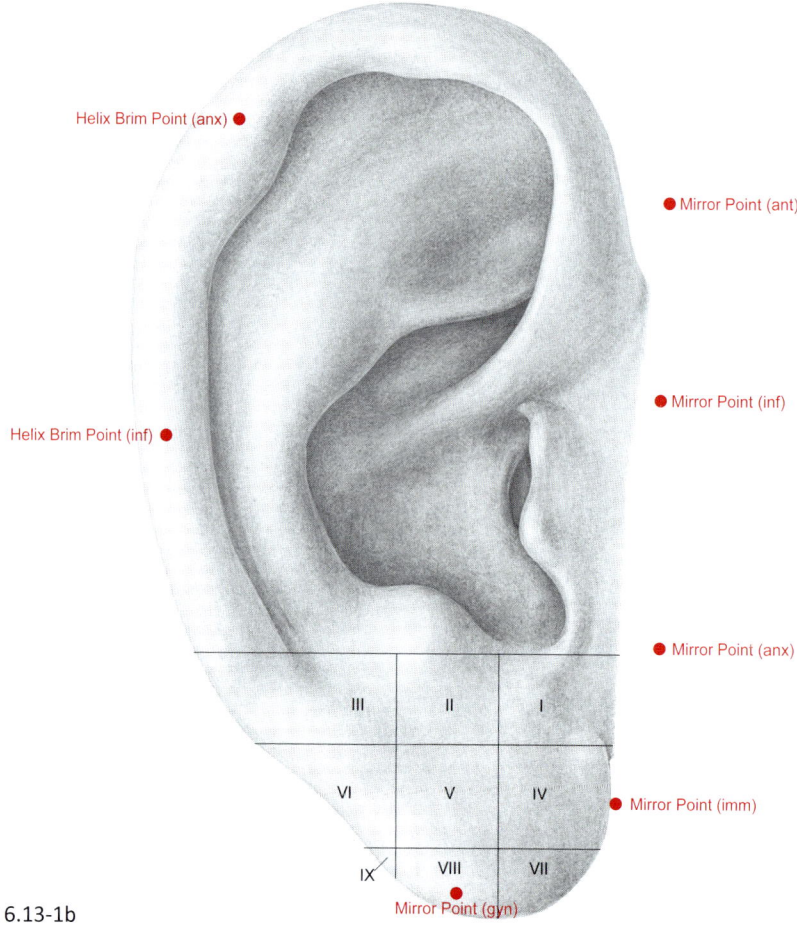

Fig. 6.13-1b

6.13.2 New Point Locations after Rubach (› Fig. 6.13-2)

Axel Rubach describes four psychologically relevant points as psychotropic points PT 1–4:

- **PT 1:** Anti-Aggression Point (› 6.8.5)
- **PT 2:** Anxiety/Worry (› 6.8.5)
- **PT 3:** Antidepressant Point/TMJ (› 6.8.3)
- **PT 4:** Sorrow/Joy (› 6.8.5)

Location: on an imaginary extension of the Vegetative Groove, on a horizontal line with the point pair **Anxiety/Worry**, level with the insertion of the lobe. **Joy** is located on the dominant ear, **Sorrow** on the non-dominant ear

Indication: lethargy, reduced vitality

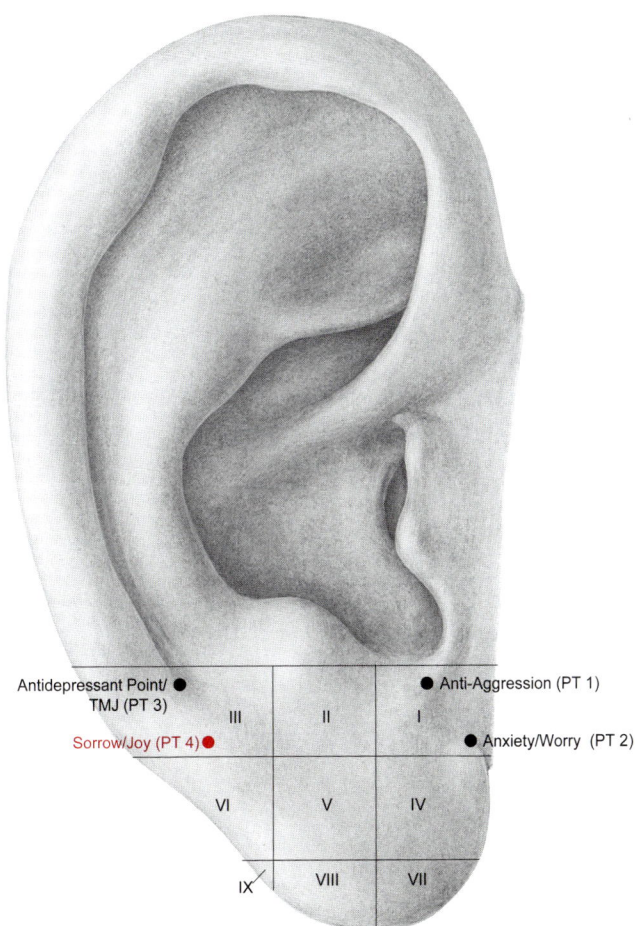

Fig. 6.13-2

6.13.3 New Point Locations after Bahr (› Fig. 6.13-3a)

Dr Frank Bahr distinguishes between the Bridging Point and various Chakra Points:

- **Bridging Point:** between the **Master Ω Point** and the **Anti-Aggression** point; indication: reinforces the point combination **Master Ω Point** and **Anti-Aggression**, e.g. for addiction therapy, also in combination with the addiction axis (› 6.12.2)
- **Chakra 1, Root Chakra:** on the helix brim, slightly superior to Darwin's tubercle; indication: blockage of the root chakra, intestinal disorders, sciatica, lower extremities, emotional disturbances (inferiority complex, narcissism, perfectionism)
- **Chakra 2, Sacral Chakra:** in the scapha, medial to the tip of Darwin's Tubercle, in the area of the point **Wrist**; indication: bladder and kidney disorders, sexual dysfunction, vaginal candidiasis, menstrual disorders, lower back pain
- **Chakra 3, Solar Plexus Chakra:** in the area of **Point Zero**; indication: strengthens the Middle, disorders of the stomach, liver, gallbladder, and spleen, eating disorders
- **Chakra 4, Heart Chakra:** on the posterior ear, in the antihelix groove, inferior to the dividing point of the superior and anterior crus; indication: heart and lung disorders, skin disorders, disorders of the shoulder and thoracic spine
- **Chakra 5, Throat Chakra:** on the antihelix, at the junction between the zone representing the cervical and thoracic spine respectively; indication: dysphonia, problems communicating, disorders of the larynx/pharynx, thyroid disorders, dental disorders
- **Chakra 6, Brow Chakra:** on the lateral antitragus (at the junction to the antihelix), slightly medial to the point **Occiput (29)**; indication: visual and auditory disorders, difficulty concentrating, neurological disorders of the central nervous system, e.g. Alzheimer's disease
- **Chakra 7, Crown Chakra:** in the centre of the lobe; indication: headaches, sleeping disorders, multiple sclerosis, emotional disorders such as depression and loss of sense of reality

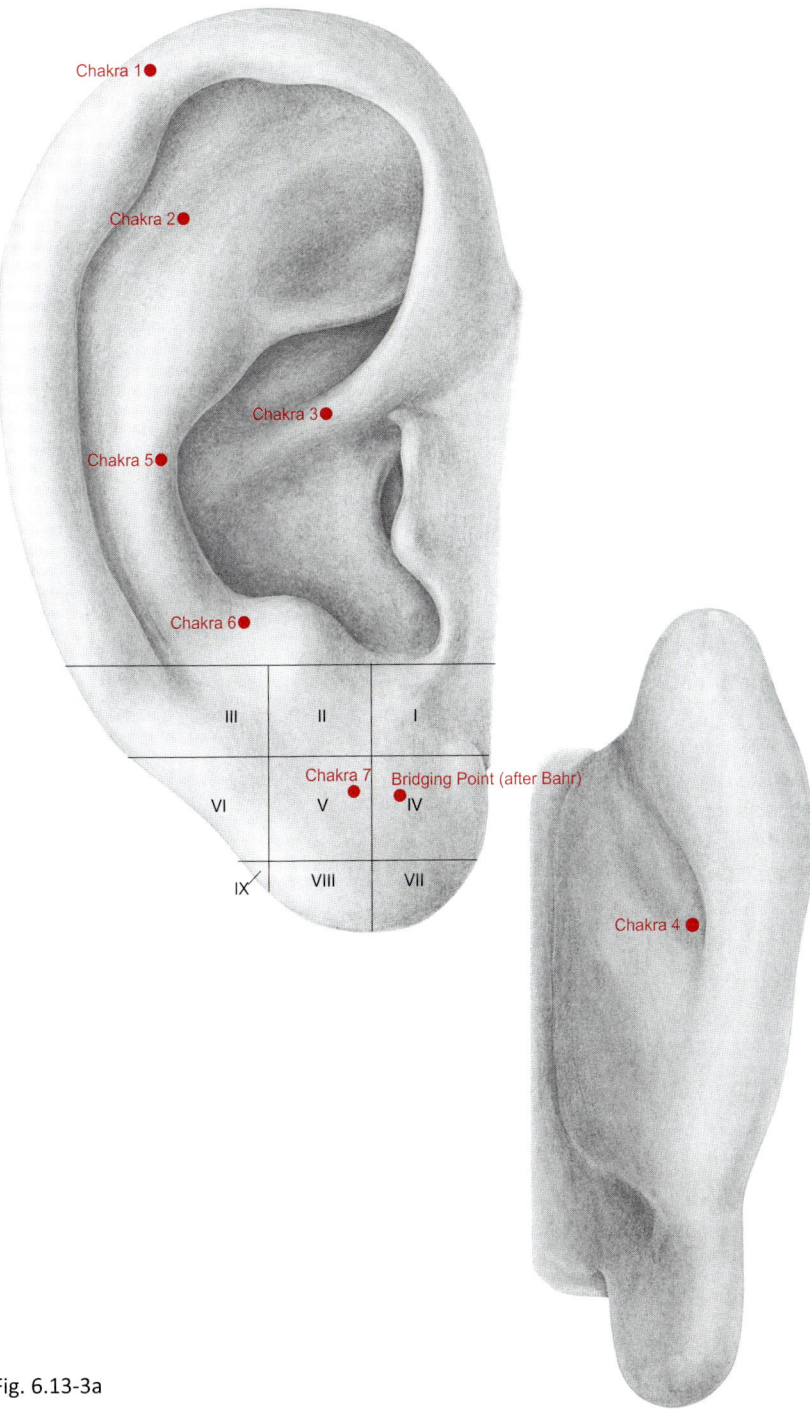

Fig. 6.13-3a

6.13.3 New Point Locations after Bahr *(ctd.)* (› Fig. 6.13-3b+c)

- **Chakra 8, 'Source of Sacred' (extra-corporeal):** on the face, medial and inferior to the tip of the earlobe, inferior to the Mirror Point (imm); indication: softens hard-heartedness, reaching love, kindness, and perfection
- **Chakra 9, 'Cosmos', 'Universe' (extra-corporeal):** on the face, inferior to the point Chakra 8, at the intersecting point of an imaginary extension of the Vegetative Groove; indication: inner restlessness and tension, impatience, attaining transcendental knowledge
- **Chakra 10, 'Protective Chakra' (primary):** on the face, on a slightly curved line inferior to the point Chakra 9, on the intersecting point of an imaginary extension of the outer helix brim; indication: emotional stress, desperation, support in life-threatening illnesses
- **Chakra 11, Energy Point:** inferior to the point Chakra 10, on the extension of the omega line; indication: immunisation side effects, genetic disorders, hereditary predisposition
- **Chakra 12, Energy Point:** in the face, inferior to the point Chakra 11; indication: family history of the patient's complaint, strengthening point for pandemics
- **Chakra 13, Energy Point:** corresponds to the point Thymus on the Hormonal Line on the concha wall, level with T2/3; indication: strengthens the immune system, also against radiation
- **Turning Point Chakra:** on the face, slightly lateral to the tragus groove (the fold between the ear and the face) level with the tragus tip; indication: lack of self-confidence, 'acidosis'
- **Chakra Minus-1:** on the edge of the ascending helix, slightly superior to the intersecting point with an imaginary extension of the antihelix; indication: exhaustion due to severe illness (e.g. cancer), burnout syndrome
- **Chakra Minus-2:** on the hairline, on a straight line superior to the point 'Chakra Minus-1'; indication: possible sign of cancer, strengthens the immune system, analgesic
- **Chakra Minus-3:** on the face, slightly outside of the superior helix and slightly medial to the point Ω_2; indication: posttraumatic stress disorder, pessimism

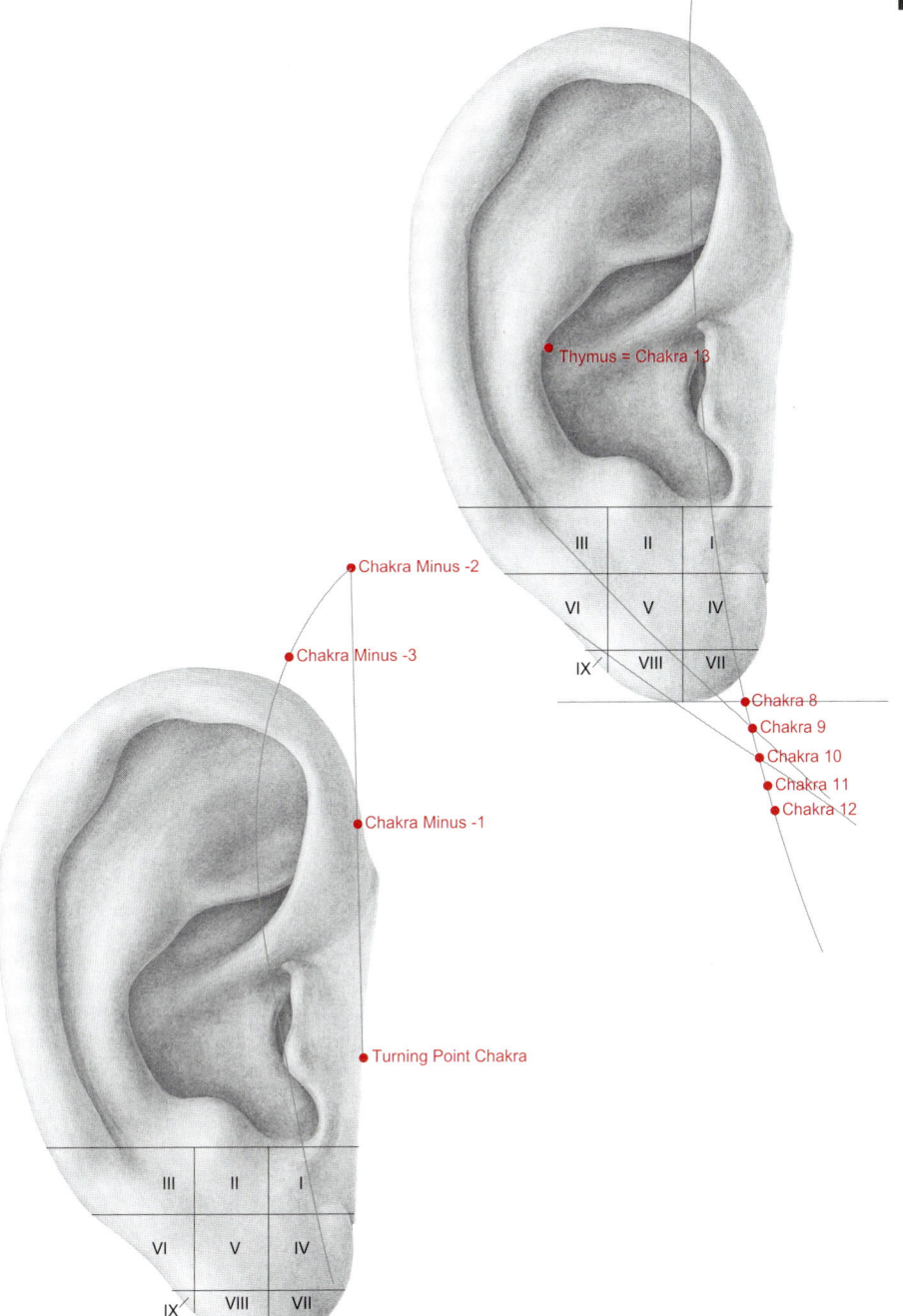

Thymus = Chakra 13

Chakra Minus -2

Chakra Minus -3

Chakra Minus -1

Turning Point Chakra

Chakra 8
Chakra 9
Chakra 10
Chakra 11
Chakra 12

Fig. 6.13-3b+c

6.13.4 Further New Point Locations after Dr Bahr *(ctd.)* (› Fig. 6.13-4a+b)

- **Acomplia:** on the lobe, superior to **Eye (8)** in the centre of the lobe; indication: obesity, weight loss
- **Champix:** on the lobe, medial to the point **Acomplia**, corresponds to the **Bridging Point** (› 6.13.3) indication: nicotine abuse
- **Detox:** a point on the lateral and of the antitragus, located towards the inside, at the junction with the antihelix; indication: detoxification, especially for skin disorders
- **CNS-Memory for the Trigeminal Nerve:** a point inferior to the intertragic notch, medial to the point **Anti-Aggression**; indication: clears pathological memory from the mind once symptoms have resolved
- **CNS-Memory for the Lungs:** point on the upper border of the lobe, lateral to the insertion of the lobe; indication: clears pathological memory from the mind once symptoms have resolved
- **CNS-Memory for the Kidneys:** point on the upper border of the lobe, inferior to the medial end of the antitragus, superior and medial to the CNS-Memory point for the Lungs; indication: clears pathological memory from the mind once symptoms have resolved
- **CNS-Memory for the Stomach:** a point on the left ear, at the junction of the lobe to the antitragus, vertically below the midpoint of the antitragus, superior and medial to the CNS-Memory point for the Kidneys; indication: clears pathological memory from the mind once symptoms have resolved
- **COX-2-Inhibitor:** a point on the posterior ear, medial to the projection of the upper cervical spine; indication: anti-inflammatory point
- **Resveratrol:** a point at the midpoint of the antitragus edge, between the points **Pituitary Gland** (28) and **Parotid Gland** (30); indication: antioxidant effect
- **Acidosis:** a point on the face, slightly medial to the tragus fold, on the midline extending from the tragus tip to the **Laterality Point**; indication: resolves acidosis

The point locations after Dr Frank Bahr presented above could be verified by the author. In addition, there is a multitude of further points which are attributed to Dr Bahr. Since they were discovered only very recently the author has not been able to verify these points with a statistically significant number of patients. For more information on further points after Dr Bahr see Strittmatter and Bahr (2010, › 12.3).

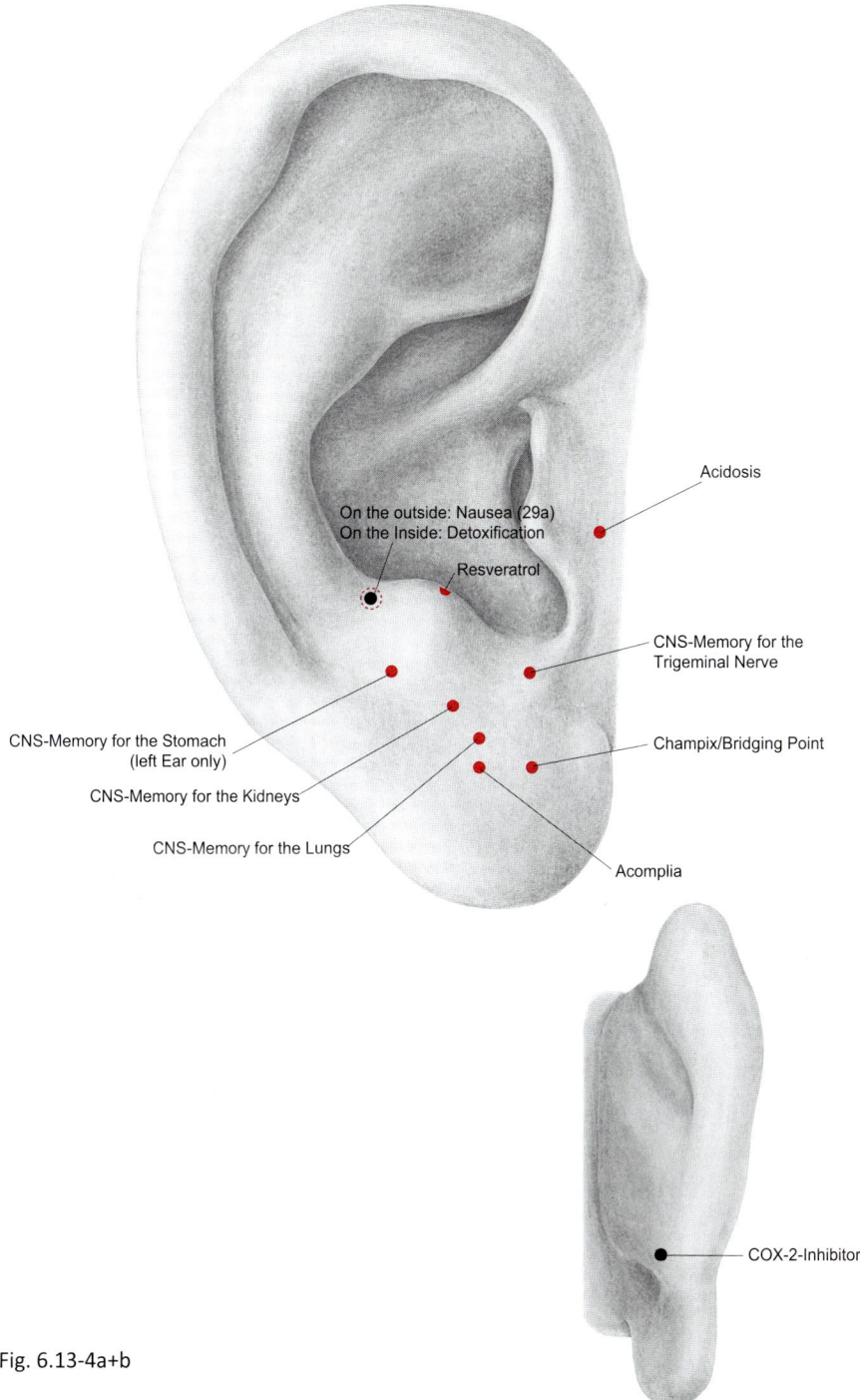

On the outside: Nausea (29a)
On the Inside: Detoxification

Resveratrol

Acidosis

CNS-Memory for the
Trigeminal Nerve

CNS-Memory for the Stomach
(left Ear only)

CNS-Memory for the Kidneys

CNS-Memory for the Lungs

Champix/Bridging Point

Acomplia

COX-2-Inhibitor

Fig. 6.13-4a+b

6.13.5 New Point Locations after other Authors (› Dr Rudolf Bucek, Dr Ulrich Werth) (› Fig. 6.13-5a+b)

- **Substantia Nigra (after Bucek):** on a line perpendicular to the point **Atlanto-occipital Joint** and the edge of the ear, between the points **Point de Jérome** and **Desire** (29c), slightly lateral to where the **Vegetative Groove** gradually terminates; indication: Parkinson's disease

- **Substantia Nigra, posterior ear (after Werth):** slightly superior and a few millimetres lateral to the insertion of the lobe (if the lobe is completely attached in the area of the cartilaginous tissue superior to the soft part of the lobe): indication: Parkinson's disease

- **Hypothalamus (after Werth):** on the edge of the lateral aspect of the antitragus, slightly medial to the junction with the antihelix; this means the point is located adjacent to the more medial point **Pituitary Gland**; indication: Parkinson's disease, especially tremors

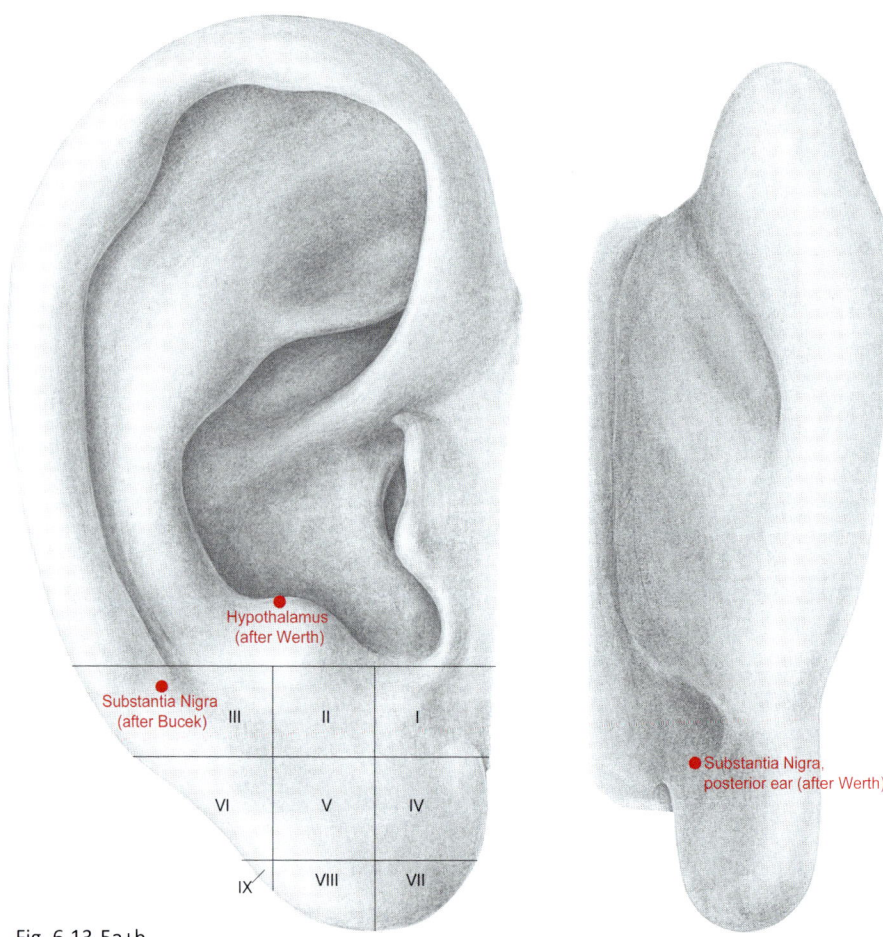

Fig. 6.13-5a+b

6.13.6 Additional Point Locations (› Fig. 6.13-6)

- **Lower Abdomen (109)** Xiafu **(after Bernd Lange):** at the top of the ear canal; indication: abdominal pain, acute chest syndrome
- **Epigastrium (110)** Shangfu **(after Bernd Lange):** at the bottom of the ear canal; indication: epigastric pain, acute chest syndrome

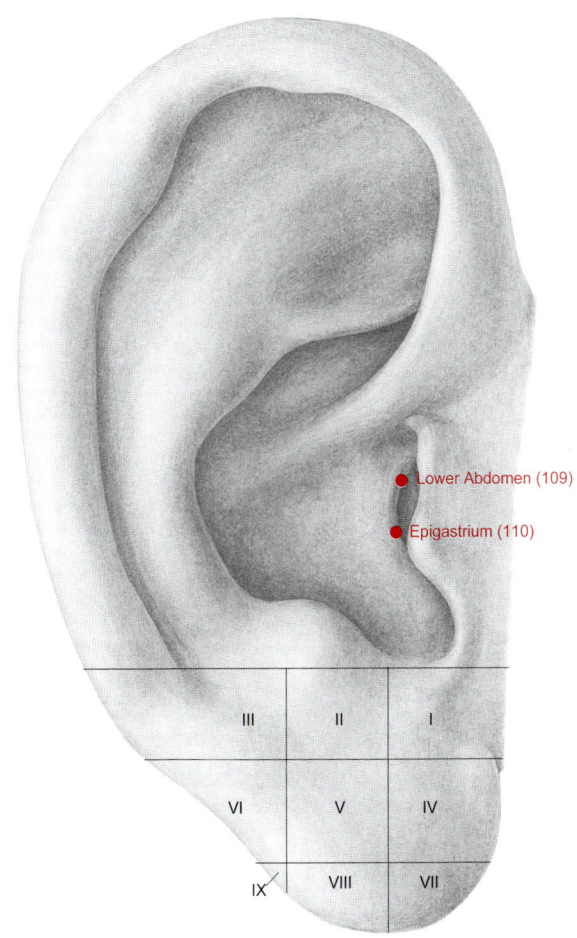

Fig. 6.13-6

7 The Treatment of Pain with Auricular Acupuncture

7.1 Acute Musculoskeletal Pain

7.1.1 Acute Cervical Myalgia

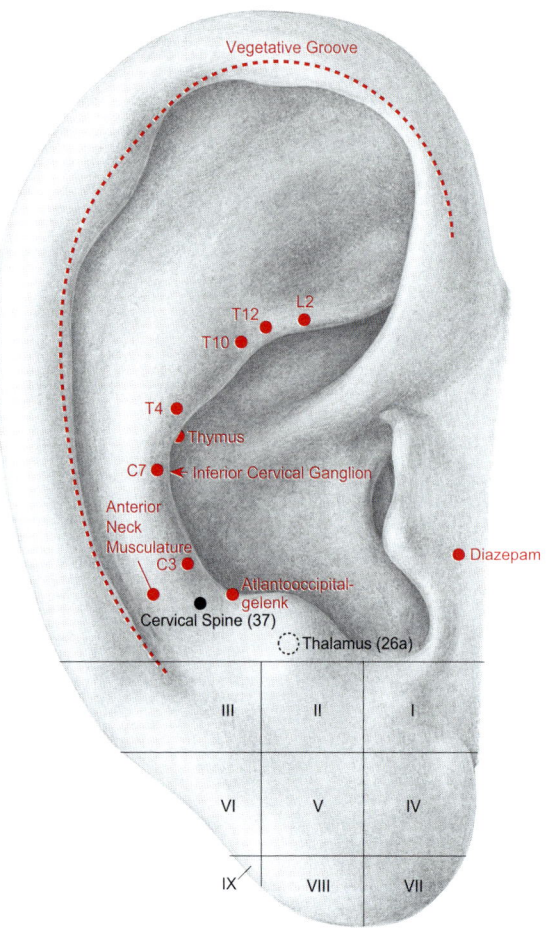

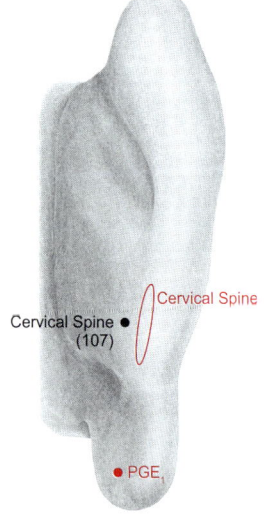

Fig. 7.1-1a+b

Description

- Paravertebral, segment-specific pain, may radiate to the shoulders and occipital region
- No motor deficits, rarely sensory deficits
- Most common form: cervical myalgia following whiplash (car accident)

Signs and symptoms requiring a referral to a neurologist/neurosurgeon:
- progressive sensory and motor deficits (especially with prolapsed disc)
- difficulty swallowing.

While further treatment with exclusively auricular acupuncture may alleviate the pain, this might mask the underlying disorder and therefore result in the delay of necessary surgery.

Point Prescription

French points

- Local points: **Atlanto-occipital Joint, C3, C7** (› 6.1.1), **Anterior Neck Musculature** (› 6.2.1), **Inferior Cervical Ganglion** (› 6.9.2) on the anterior ear; **Cervical Spine** (› 6.11.1) on the posterior ear
- Points in the **Vegetative Groove** (› 6.9.1)
- Analgesic points: **Diazepam** (› 6.7.3), **PGE₁/Thymus** (› 6.7.6)
- For restricted movement: relevant cervical spine points on the anterior ear; restricted movement in one area of the spine often results in (compensatory) counter-blockages in other parts of the spine; needling these points is therefore recommended: e.g. **T4, T10, T12, L2** (› 6.1.1)

Chinese points

- Local points: **Cervical Spine (37)** (› 6.1.1) on the anterior ear; **Cervical Spine (107)** (› 6.11.1) on the posterior ear
- Analgesic point: **Thalamus (26a)** (› 6.7.4)

Treatment Intervals

- Once daily until the pain has reduced significantly
- Then once weekly until symptoms have subsided completely

Treatment Course and Prognosis

- The sooner treatments commence after onset of the pain, the sooner there will be treatment results, and, in case of whiplash, the lower the risk of long-term complications.
- Generally, the pain diminishes or completely subsides within minutes to hours after acupuncture but this effect tends to be short-lived; daily repeat treatments are necessary for approximately 3 days.
- The pain usually subsides completely after 4 weeks at the latest.

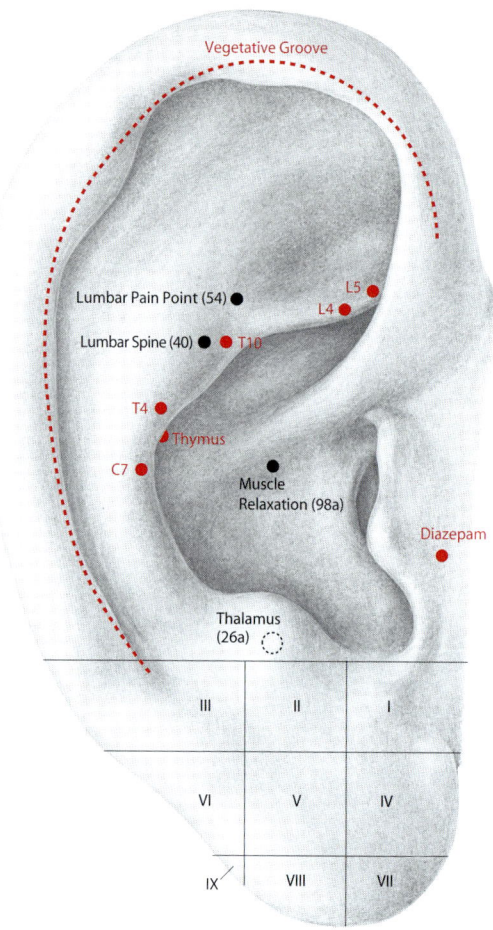

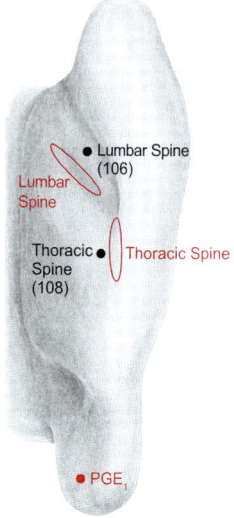

Fig. 7.1-2a+b

7.1.2 Acute Lower Back Pain (Lumbago)

Description

- Muscle pain in the lumbar area (longissimus dorsi, iliopsoas, and quadratus lumborum); with or without radicular pain towards lateral (differential diagnosis: kidney pain), but no pain radiating to the thigh (acute sciatica)
- Causes: generally degenerative changes of the spine and especially of the discs
- No motor deficits, rarely sensory deficits

- Signs and symptoms requiring a referral to a neurologist/neurosurgeon:
  - progressive sensory and motor deficits (especially with prolapsed disc)
  - difficulty swallowing
  - sensory deficits in the segments S1–S5 (in particular cauda equina syndrome).
- While further treatment exclusively with auricular acupuncture may alleviate the pain, this might mask the underlying disorder and therefore result in the delay of necessary surgery.

Point Prescription

French points
- Local points: e.g. **L4** and/or **L5** (› 6.1.1) on the anterior ear; **Lumbar Spine** (› 6.11.1) on the posterior ear
- Points in the **Vegetative Groove** (› 6.9.1)
- Analgesic points: **Diazepam** (› 6.7.3), **PGE$_1$/Thymus** (› 6.7.6)
- For restricted movement: relevant points of the lumbar spine on the anterior ear, for example **L4/5** (› 6.1.1); restricted movement in one area of the spine often results in (compensatory) counter-blockages in other parts of the spine; needling these points is therefore recommended: e.g. **C7, T4, T10** (› 6.1.1); **Thoracic Spine** (› 6.11.1) on the posterior ear

Chinese points
- Local points: **Lumbar Spine (40)** (› 6.1.1) on the anterior ear; **Lumbar Spine (106), Thoracic Spine (108)** (› 6.11.1) on the posterior ear
- Analgesic points: **Lumbar Pain Point (54)** (› 6.1.1), **Thalamus (26a)** (› 6.7.4)
- Relaxing point: **Muscle Relaxation (98a)** (› 6.1.3)

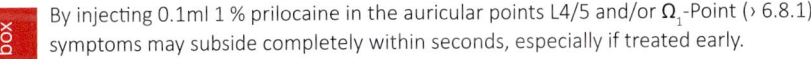

By injecting 0.1ml 1 % prilocaine in the auricular points L4/5 and/or Ω_1-Point (› 6.8.1) symptoms may subside completely within seconds, especially if treated early.

Treatment Intervals
- Once daily until the pain has reduced significantly
- Then once weekly until symptoms have subsided completely

Treatment Course and Prognosis
- The sooner treatments commence after the onset of the pain, the sooner there will be results.
- Generally the pain will diminish or subside completely within minutes to hours after acupuncture but this tends to be temporary; repeat treatments will be necessary until there is a sustained subsidence of symptoms.
- The pain usually subsides completely after 4 weeks at the latest.

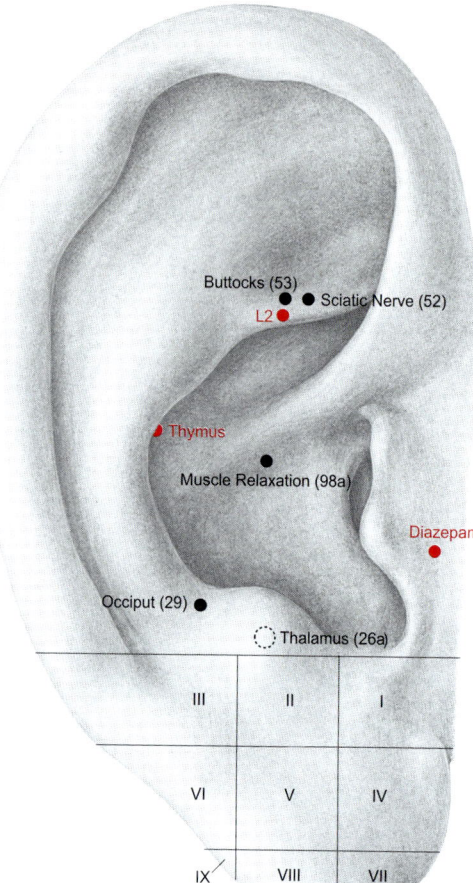

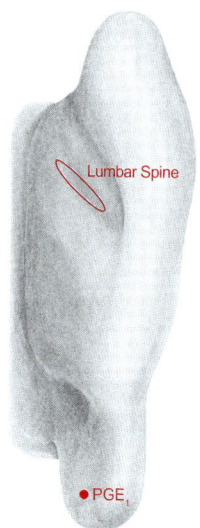

Fig. 7.1-3a+b

7.1.3 Acute Sciatica

Description

- Pain radiating from the buttock to the leg along the course of the sciatic nerve
- Generally one-sided (nearly always on both sides with diabetes mellitus), sudden exacerbations of the pain; sensory deficits are rare
- Causes: injuries caused by heavy lifting or compression, especially in cases of a prolapsed disc
- A prolapsed disc generally manifests with sensory deficits and is only rarely accompanied by motor deficits; compare with acute lower back pain (> 7.1.2).

Point Prescription

French points

- Local points: points on the lumbar spine on the anterior ear; most commonly **L2** (> 6.1.1); **Lumbar Spine** (> 6.11.1) on the posterior ear
- Analgesic points: **Diazepam** (> 6.7.3), **PGE$_1$/Thymus** (> 6.7.6)

Chinese points

- Local points: **Sciatic nerve (52), Buttocks (53)** (> 6.1.1)
- Analgesic points: **Occiput (29), Thalamus (26a)** (> 6.7.4)
- Relaxing point: **Muscle Relaxation (98a)** (> 6.1.3)

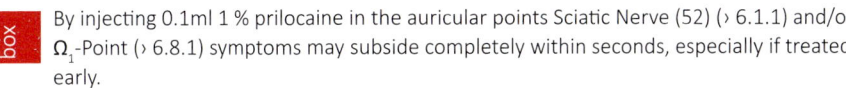

box — By injecting 0.1ml 1 % prilocaine in the auricular points Sciatic Nerve (52) (> 6.1.1) and/or Ω_1-Point (> 6.8.1) symptoms may subside completely within seconds, especially if treated early.

Treatment Intervals

- Once daily until the pain has reduced significantly
- Then once weekly until symptoms have subsided completely

Treatment Course and Prognosis

- When treated early only 2–5 daily treatments are necessary.
- The pain will generally subside or disappear completely after the first treatment but repeat treatments will be necessary for sustained results.
- The pain generally subsides completely within 2–4 weeks at the latest.

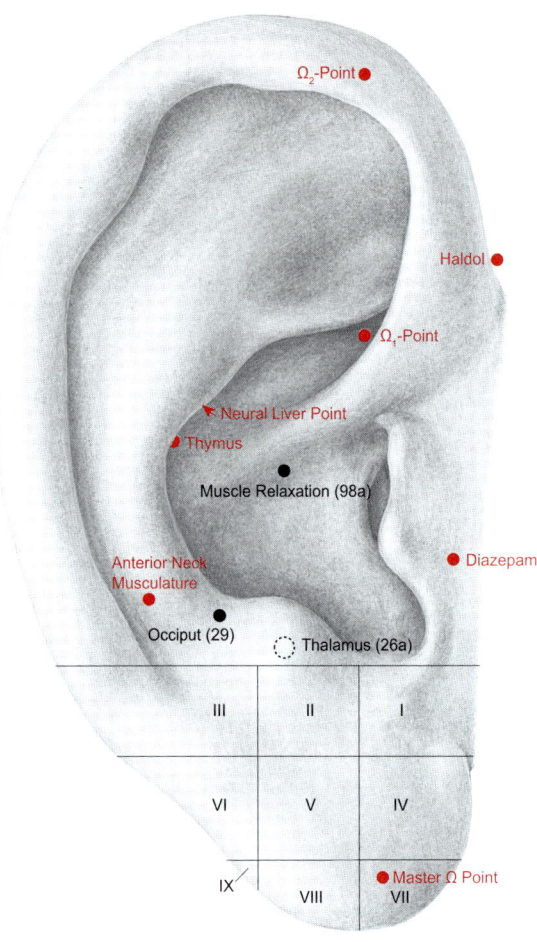
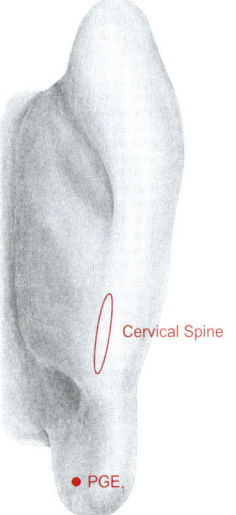

Fig. 7.1-4a+b

7.1.4 Torticollis (Wry Neck)

Description

- One-sided cramp or shortening of the sternocleidomastoideus; this results in a poor posture with lateral flexion and rotation of the head
- Causes:
  - generally muscular
  - others, such as neurogenic (with damage to the extrapyramidal system) or ocular (with trochlear palsy) are rare; in these cases auricular acupuncture is of no benefit

Point Prescription

French points

- Local points: **Anterior Neck Musculature** (> 6.2.1) on the anterior ear; **Cervical Spine** (> 6.11.1) on the posterior ear
- Analgesic points: **Diazepam** (> 6.7.3), **PGE$_1$/Thymus** (> 6.7.6)
- Psycho-emotional points: **Omega Axis** (> 6.12.1), **Neural Liver Point (Resentment)** (> 6.8.1), **Haldol** (> 6.8.6)

Chinese points

- Analgesic points: **Occiput (29), Thalamus (26a)** (> 6.7.4)
- Relaxing point: **Muscle Relaxation (98a)** (> 6.1.3)

Treatment Intervals

- **Acute symptoms:** once daily until the pain has reduced significantly – existing analgesic medication can then be discontinued; then once weekly until symptoms have subsided completely
- **Chronic symptoms:** 2–3 times weekly for approximately 4 weeks; then 1–2 times weekly until symptoms have subsided completely

> **box** By injecting 0.1ml 1 % prilocaine in the auricular points Anterior Neck Musculature (> 6.2.1) and/or Ω_1-Point (> 6.8.1) symptoms may subside completely within seconds, especially if treated early.

Treatment Course and Prognosis

- **Acute symptoms:** symptoms generally resolve within 4 weeks
- **Chronic symptoms:** complete remission is generally not possible but a significant relaxation and reduction in pain can be achieved within 4–6 weeks; analgesic medication will then be no longer necessary

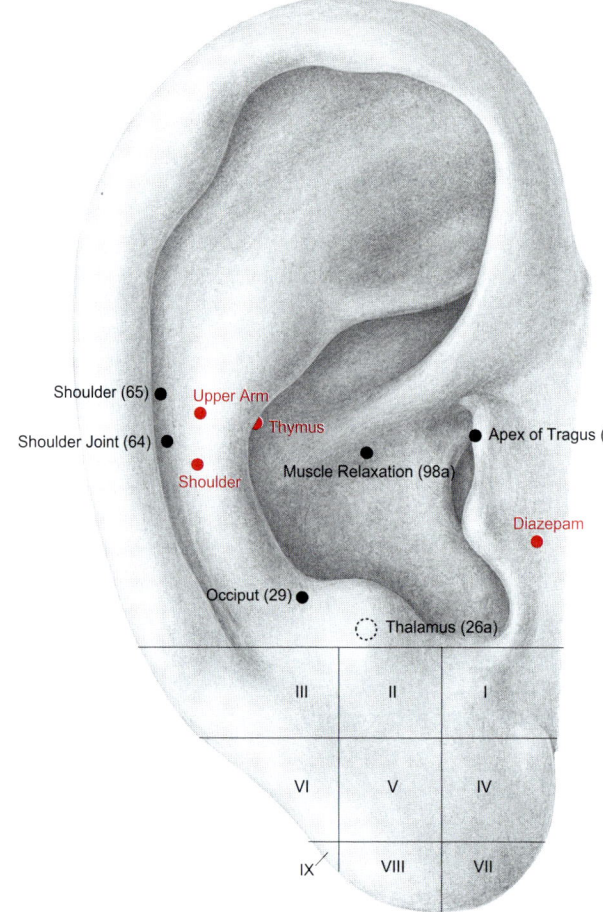

Shoulder (65)

Upper Arm

Thymus

Apex of Tragus (12)

Shoulder Joint (64)

Muscle Relaxation (98a)

Shoulder

Diazepam

Occiput (29)

Thalamus (26a)

III II I

VI V IV

IX VIII VII

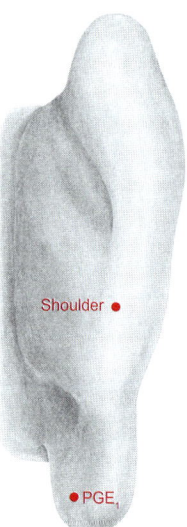

Shoulder

PGE₁

Fig. 7.1-5a+b

7.1.5 Cervicobrachial Syndrome

Description

- Pain in the shoulder area, often radiating to the upper arm
- Various forms: humeroscapular periarthritis, adhesive capsulitis ('frozen shoulder'), degenerative arthritis of the shoulder
- Causes: often trauma (e.g. falls, sports injuries) which over time becomes chronic
- Exacerbation of the pain during the night

Point Prescription

The same point prescription applies to all forms of cervicobrachial syndrome mentioned above.

French points

- Local points: **Shoulder** and **Upper Arm** (› 6.2.1) on the anterior ear; **Shoulder** (› 6.11.2) on the posterior ear
- Relaxing point: **Diazepam** (› 6.7.3)
- Analgesic point: **PGE$_1$/Thymus** (› 6.7.6)

Chinese points

- Local points: **Shoulder (65)**, **Shoulder Joint (64)** (› 6.2.1)
- Relaxing point: **Muscle Relaxation (98a)** (› 6.1.3)
- Analgesic points: **Occiput (29), Thalamus (26a)** (› 6.7.4), **Apex of Tragus (12)** (› 6.7.3)

Treatment Intervals

- **Acute stage:** twice weekly
- Pain for > 4 weeks: once weekly until the pain has resolved completely

Treatment Course and Prognosis

- Start of treatments during the **acute stage:** symptoms generally subside after 4 weeks
- **Degenerative disorder:** symptoms may subside completely but treatments are required for at least 3 months

> **box**
> With increasing age degenerative changes tend to be of a physiological nature and even in advanced stages there may be only little or no pain. Therefore X -rays provide no information about the necessity or duration of the treatment.

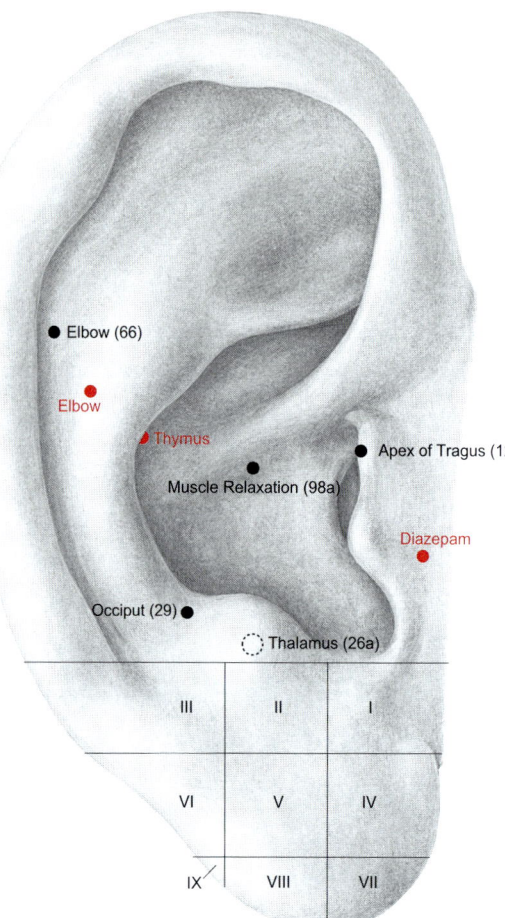

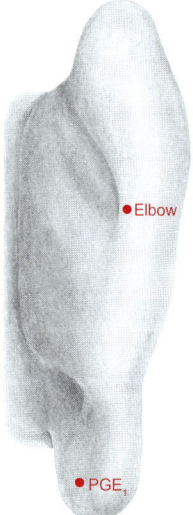

Fig. 7.1-6a+b

7.1.6 Epicondylitis

Description

- Two forms can be distinguished:
  - lateral epicondylitis: local pressure pain at the insertion of the extensor digitorum communis and extensor carpi radialis; most common form
  - medial epicondylitis: local pressure pain at the insertion of the flexor digitorum communis and flexor digitorum sublimis; less common form
- Often movement-induced pain after overexertion
- With the muscles flexed the pain radiates towards distal and proximal

Point Prescription

The same point prescription applies to both lateral and medial epicondylitis.

French points

- Local points: **Elbow** (› 6.2.1) on the anterior ear; **Elbow** (› 6.11.2) on the posterior ear
- Relaxing point: **Diazepam** (› 6.7.3)
- Analgesic point: **PGE₁/Thymus** (› 6.7.6)

Chinese points

- Local point: **Elbow (66)** (› 6.2.1)
- Relaxing point: **Muscle Relaxation (98a)** (› 6.1.3)
- Analgesic points: **Thalamus (26a), Occiput (29)** (› 6.7.4), **Apex of Tragus (12)** (› 6.7.3)

Treatment Intervals

- **Acute stage:** twice weekly
- With pain for > 4 weeks: once weekly until symptoms have completely subsided

Treatment Course and Prognosis

- Start of treatments during the **acute stage:** symptoms generally subside after 4 weeks
- Start of treatments during the **chronic stage** (pain for > 4 weeks): symptoms may subside completely but treatments required for at least 3 months

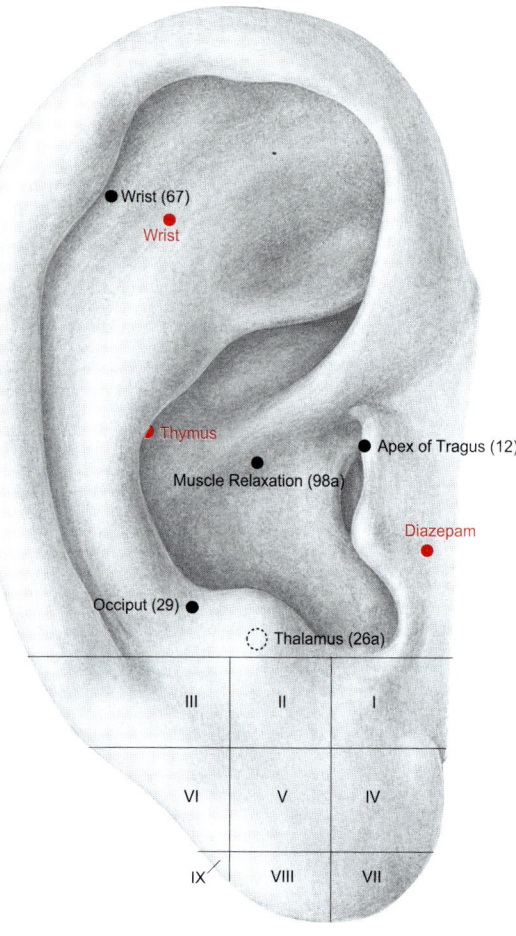
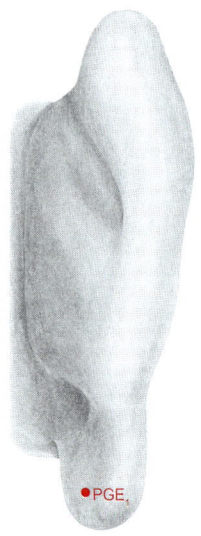

Fig. 7.1-7a+b

7.1.7 Carpal Tunnel Syndrome (CTS)

Description

- Mechanic compression of the median nerve in the carpal tunnel
- Pain in the wrist and hand, may radiate to the upper arm or shoulder
- Numbness, tingling, and/or paraesthesia of the fingers I–III and the radial side of finger IV, in chronic cases atrophy of the thenar eminence
- Acute onset through overuse of the hand
- Often exacerbation during the night

Point Prescription

French points
- Local point: **Wrist** (› 6.2.1)
- Relaxing point: **Diazepam** (› 6.7.3)
- Analgesic point: **PGE₁/Thymus** (› 6.7.6)

Chinese points
- Local point: **Wrist (67)** (› 6.2.1)
- Relaxing point: **Muscle Relaxation (98a)** (› 6.1.3)
- Analgesic points: **Thalamus (26a)**, **Occiput (29)** (› 6.7.4), **Apex of Tragus (12)** (› 6.7.3)

Treatment Intervals

- **Acute stage:** 3 times weekly
- Pain for > 4 weeks: once or twice weekly until symptoms have subsided completely, provided there is progressive improvement

- During the treatment course the patient should use the affected hand as little as possible.
- If there is no improvement after 4 weeks of treatment the patient should be referred to an orthopaedic consultant for endoscopic surgery in order to avoid permanent nerve damage. In such cases acupuncture can provide peri/postoperative support.

Treatment Course and Prognosis

- Significant reduction of symptoms within 1–2 weeks
- Start of treatments during the **acute stage**: symptoms generally resolve within 4 weeks

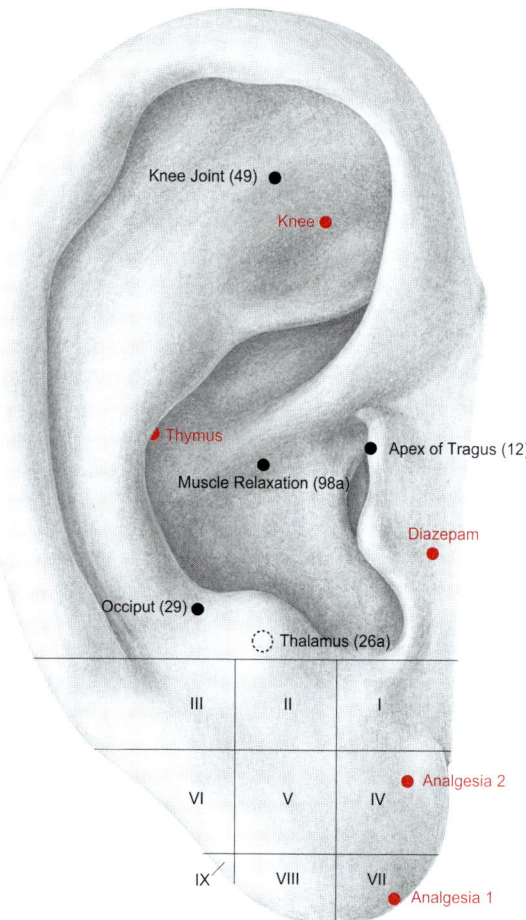
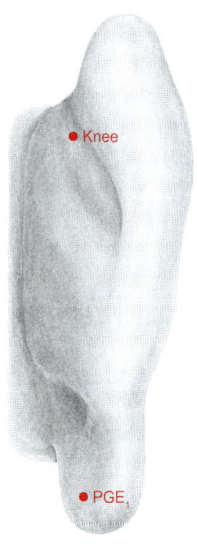

Fig. 7.1-8a+b

7.1.8 Knee Pain

Description

- Pain in the area of the knee
- Auricular acupuncture is indicated for the following disorders:

- osteoarthritis of the knee: degenerative changes of the knee joint
- inflammatory arthritis of the knee, e.g. gouty arthritis (› 7.1.2)
- patellar chondropathy: degenerative changes of the cartilage under the patella
- distorsion (after excluding the possibility of ligament lesions or a fracture)
- Depending on the cause, the pain may return periodically; there may also be pain after putting weight on the knee joint or there may be constant pain; swelling and overheating may occur as accompanying symptoms

- Before starting acupuncture treatments the affected knee should be examined by an orthopaedic consultant in order to exclude ligament or meniscus lesions. In these cases conventional treatment is necessary.
- Acupuncture is beneficial as after-care and accelerates the postoperative recovery

Point Prescription

The same treatment protocol applies to all forms of knee pain mentioned above; the determining factor is in all cases RAC-palpation.

French points
- Local points: **Knee** (› 6.2.3) on the anterior ear; **Knee** (› 6.11.2) on the posterior ear
- Relaxing point: **Diazepam** (› 6.7.3)
- Analgesic points: **PGE$_1$/Thymus, Valoron (Analgesia 2 and Thalamus)** (26a) (› 6.7.6), **Analgesia 1** (› 6.7.5)

Chinese points
- Local point: **Knee Joint (49)** (› 6.2.2)
- Relaxing point: **Muscle Relaxation (98a)** (› 6.1.3)
- Analgesic points: **Apex of Tragus (12)** (› 6.7.3), **Occiput (29)** (› 6.7.4)

Treatment Intervals
- **Acute stage:** once daily or every other day
- Pain for > 4 weeks: once to twice weekly until symptoms have subsided completely

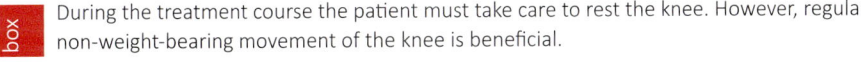

During the treatment course the patient must take care to rest the knee. However, regular non-weight-bearing movement of the knee is beneficial.

Treatment Course and Prognosis
- Significant pain reduction within 1–2 weeks
- Start of treatments during the **acute stage:** symptoms clear completely after up to 4 weeks
- Inflammatory knee pain generally responds better and quicker to auricular acupuncture
- In cases of pronounced degeneration a complete remission is generally not possible

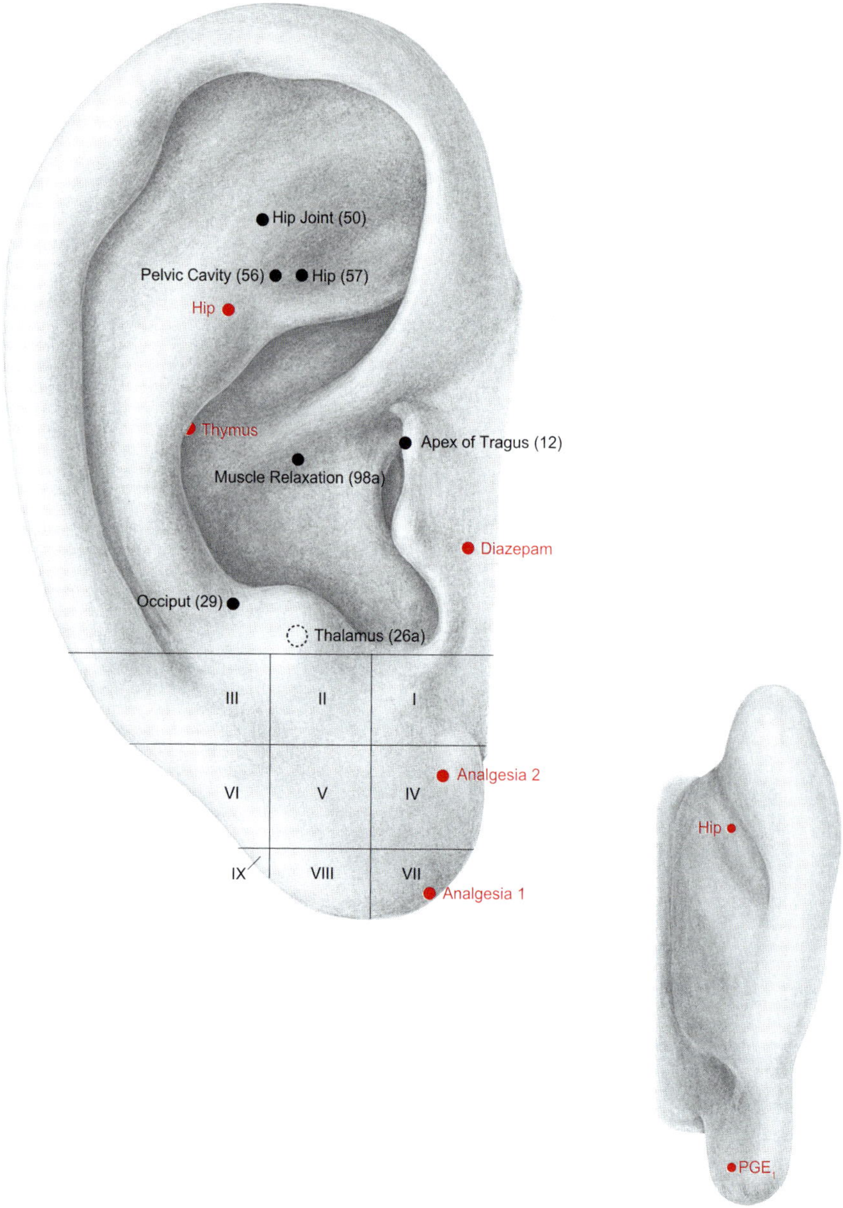

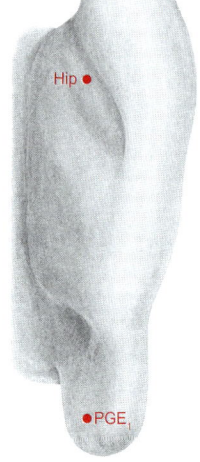

Hip Joint (50)

Pelvic Cavity (56) ● ● Hip (57)

Hip ●

Thymus

Apex of Tragus (12)

Muscle Relaxation (98a)

Diazepam

Occiput (29) ●

Thalamus (26a)

III   II   I

Analgesia 2

VI   V   IV

IX   VIII   VII

Analgesia 1

Hip ●

●PGE₁

Fig. 7.1-9a+b

7.1.9 Hip Pain (Coxalgia)

Description

- Pain in the hip area
- The following disorders represent an indication for auricular acupuncture:

- osteoarthritis of the hip: degenerative changes of the joint, also as a result of trauma; most common cause
- inflammatory arthritis of the hip
- periarthritis of the hip: generally chronically recurrent inflammatory processes of the hip with bursitis, calcification etc.
- Pain unrelated to the pathogenesis, especially during weight-bearing movements, e.g. using stairs – particularly when descending

 In cases of hip pain after a traumatic injury the patient should be X-rayed before starting acupuncture treatments in order to exclude the possibility of a fracture.

Point Prescription

The same point prescription applies to the various forms of hip pain.

French points
- Local points: **Hip** (› 6.2.3) on the anterior ear; **Hip** (› 6.11.2) on the posterior ear
- Relaxing point: **Diazepam** (› 6.7.3)
- Analgesic points: **PGE$_1$/Thymus, Valoron (Analgesia 2 and Thalamus [26a])** (› 6.7.6), **Analgesia 1** (› 6.7.5)

Chinese points
- Local points: **Hip (57), Hip Joint (50)** (› 6.2.2), **Pelvic Cavity (56)** (› 6.2.3, › 6.7.2)
- Relaxing point: **Muscle Relaxation (98a)** (› 6.1.3)
- Analgesic points: **Occiput (29)** (› 6.7.4), **Apex of Tragus (12)** (› 6.7.3)

Treatment Intervals
- **Acute stage:** three times weekly
- Pain for > 4 weeks: once or twice weekly until symptoms have subsided completely

 While treatments are ongoing the patient should not put any weight on the affected hip, and should avoid carrying heavy loads or working in a bent-over position. Light active or passive exercise (e.g. physiotherapy) supports the acupuncture treatments.

Treatment Course and Prognosis
- **Posttraumatic and inflammatory causes:** significant pain reduction within 1–2 weeks; if treatments start during the acute stage or immediately after the trauma, symptoms generally subside completely within 4 weeks
- **Chronic degenerative causes:** significant reduction of symptoms within 4 weeks; symptoms generally subside completely after approximately 6 months

 In very advanced degenerative cases auricular acupuncture can provide pain relief only to a certain extent. These cases generally require surgery (hip replacement). Auricular acupuncture can be administered postoperatively to support the healing process.

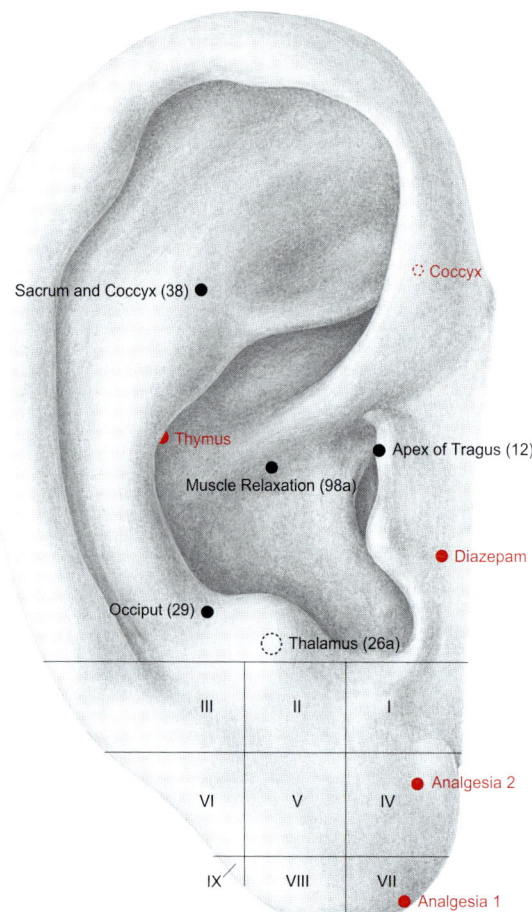

Sacrum and Coccyx (38) ●

◌ Coccyx

◖ Thymus

● Apex of Tragus (12)

Muscle Relaxation (98a) ●

● Diazepam

Occiput (29) ●

◌ Thalamus (26a)

III	II	I
VI	V	IV
IX	VIII	VII

● Analgesia 2

● Analgesia 1

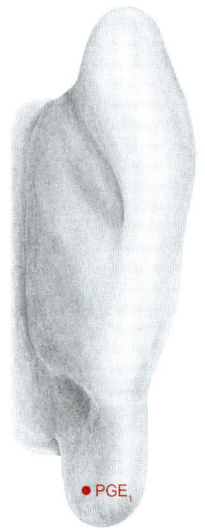

● PGE₁

Fig. 7.1-10a+b

7.1.10 Coccydynia (Coccyx Pain)

Description

- Pain in the area of the coccyx
- Causes:
  - trauma due to a fall on the coccyx
  - inflammatory changes due to excessive strain (e.g. horse riding)
  - neuralgia of the coccygeal nerve
- Pain, especially when sitting; generally this does not radiate
- Neuralgic forms are more common in women, often psycho-emotional component (stress etc.)

Point Prescription

The following points may respond to RAC-palpation for the forms of coccydynia described above:

French points
- Local point: **Coccyx** (› 6.1.1)
- Relaxing point: **Diazepam** (› 6.7.3)
- Analgesic points: **PGE$_1$/Thymus, Valoron (Analgesia 2 and Thalamus [26a])** (› 6.7.6), **Analgesia 1** (› 6.7.5)

Chinese points
- Local point: **Sacrum and Coccyx (38)** (› 6.1.1)
- Relaxing point: **Muscle Relaxation (98a)** (› 6.1.3)
- Analgesic points: **Apex of Tragus (12)** (› 6.7.3), **Occiput (29)** (› 6.7.4)

Treatment Intervals
- **Acute stage:** once daily or every other day
- Pain for > 1 week: twice weekly until symptoms have subsided completely

Treatment Course and Prognosis
- Generally significant reduction of symptoms within 1 week
- Start of treatments during the **acute stage:** generally symptoms subside completely after approximately 2 weeks

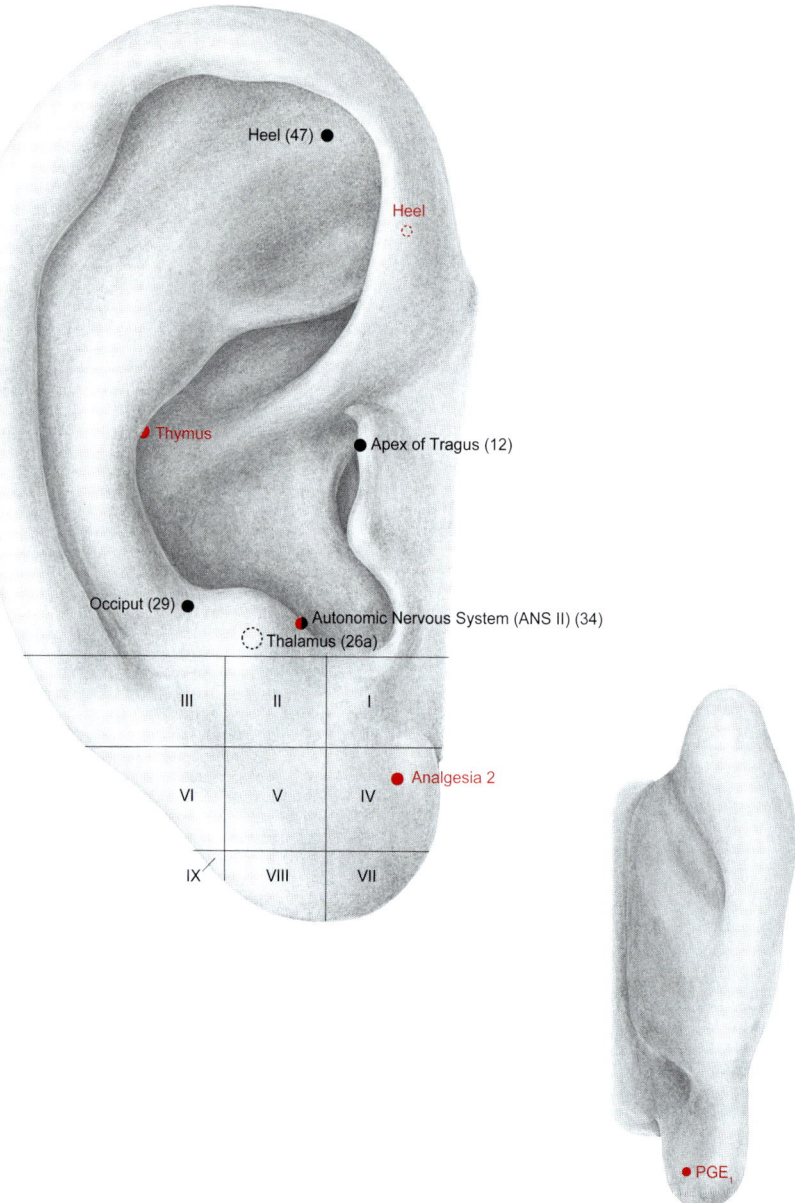

Heel (47)

Heel

Thymus

Apex of Tragus (12)

Occiput (29)

Autonomic Nervous System (ANS II) (34)

Thalamus (26a)

III   II   I

VI   V   IV   Analgesia 2

IX   VIII   VII

PGE₁

Fig. 7.1-11a+b

7.1.11 Heel Spur (Calcaneal Spur)

Description

- A spur-like bony protrusion on the lower surface of the calcaneal tuber at the insertion point of the tendons and aponeurotic fibres with heel pain exacerbated by weight-bearing
- Causes:
  - excessive strain, in particular associated with foot deformities such as flat foot and skew foot deformities; most common cause
  - degenerative changes, common in standing professions and in overweight persons
  - inflammation, e.g. with rheumatoid arthritis
- May occur in one or both heels, flare-ups are common

Point Prescription

French points

- Local point: **Heel** › 6.2.3)
- Analgesic points: **PGE$_1$/Thymus** (› 6.7.6), **Analgesia 2** (› 6.7.5)

Chinese points

- Local point: **Heel (47)** (› 6.2.2)
- Analgesic points: **Thalamus (26a)**, **Occiput (29)** (› 6.7.4), **Apex of Tragus (12)** (› 6.7.3), **ANS II (34)** (› 6.7.4)

Treatment Intervals

- **Acute stage:** three times weekly
- With pain for > 4 weeks: once or twice weekly until symptoms have subsided completely

> **box** During the treatment course it is essential that the patient rests his/her foot. Insoles that ease the pressure on the heel spur are beneficial.

Treatment Course and Prognosis

- Significant reduction of symptoms mostly within 1–2 weeks
- Start of treatments during the **acute stage:** symptoms often subside completely after up to 4 weeks

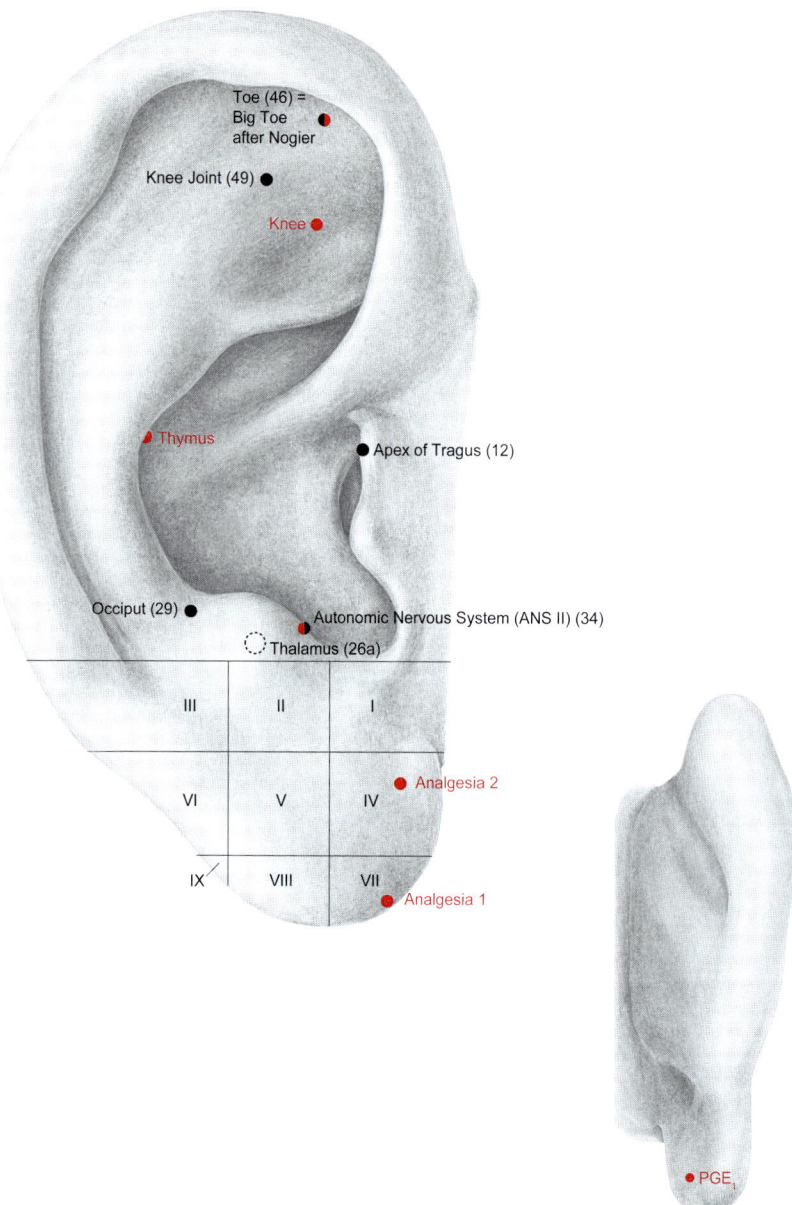

Toe (46) =
Big Toe
after Nogier

Knee Joint (49) ●

Knee ●

● Thymus

● Apex of Tragus (12)

Occiput (29) ●

Autonomic Nervous System (ANS II) (34)

◌ Thalamus (26a)

III | II | I

VI | V | IV ● Analgesia 2

IX | VIII | VII

● Analgesia 1

● PGE₁

Fig. 7.1-12a+b

7.1.12 Gout

Description

- Acute intense pain, erythema, and overheating of the affected joint due to hyperuricaemia; onset mostly during the night or early morning
- Forms: mostly primary (hereditary); secondary forms with an increase in cell death (e.g. polycythaemia or as a side-effect of chemotherapy) or with functional disorders of the kidneys are less common
- Triggers: high-purine foods, alcohol, physical exertion, or hypothermia
- Typical pattern: the metatarsophalangeal joint of the big toe (podagra) is affected in ⅔ of cases, more rarely the knee joint (gonagra, gonalgia)

Point Prescription

French points
- Local points: **Big Toe** (› 6.2.1), **Knee** (› 6.2.3)
- Anti-inflammatory points: PGE_1/**Thymus** (› 6.7.6)
- Analgesic points: **Valoron (Analgesia 2 and Thalamus [26a])** (› 6.7.6), **Analgesia 1** (› 6.7.5)

Chinese points
- Local points: **Toes (46)** (› 6.2.1), **Knee Joint (49)** (› 6.2.2)
- Analgesic points: **Thalamus (26a)**, **Occiput (29)**, **ANS II (34)** (› 6.7.4), **Apex of Tragus (12)** (› 6.7.3)

Treatment Intervals

- Once daily until symptoms improve
- Once inflammatory symptoms have subsided, twice weekly until symptoms disappear completely

- With elevated levels of uric acid (e.g. due to poor dietary habits) acupuncture treatments should be complemented by changes in diet.
- Conventional analgesic medication for 1-2 days tends to be beneficial during an acute attack since acupuncture can often alleviate pain only after this period.

Treatment Course and Prognosis

- Significant reduction of symptoms generally within 1–2 weeks
- Start of treatments during the **acute stage:** symptoms often subside completely after up to 4 weeks
- Depending on the pain intensity and uric acid levels the dosage of both analgesic (e.g. anti-inflammatory medication, colchicine) and uricosuric drugs (e.g. allopurinol, probenecid, sulfinpyrazone) can be reduced or they can be discontinued completely at an earlier stage.

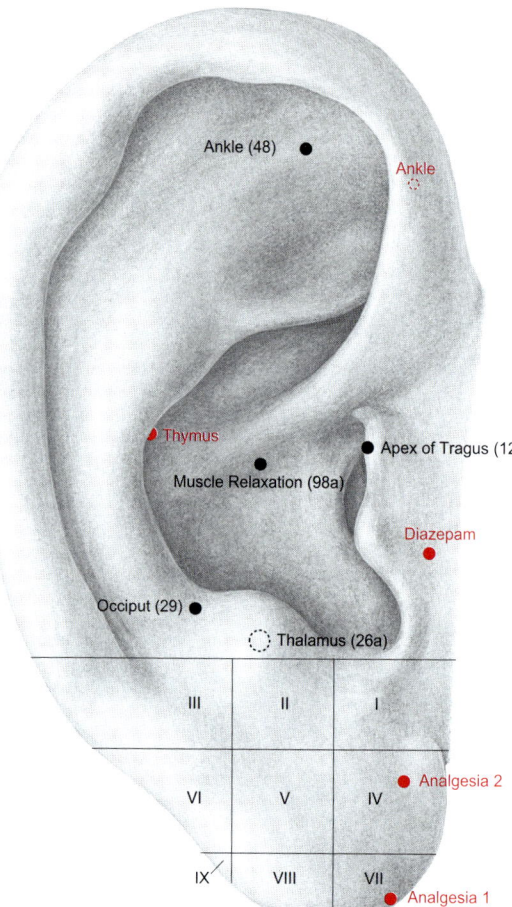

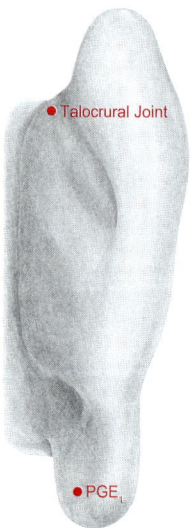

Fig. 7.1-13a+b

7.1.13 Sprained Ankle

Description

- Pain in the area of the ankle joint (talocrural joint), mostly at the lateral malleolus
- Accompanied by swelling and haematoma, even if the ligament is not ruptured
- Post-traumatic, an unstable ankle joint is often more prone to sprain injuries (repeatedly 'twisting' one's ankle)

Point Prescription

French points

- Local points: **Ankle** (› 6.2.3) on the anterior ear; **Talocrural Joint** (› 6.11.2) on the posterior ear
- Relaxing point: **Diazepam** (› 6.7.3)
- Analgesic points: **PGE$_1$/Thymus** (› 6.7.6), **Analgesia 1** and **Analgesia 2** (› 6.7.5)

Chinese points

- Local point: **Ankle (48)** (› 6.2.2)
- Relaxing point: **Muscle Relaxation (98a)** (› 6.1.3)
- Analgesic points: **Thalamus (26a)**, **Occiput (29)** (› 6.7.4), **Apex of Tragus (12)** (› 6.7.3)

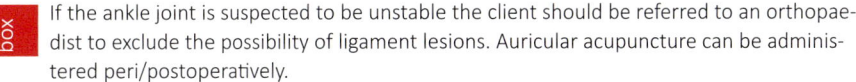

box If the ankle joint is suspected to be unstable the client should be referred to an orthopaedist to exclude the possibility of ligament lesions. Auricular acupuncture can be administered peri/postoperatively.

Treatment Intervals

- **Acute stage:** once daily or every other day
- Pain for > 4 weeks: once or twice weekly until symptoms have subsided completely

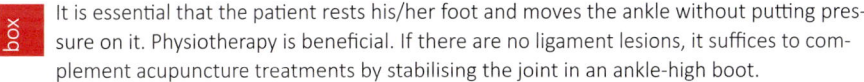

box It is essential that the patient rests his/her foot and moves the ankle without putting pressure on it. Physiotherapy is beneficial. If there are no ligament lesions, it suffices to complement acupuncture treatments by stabilising the joint in an ankle-high boot.

Treatment Course and Prognosis

- Significant reduction of symptoms within a few days
- If treatments start during the acute stage symptoms tend to subside completely after 1–2 weeks; in exceptional cases, depending on the severity of the trauma, only after up to 4 weeks

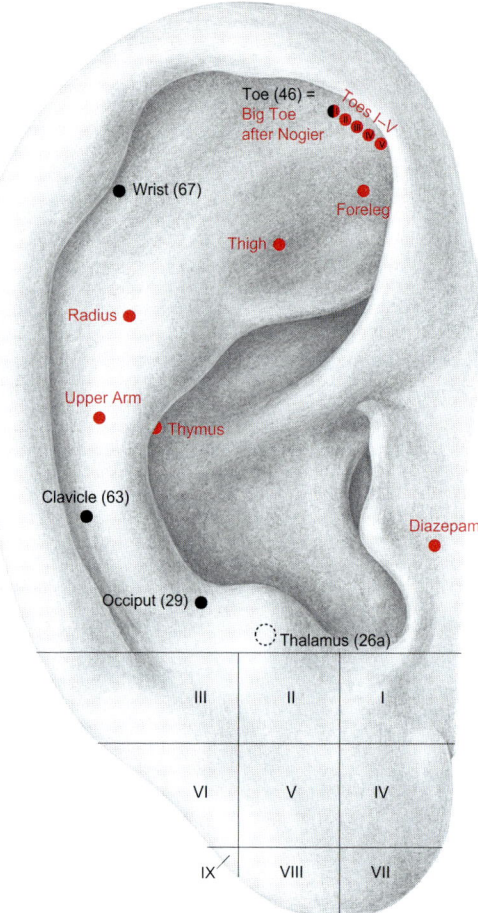

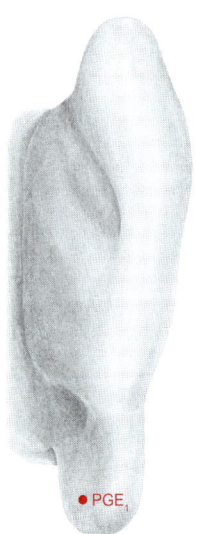

Toe (46) =
Big Toe
after Nogier

Toes I–V

Wrist (67)

Foreleg

Thigh

Radius

Upper Arm

Thymus

Clavicle (63)

Diazepam

Occiput (29)

Thalamus (26a)

III   II   I

VI   V   IV

IX   VIII   VII

PGE₁

Fig. 7.1-14a+b

7.1.14 Pain Treatment for Fractures

Description

- Posttraumatic pain, swelling, and/or haematoma
- Auricular acupuncture may alleviate pain as well as improve and accelerate healing

 Acupuncture should always be preceded by a conventional diagnosis and primary medical care!

Point Prescription

French points
- Local points: e.g. **Upper Arm**, **Radius**, **Toes** (› 6.2.1), **Foreleg**, **Thigh** (› 6.2.3)
- Analgesic points: **Diazepam** (› 6.7.3), **PGE$_1$/Thymus** (› 6.7.6)

Chinese points
- Local points: **Clavicle (63)** (› 6.2.1), **Wrist (67)** (› 6.2.1)
- Analgesic points: **Occiput (29), Thalamus (26a)** (› 6.7.4)

Treatment Intervals

- Initially once daily until the pain has reduced significantly
- Then once weekly until symptoms have subsided completely

Treatment Course and Prognosis

- The sooner treatments start after the fracture, the sooner there will be results
- The pain diminishes mostly within minutes to hours after acupuncture; for a sustained reduction in pain daily treatments should be continued for several days
- Generally the pain subsides completely after 1–3 weeks, in rare cases only after up to 6 weeks

 For acute injuries local laser therapy (› 4.2.3) can significantly accelerate the reduction in swelling and promote healing.

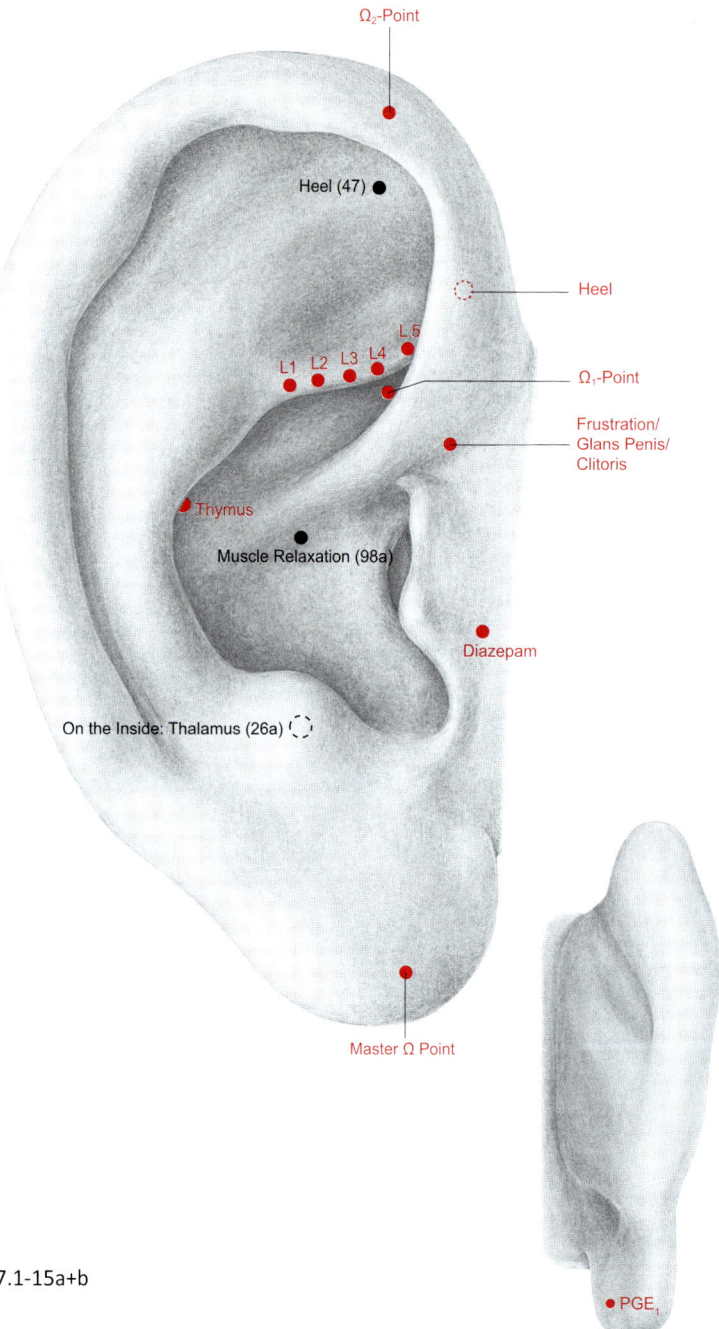

Fig. 7.1-15a+b

7.1.15 Achillodynia

Description

- Pain in the area of the Achilles tendon insertion at the calcaneus, approximately 2–6 cm superior to the insertion of the tendon
- Often Achilles insertional tendinopathy (compare epicondylitis › 7.1.6)
- Causes:
  - initially mostly irritation due to excessive strain
  - microtrauma in the area of the tendon due to mechanical irritation

Point Prescription

French points

- Local points: **Heel** (› 6.2.3) **L1–5** (› 6.1.1)
- Analgesic points: **Diazepam** (› 6.7.3), **PGE$_1$/Thymus** (› 6.7.6)
- Psychological points: **Omega Axis** (› 6.12.1), **Frustration** (› 6.8.3)

Chinese points

- Local point: **Heel (47)** (› 6.2.2)
- Analgesic point: **Thalamus (26a)** (› 6.7.4)
- Relaxing point: **Muscle Relaxation (98a)** (› 6.1.3)

Treatment Intervals

- **Acute symptoms or acute progression:** once daily until the pain has reduced significantly, then stop analgesic medication; then once weekly until symptoms have improved or disappeared completely
- **Chronic symptoms:** once weekly until symptoms have improved significantly; then every 2–3 weeks until symptoms have subsided completely

- Analgesic medication or locally injected cortisone often results in a short-lived period without symptoms. However, this may not prevent future damage to the tendinous tissue and even subsequent rupture of the tendon.
- Osteopathy is recommended as adjuvant therapy.

Treatment Course and Prognosis

- **Acute symptoms:** symptoms generally improve within 4 weeks
- **Chronic symptoms:** complete remission often only after extended therapy, depending on the severity of symptoms up to half a year or longer; however, a significant relaxation and pain reduction can be expected within 4–6 weeks

7.2 Chronic Musculoskeletal Pain

7.2.1 Chronic Polyarthritis

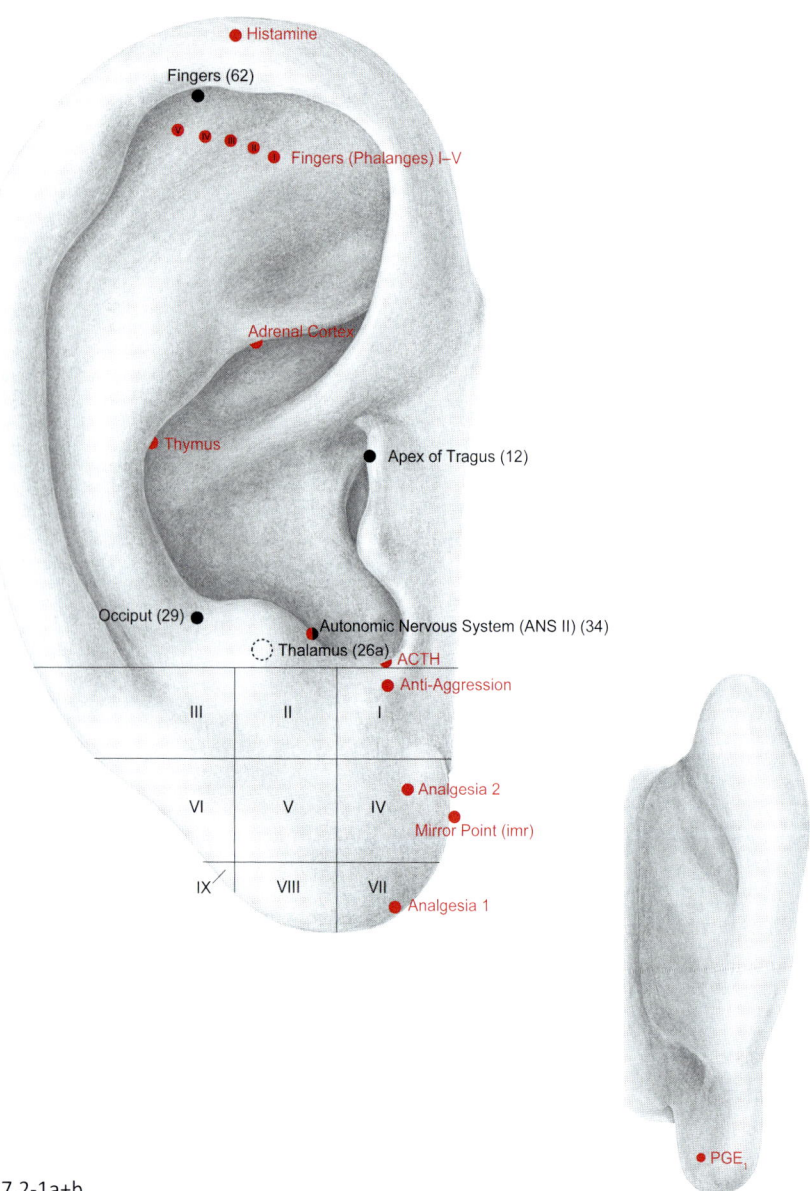

Fig. 7.2-1a+b

- Most common rheumatic disorder; autoimmune disorder affecting the synovial membranes with inflammatory-degenerative changes in the joints; three times more common in females than in males
- Pattern: initially affects mainly the small joints (hands and/or toes), but the clinical picture can vary significantly
- Symptoms: pain, overheating, and swelling of joints, morning stiffness (principal symptom during early stages), increased sweating, loss of appetite, paraesthesia
- Course of disease: onset generally at age 20–50; gradual progression or intermittent attacks

Point Prescription

French points
- Local points: e.g. **Fingers (Phalanges)** (› 6.2.1)
- Immunostimulant points: **ACTH** (› 6.6.6), **Adrenal cortex** (› 6.6.1), **Immune Axis** (› 6.12.3)
- Anti-inflammatory point: **PGE$_1$/Thymus** (› 6.7.6)
- Analgesic points: **Valoron (Analgesia 2 and Thalamus [26a])** (› 6.7.6), **Analgesia 1** (› 6.7.5)
- Psychological point: **Anti-Aggression** (› 6.8.5)

Chinese points
- Local point: e.g. **Fingers (62)** (› 6.2.1)
- Analgesic points: **Thalamus (26a), Occiput (29), ANS II (34)** (› 6.7.4), **Apex of Tragus (12)** (› 6.7.3)

 The Anti-Aggression Point is considered the most effective point for polyarthritis. Intradermal needles are the preferred method as they can remain in situ for one week up to a maximum of two weeks. If a needle falls out a new intradermal needle can be inserted after 1–2 days.

Treatment Intervals

- Treatment intervals are determined by the duration of the pain reduction; initially generally every 2–3 days, later once weekly; once there is no worsening of symptoms after several days without acupuncture the treatment intervals can be extended to twice monthly
- During or following steroid treatment: initially twice weekly until symptoms no longer worsen after the treatment
- Treatments should be given during acute episodes but also during remission when there is little or no pain
- **Caution:** during or after steroid treatment immunostimulant points can lead to an exacerbation of symptoms after the treatment; if necessary, this can be prevented with conventional analgesic (non-steroidal) medication.

Treatment Course and Prognosis

The treatment course and prognosis depend on the duration, severity and previous treatments (steroids?):

- No previous treatment with steroids: with start of treatments during the early stage symptoms will subside completely after 3 months at the latest
- No previous treatment with steroids: with start of treatments during the chronic stage symptoms will subside completely after approximately 1 year
- Previous treatment with steroids: with start of treatments during the chronic stage symptoms will subside completely after > 1 year

7.2.2 Complex Regional Pain Syndrome (CRPS)

Description

- Localised circulatory and metabolic disorder with secondary painful dystrophy, followed later by atrophy of the affected extremity; occurs as a complication after a fracture or other trauma, surgery, or inflammation; mainly affecting the hands or feet
- Affects all tissue layers of both soft and bony tissue
- Generally develops several weeks after the initial trauma; divided into inflammatory acute stage, dystrophy stage, and atrophy stage
- Mostly in emotionally unstable and nervous patients

Point prescription

The same point prescription applies to all three stages; RAC-palpation is the determining factor.

French points
- Local point: e.g. **Wrist** (› 6.2.1)
- Analgesic point: **PGE$_1$/Thymus** (› 6.7.6)
- Psychological points: **Omega Axis** (› 6.12.1), **Antidepressant Point** (› 6.8.5), **Haldol** (› 6.8.6)
- Stabilising points: **Point Zero** (› 6.10.3), **Laterality Point** (› 6.8.6)

Chinese points
- Local point: **Wrist (67)** (› 6.2.1)
- Analgesic points: **Thalamus (26a)**, **Occiput (29)** (› 6.7.4)

> **box**
> In cases of CRPS psycho-emotional support has an analgesic affect. For this reason particular attention should be paid to psychological and stabilising points. It is therefore recommended to insert intradermal needles in one or two of these points.

Treatment Intervals
- Initially once or twice weekly
- Once symptoms improve 2–4 times monthly
- After 3 months intervals can be extended to twice monthly

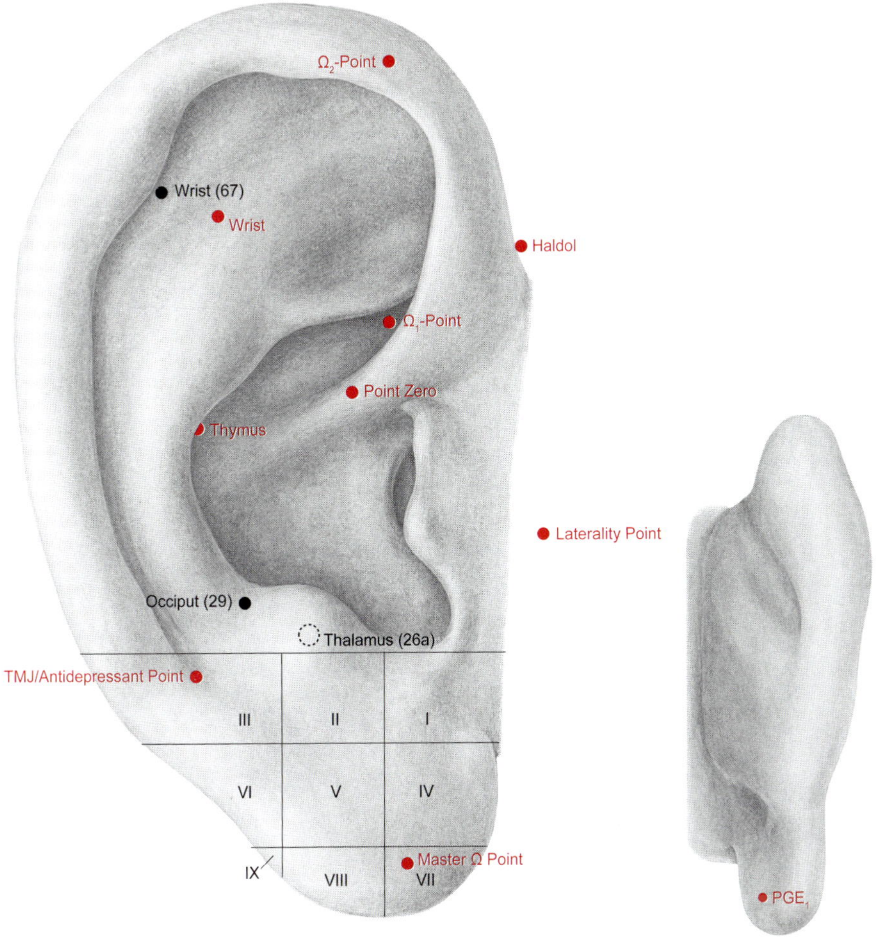

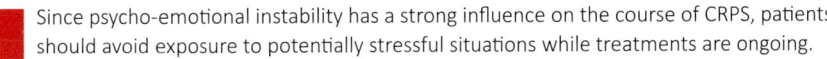

Ω₂-Point ●
Wrist (67) ●
● Wrist
● Haldol
● Ω₁-Point
● Point Zero
● Thymus
● Laterality Point
Occiput (29) ●
◌ Thalamus (26a)
TMJ/Antidepressant Point ●
III | II | I
VI | V | IV
IX | VIII | VII
● Master Ω Point
● PGE₂

Fig. 7.2-2a+b

- **Intradermal needles** should be removed after one week and new needles inserted after a few days; repeat this procedure until symptoms have improved

Treatment Course and Prognosis

- Start of treatments during the **inflammatory acute stage:** generally only short-term treatments required with symptoms subsiding completely within 4 weeks
- Start of treatments during the **dystrophy or atrophy stage:** generally treatments over a long period of time necessary:
  - short-term (weeks): reduction in pain
  - medium-term (months): preventing long-term damage
  - long-term (up to 1 year): full recovery

> **box** Since psycho-emotional instability has a strong influence on the course of CRPS, patients should avoid exposure to potentially stressful situations while treatments are ongoing.

7.2.3 Osteoarthritis

Description

- Degenerative joint disorder
- Characterised by joint stiffness during the early stages, followed later by pain when starting to move, then by pain during movement, and eventually by continuous pain
- The degree of degenerative changes (X-ray findings) does not necessarily correlate with the pain intensity and/or the extent to which the range of motion is limited

Point Prescription

French points

- Local points: e.g. **Hip** (› 6.2.3), **Knee, Ankle Joint** (› 6.2.3) on the anterior ear; **Hip, Knee, Talocrural Joint** (› 6.11.2) on the posterior ear
- Analgesic points: **PGE₁/Thymus** (› 6.7.6), **Analgesia 1 and 2** (› 6.7.5)

Chinese points

- Local points: **Hip (57), Knee Joint (49), Ankle (48)** (› 6.2.2)
- Analgesic point: **Thalamus (26a)** (› 6.7.4)

> **box**
> X-ray findings do not allow a direct conclusion as to what extent recovery from the joint pain is possible. Joint pain is often of a functional nature and occurs in addition to arthritis while not being caused by it. In such cases it is possible to alleviate symptoms with acupuncture even if the degenerative changes remain.

Treatment Intervals

- Regardless of the severity: once weekly until symptoms have subsided completely

> **box**
> In very advanced cases of arthritis surgical intervention is sometimes unavoidable. However, acupuncture can support the post-operative healing process.

Treatment Course and Prognosis

- **Recurrent pain:** 5–10 treatments until symptoms have subsided completely
- **Constant pain:** treatments for about 3 months until regular pain medication can be reduced or discontinued; repeat treatment courses may be necessary

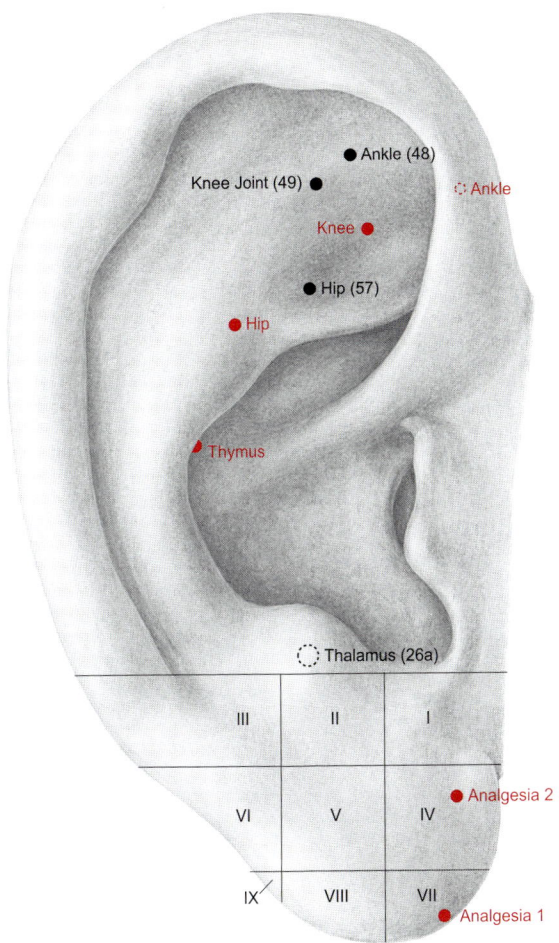

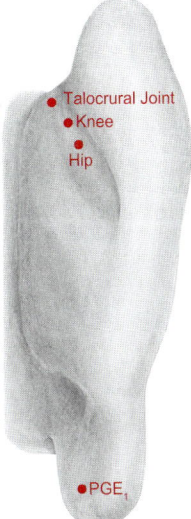

Fig. 7.2-3a+b

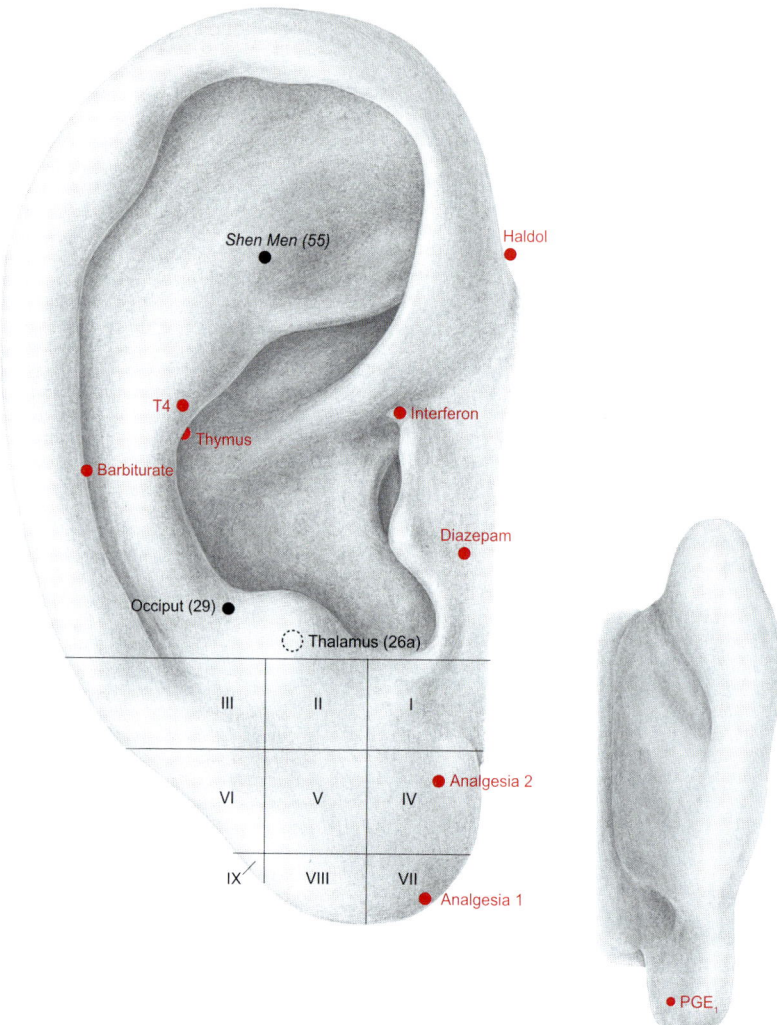

Fig. 7.2-4a+b

7.2.4 Intercostal Neuralgia

Description

- Pain along the course of one or more intercostal nerves, mostly in the form of acute flare-ups; often accompanied by hyperaesthesia of the affected intercostals spaces
- Causes: e.g. herpes zoster (› 8.5.3), rib injuries, or disorders of the spine

Point Prescription

French points

- Local points: e.g. if the 4th intercostal space is affected **T4** should be treated (› 6.1.1)
- Analgesic points: PGE_1/**Thymus** (› 6.7.6), **Analgesia 1** and **Analgesia 2** (› 6.7.5)

- Immunostimulant points: **Interferon** (› 6.7.3), **Thymus** (› 6.6.1)
- Psychological points: **Diazepam** (› 6.7.3), **Barbiturate** (› 6.7.1), **Haldol** (› 6.8.6)

Chinese points
- Analgesic points: **Thalamus (26a)**, **Occiput (29)** (› 6.7.4), *Shen Men* **(55)** (› 6.7.2)

 By injecting 0,1ml 1 % prilocaine in the auricular points pertaining to the affected spinal segment and/or Ω_1-Point (› 6.8.1 and › 6.12.1) symptoms may subside completely within seconds, especially during the acute stage.

Treatment Intervals
- **Acute stage:** once daily until the pain has reduced significantly (analgesic medication no longer necessary); then once weekly until symptoms have subsided completely
- **Chronic stage:** 2–3 times weekly for about 4 weeks, then once or twice weekly until symptoms have subsided completely
- Until the pain has reduced significantly it is beneficial to combine acupuncture with non-steroidal anti-inflammatory drugs (NSAIDs). Alternatively, neural therapy can provide short-term pain relief and thus support auricular acupuncture treatments which are slower in giving pain relief but provide more sustained long-term support.

Treatment Course and Prognosis
- Start of treatments during the **acute stage:** symptoms usually subside within 4 weeks
- Start of treatments during the **chronic stage:** treatments for up to 6 months; generally there is a significant relaxation and pain reduction within 4–6 weeks; additional analgesic medication is then no longer necessary

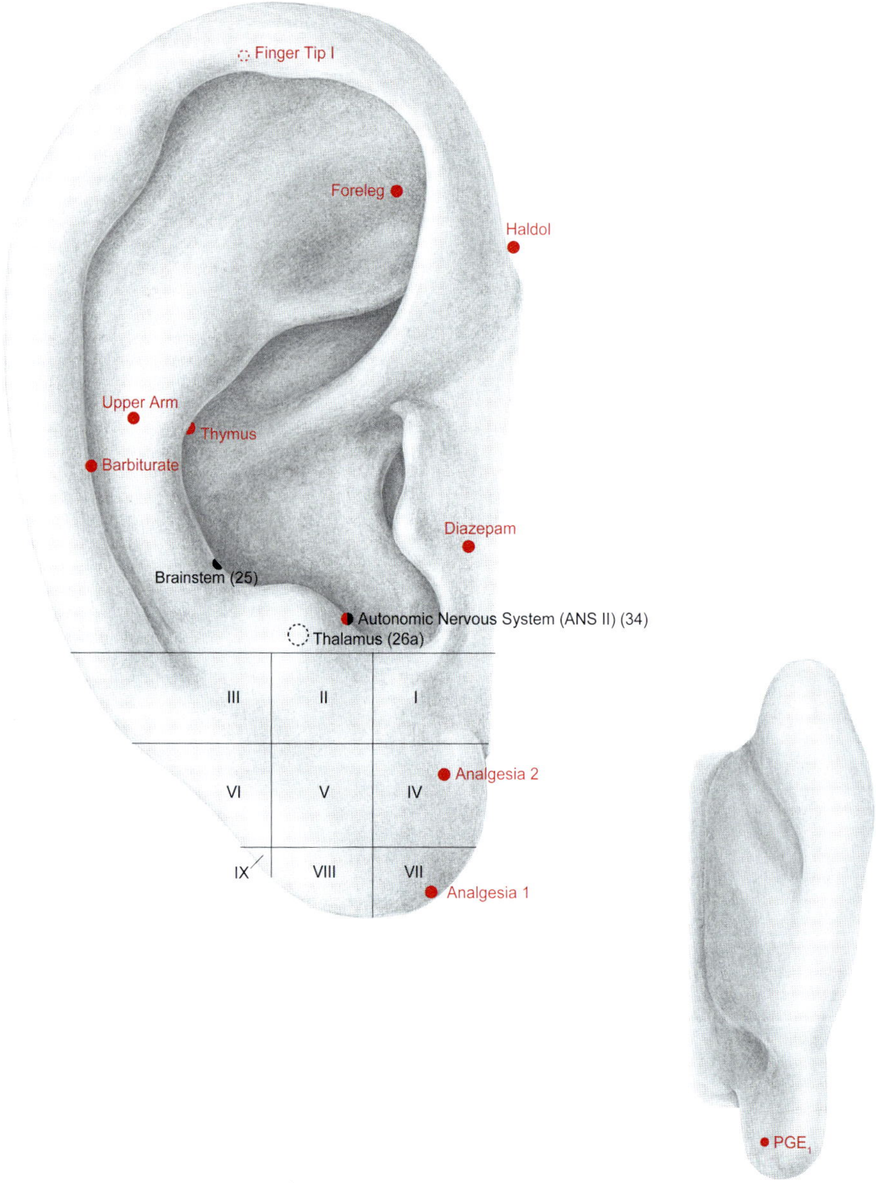

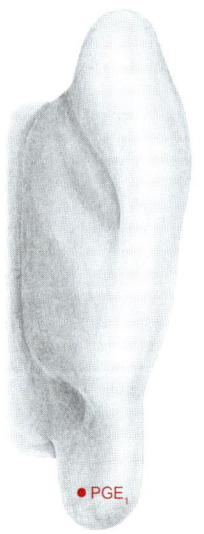

Finger Tip I

Foreleg

Haldol

Upper Arm

Thymus

Barbiturate

Diazepam

Brainstem (25)

Autonomic Nervous System (ANS II) (34)

Thalamus (26a)

III | II | I

Analgesia 2

VI | V | IV

IX | VIII | VII

Analgesia 1

PGE₁

Fig. 7.2-5a+b

7.2.5 Phantom Pain

Description

- Pain which can occur after the amputation of a limb in that part of the body that is no longer there
- Often occurs together with pain in the remaining part of the limb
- Phantom pain is more likely to occur if there has been pain in the affected extremity before the amputation

Point Prescription

French points

- Local points: depending on the amputated extremity, e.g. **Upper Arm**, **Fingertips I** (› 6.2.1) or **Foreleg** (› 6.2.3)
- Analgesic points: **PGE$_1$/Thymus** (› 6.7.6), **Analgesia 1** and **Analgesia 2** (› 6.7.5)
- Psychological points: **Diazepam** (› 6.7.3), **Barbiturate** (› 6.7.1), **Haldol** (› 6.8.6)

Chinese points

- Analgesic points: **Brainstem (25)** (› 6.10.4), **ANS II (34)**, **Thalamus (26a)** (› 6.7.4)

Treatment Intervals

- Every 3 days in combination with (often) existing analgesic medication until the pain has reduced significantly; painkillers can then be discontinued; then acupuncture only once weekly until symptoms have subsided completely

Treatment Course and Prognosis

- Approximately 3 months until symptoms subside completely
- If symptoms persist after 3 months of acupuncture treatments, expecting a complete recovery is no longer realistic; however, a long-term reduction of pain may be possible with regular acupuncture (e.g. twice monthly) so that painkillers are not required.

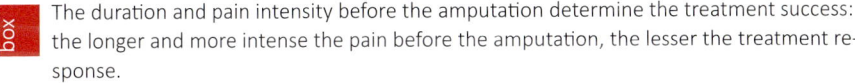

The duration and pain intensity before the amputation determine the treatment success: the longer and more intense the pain before the amputation, the lesser the treatment response.

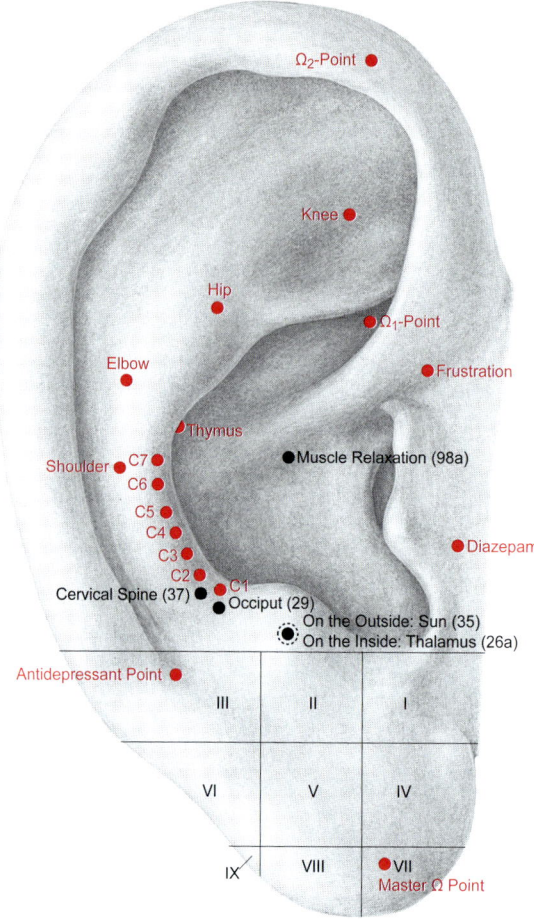
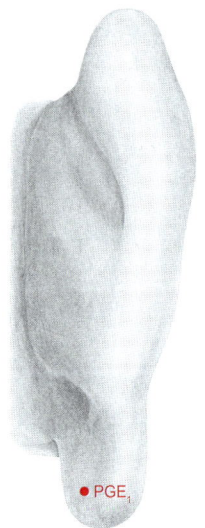

Fig. 7.2-6a+b

7.2.6 Fibromyalgia

Description

- Extra-articular rheumatic disorder; test results and X-ray findings are normal
- Bilateral pain persisting for at least 3 months and affecting at least 11 of 18 pressure points on the anterior and posterior aspect of the body, both above and below the hip
- Often in combination with stress or emotional tension
- Often improvement with age
- Causes:
  - if primary: unclear aetiology
  - if secondary: often in conjunction with traumas and rheumatic or malignant diseases

Point Prescription

French points

- Local points: **Cervical Spine 1–7** (› 6.1.1), **Shoulder** (› 6.2.1) **Elbow** (› 6.2.1); **Hip** (› 6.2.3), **Knee** (› 6.2.3)
- Analgesic points: **Diazepam** (› 6.7.3), **PGE₁/Thymus** (› 6.7.6)
- Psychological points: **Omega Axis** (› 6.12.1), **Frustration** (› 6.8.3), **Antidepressant Point** (› 6.8.5)

Chinese points

- Local point: **Cervical Spine (37)** (› 6.1.1)
- Analgesic points: **Sun (35), Occiput (29), Thalamus (26a)** (› 6.7.4)
- Relaxing point: **Muscle Relaxation (98a)** (› 6.1.3)

Treatment Intervals

- **Acute symptoms or acute progression:** once daily until the pain has reduced significantly so that existing analgesic medication can be discontinued; then further weekly treatments until symptoms have improved or disappeared completely
- **Chronic symptoms:** once weekly until symptoms have improved significantly; then every 2–3 weeks until symptoms have subsided completely

- Generally, analgesic or steroidal medication does not alleviate the pain so that acupuncture is one of the few options for pain reduction.
- Sufficient sleep and relaxation support the therapy.
- Feldenkrais, autogenic training, or osteopathy are recommended as adjuvant therapeutic methods.

Treatment Course and Prognosis

- **Acute symptoms:** symptoms often improve within 4 weeks
- **Chronic symptoms:** generally complete remission only after extended treatments (depending on the severity of symptoms treatments may be necessary for several years) but often a significant relaxation and pain reduction within 4–6 weeks

7.3 Headaches

7.3.1 Tension Headaches

Description

- Diffuse, generally moderately severe headaches
- Dull pain with intermittent throbbing sensations, occasionally accompanied by dizziness and nausea
- Chronic (> 15 days/month) or episodic forms
- Triggers include: changes in the weather, premenstrual, menopausal

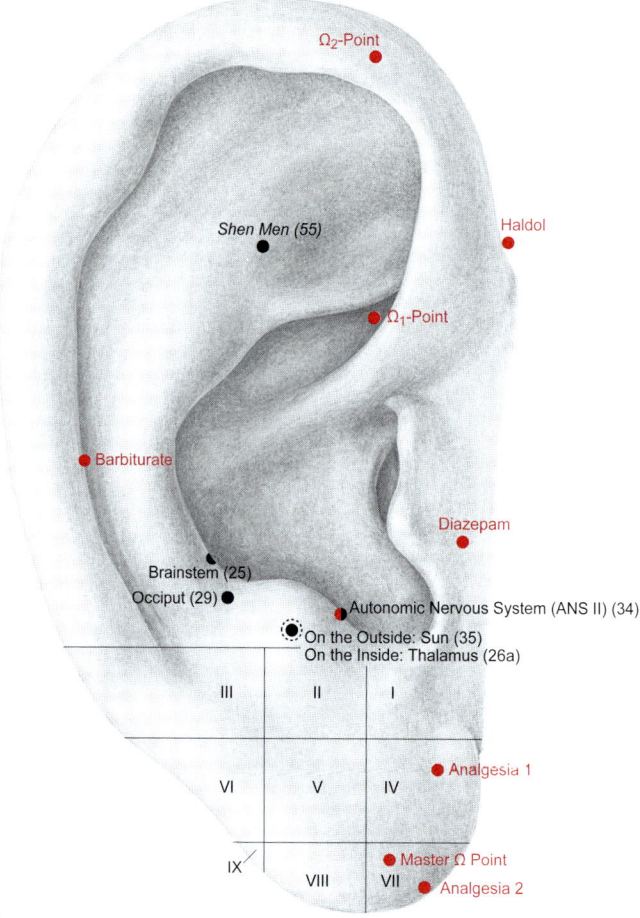

Fig. 7.3-1a+L

Point Prescription

French points
- Analgesic points: **Analgesia 1** and **Analgesia 2** (› 6.7.5)
- Psychological points: **Diazepam** (› 6.7.3), **Barbiturate** (› 6.7.1), **Haldol** (› 6.8.6), **Omega Axis** (› 6.12.1)

Chinese points
- Analgesic points: **Sun (35)**, **Thalamus (26a)**, **Occiput (29)**, **ANS II (34)** (› 6.7.4), *Shen Men* **(55)** (› 6.7.2), **Brainstem (25)** (› 6.10.4)

Treatment Intervals
- **Acute** (non-chronic recurrent) **tension headaches:** one treatment is often sufficient
- **Chronic tension headaches:** initially (depending on the frequency of the headaches) every 2–7 days, later twice monthly until symptoms have subsided completely

Treatment Course and Prognosis

The longer the headaches have been occurring, the longer the required treatment course:
- **short-term:** reduction of analgesic medication, reduced pain intensity
- **medium-term:** extended symptom-free intervals
- **long-term:** complete recovery

 In cases of rebound headaches (headaches due to medication overuse) it is necessary to gradually reduce the analgesic medication during the treatment course. Patient-compliance is required for good therapeutic results.

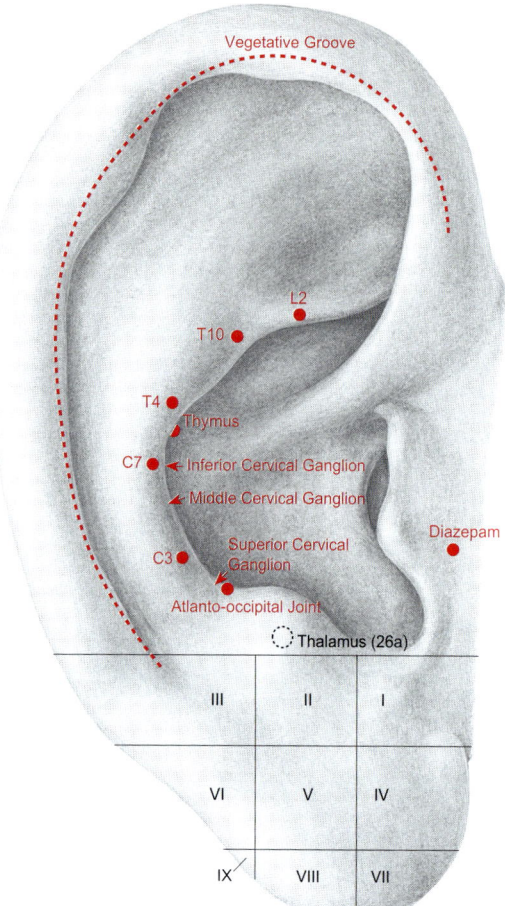

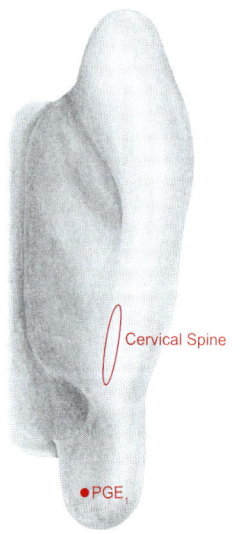

Fig. 7.3-2a+b

7.3.2 Occipital Neuralgia

Description
- Mostly paroxysmal pain along the course of the major occipital nerve (occiput), generally bilateral
- Radiates across the occiput to the vertex (acute cervical myalgia)
- Triggers include: draft, poor posture at the workplace, sleeping in a bad position, or injuries (e.g. cervical spine distorsion)
- May become chronic

Point Prescription

French points
- Local points: **Atlanto-occipital Joint**, **C3**, **C7** (› 6.1.1), **Superior, Medial, and Inferior Cervical Ganglion** (› 6.9.2) on the anterior ear; **Cervical Spine** (› 6.11.1) on the posterior ear
- For restricted movement: local points on the cervical spine (see above); restricted movement of a particular part of the spine often leads to (compensatory) counter-blockages in other areas of the spine; needling these points is therefore recommended, e.g. **T4, T10, L2** (› 6.1.1)
- Points in the **Vegetative Groove** (› 6.9.1)
- Analgesic points: **Diazepam** (› 6.7.3), **PGE$_1$/Thymus** (› 6.7.6)

Chinese points
- Analgesic point: **Thalamus (26a)** (› 6.7.4)

Treatment Intervals
- Start of treatments during the **acute stage:** 1–2 treatments are often sufficient
- Start of treatments during the **chronic stage:** initially every 2–7 days depending on the frequency of the headaches; then twice monthly until symptoms have subsided completely

Treatment Course and Prognosis
The longer the headaches have been occurring, the longer the required treatment course. Patient compliance (avoiding triggers!) is important for good therapeutic results, especially during the early phase of treatments.
- **short-term:** reduction of analgesic medication, reduction of pain intensity
- **medium-term:** extended symptom-free intervals
- **long-term:** complete recovery

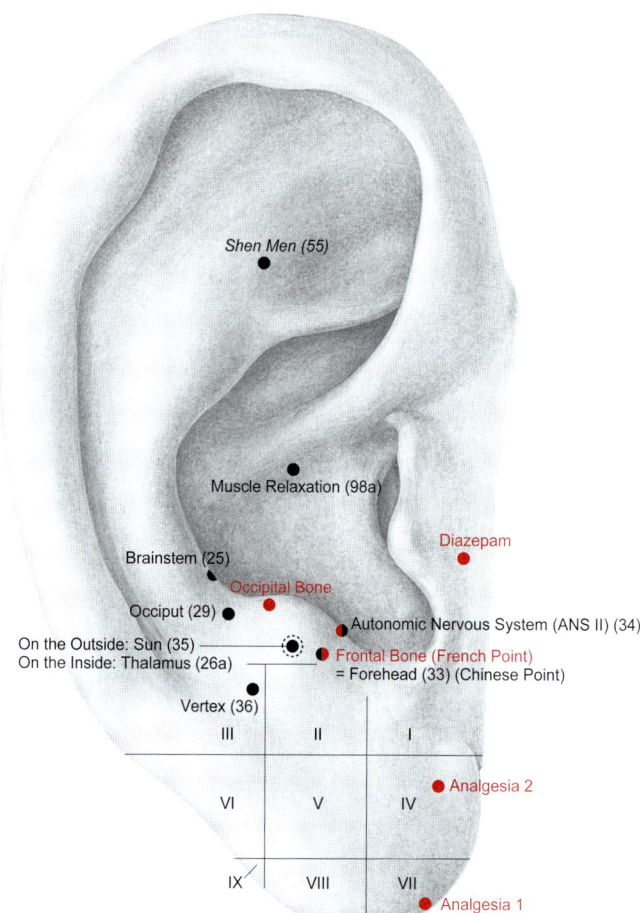

Fig. 7.3-3

7.3.3 Trauma-related Headaches

Description

- Acute, generally diffuse, occasionally localised headaches following a trauma (e.g. blow to the head, fall)

Point prescription

French points

- Local point: e.g. **Occipital Bone** (› 6.3.3)
- Analgesic points: **Analgesia 1** and **Analgesia 2** (› 6.7.5)
- Relaxing point: **Diazepam** (› 6.7.3)

Chinese points

- Local points: **Forehead (33)**, **Vertex (36)** (› 6.3.3)
- Relaxing point: **Muscle Relaxation (98a)** (› 6.1.3)
- Analgesic points: *Shen Men* **(55)** (› 6.7.2), **ANS II (34)**, **Sun (35)**, **Thalamus (26a)**, **Occiput (29)** (› 6.7.4), **Brainstem (25)** (› 6.10.4)

Treatment Intervals

- Start of treatments immediately after the trauma: once daily or every other day
- Start of treatments > 1 week after the trauma: twice weekly

Treatment Course and Prognosis

- Significant reduction of symptoms within 1 week
- Start of treatments immediately after the trauma: symptoms generally subside after approximately 2 weeks

box
Symptoms generally subside quickly if treatments are started soon after the trauma. This also prevents the headaches from becoming chronic.

7.3.4 Vascular Headaches

Description

- Characterised by continuous or paroxysmal, diffuse, dull pressure pain, often worse with postural changes
- Accompanying symptoms: dizziness, nausea
- With emotional instability, e.g. during menopause

Point Prescription

French points

- Psychological points: **Diazepam** (› 6.7.3), **Barbiturate** (› 6.7.1), **Haldol** (› 6.8.6), **Omega Axis** (› 6.12.1)

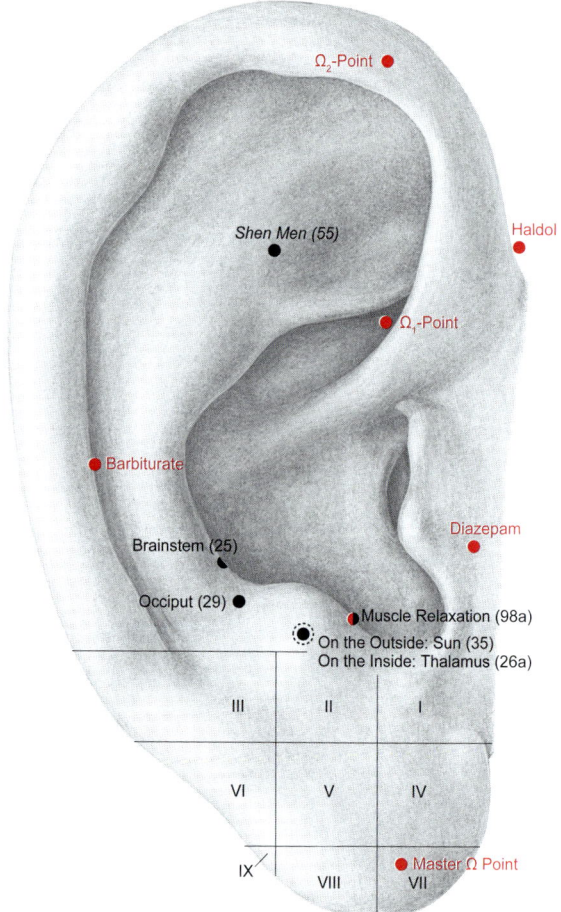

Fig. 7.3-4

Chinese points
- Analgesic points: **Sun (35)**, **Thalamus (26a)**, **Occiput (29)**, **ANS II (34)** (› 6.7.4), ***Shen Men* (55)** (› 6.7.2), **Brainstem (25)** (› 6.10.4)

Treatment Intervals

Treatment intervals depend on the frequency of the headaches:
- Headaches daily to once weekly: initially every 2–3 days until there are no symptoms for up to one week, then weekly treatments, followed by fortnightly treatments until symptoms have subsided completely
- Headaches < 3 times monthly: initially once weekly; if there are no symptoms for at least 2 weeks treatment intervals can be extended to twice monthly until symptoms have subsided completely

Treatment Course and Prognosis

- Symptoms often subside within 3 months
- In most cases symptom-free intervals will increase; acupuncture should then be given only as needed (during an acute attack)

7.4 Migraines

Auricular acupuncture distinguishes four forms of migraine:
- **Cervical migraine** (› 7.4.1): typically radiates outward from the occiput, mostly caused by degenerative changes
- **Hormonal migraine** (› 7.4.2): typically dependent on the menstrual cycle
- **'Weather migraine'** (› 7.4.3): typically triggered by changes in the weather
- **'Gallbladder migraine'** (› 7.4.4): typically triggered by stress

Often there are mixed forms of migraine. In these cases points should be chosen based on the treatment principle of the relevant form of migraine based on the patient's history and RAC palpation (› 3.1.4).

 The first treatment (or the first few treatments) may trigger a migraine attack which should be treated with analgesic medication. If this happens, fewer auricular points should be needled in the next treatment. Body acupuncture or herbal medicine can be used additionally in such cases.

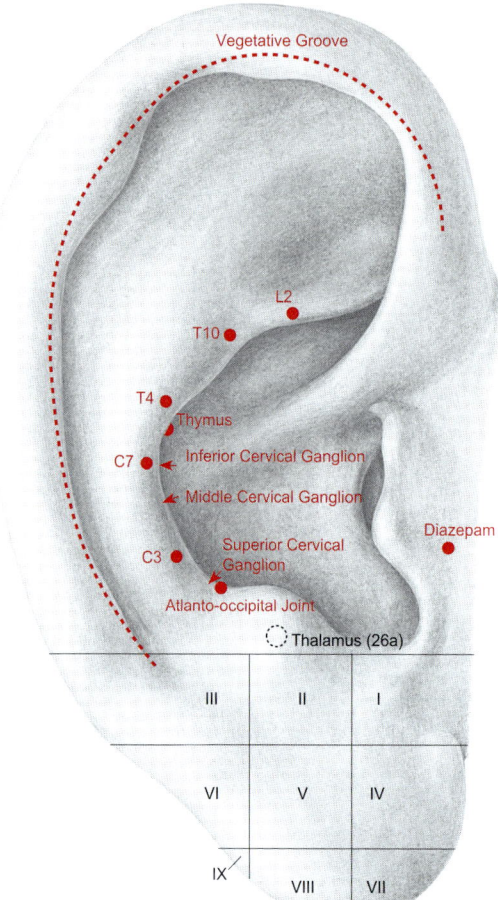

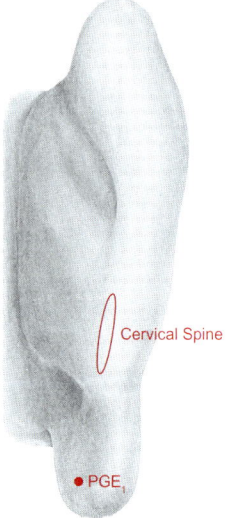

Fig. 7.4-1a+b

7.4.1 Cervical Migraine

- Can be triggered by draft, a bad position during sleep, or poor posture at the work-place; occipital paroxysmal headaches which can last for several hours
- Accompanying signs and symptoms: nausea, vomiting, sensitivity to light, visual disturbances
- Predisposition: cervical degenerative changes or trauma, e.g. neck distortion

Point prescription

French points
- Local points: Cervical Spine Points, e.g. **Atlanto-occipital Joint, C3, C7** (› 6.1.1), **Superior, Medial, and Inferior Cervical Ganglion** (› 6.9.2) on the anterior ear; **Cervical Spine** (› 6.11.1) on the posterior ear
- For restricted movement: local points on the cervical spine (see above); restricted movement in a particular part of the spine often leads to (compensatory) counter-blockages in other areas of the spine; needling these points is therefore recommended, e.g. **T4, T10, L2** (› 6.1.1)
- Points in the **Vegetative Groove** (› 6.9.1)
- Analgesic points: **Diazepam** (› 6.7.3), **PGE₁/Thymus** (› 6.7.6)

Chinese points
- Analgesic point: **Thalamus (26a)** (› 6.7.4)

Treatment Intervals

- **Acute** (not chronic recurrent) **cervical migraine:** a one-off treatment is generally sufficient
- **Chronic cervical migraine:** depending on the frequency of attacks initially every 2–7 days, later twice monthly until symptoms have subsided completely

Treatment Course and Prognosis

The longer the duration of the disorder, the longer the treatment course; the first treatment course generally lasts approximately 6 months; in particular at the start of treatments patient compliance is very important: triggers such as red wine, draft, and stress should be avoided!

- **Short-term:** reduction of analgesic medication due to decreased pain intensity
- **Medium-term:** extended symptom-free intervals
- **Long-term:** complete recovery

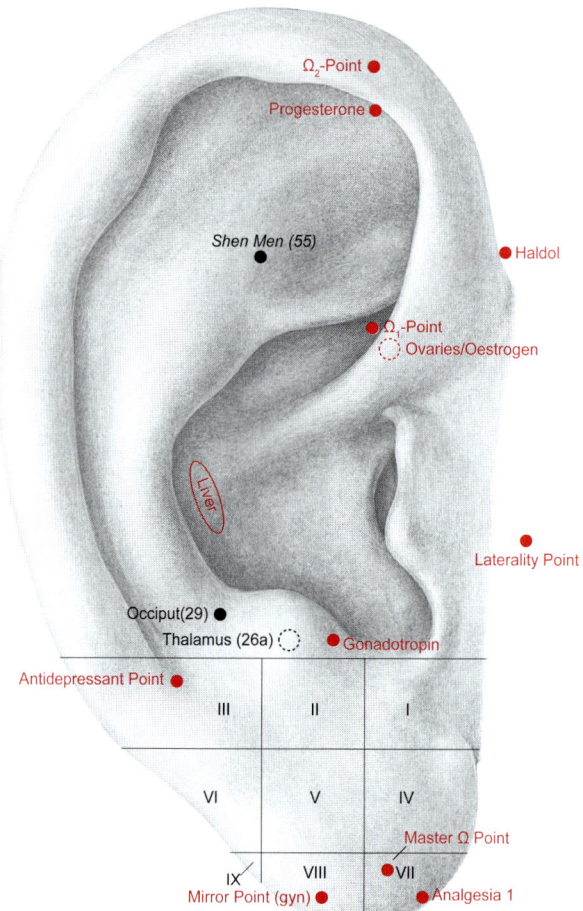

Ω₂-Point

Progesterone

Shen Men (55)

Haldol

Ω₁-Point
Ovaries/Oestrogen

Liver

Laterality Point

Occiput(29)
Thalamus (26a)
Gonadotropin

Antidepressant Point

III

II

I

Master Ω Point

VI

V

IV

IX

VIII

VII

Mirror Point (gyn)

Analgesia 1

Fig. 7.4-2

7.4.2 Hormonal Migraines

Description

- Paroxysmal, mostly one-sided headaches that can be cycle-related (often at the onset of the period)
- Accompanying symptoms include: nausea, vomiting, light sensitivity, and visual disturbances
- Onset during pregnancy or menopause rare – these are periods that are generally symptom-free
- Duration: several hours

Point Prescription

French points

- Hormonal points: **Gynaecological Axis** (› 6.12.5), **Progesterone** (› 6.6.3), **Oestrogen** (› 6.6.4) / **Ovary** (› 6.5.2), **Gonadotropin** (› 6.6.7)
- Analgesic point: **Analgesia 1** (› 6.7.5)
- Psychological points: **Antidepressant Point** (› 6.8.5) **Haldol** (› 6.8.6), **Omega Axis** (› 6.12.1)
- Stabilising points: **Liver** (› 6.4.1), **Laterality Point** (› 6.8.6)

Chinese points

- Analgesic points: *Shen Men* **(55)** (› 6.7.2), **Occiput (29)** (› 6.7.4), **Thalamus (26a)** (› 6.7.4)

 Hormone medication, e.g. the contraceptive pill, can alleviate hormonal migraines but also trigger them. Therapy with auricular acupuncture is certainly preferable to hormone therapy.

Treatment Intervals

Depending on the frequency of the migraines:
- Migraine once monthly: treat twice monthly, one of the treatments should be 2–3 days before the period is due
- Migraines > once monthly: treat once weekly, with one of the treatments 2–3 days before the period is due

Treatment Course and Prognosis

The longer the duration of the disorder, the longer the treatment course; the first treatment course is generally approximately 6 months; in particular at the start of treatments patient compliance is very important: triggers such as red wine, draft, and stress should be avoided!
- **Short-term:** reduction of analgesic medication due to decreased pain intensity
- **Medium-term:** extension of symptom-free intervals
- **Long-term:** complete recovery

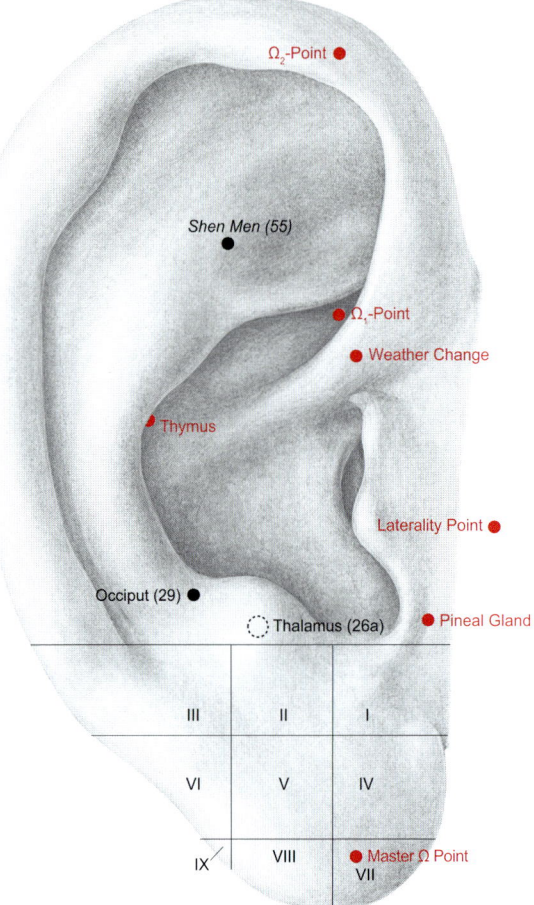

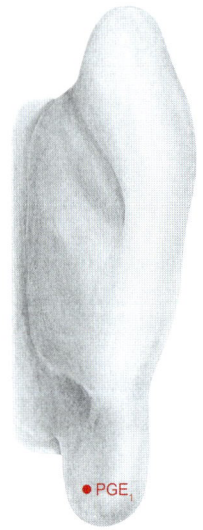

Fig. 7.4-3a+b

7.4.3 'Weather Migraine'

Description

- Migraine attacks triggered by changes in the weather or by particular weather conditions (barometric pressure), mostly one-sided with changing location
- Accompanying symptoms include: nausea, vomiting, light sensitivity, and visual disturbances
- Occurs at irregular intervals
- Duration: several hours

Point prescription

French points
- Local point: **Weather Change** (› 6.8.3)
- Primary point: **Laterality Point** (› 6.8.6)
- Psychological points: **Pineal Gland** (› 6.8.4), **Omega Axis** (› 6.12.1)
- Analgesic point: **PGE$_1$/Thymus** (› 6.7.6)

Chinese points
- Analgesic points: ***Shen Men* (55)** (› 6.7.2), **Occiput (29)** (› 6.7.4), **Thalamus (26a)** (› 6.7.4)

Treatment Intervals

- Depending on the frequency of attacks, initially every 2–7 days, then twice monthly until symptoms have subsided completely

Treatment Course and Prognosis

The longer the duration of the disorder, the longer the required therapy; the first treatment course tends to last 6 months

- **Short-term:** reduction of analgesic medication due to a reduction of the pain intensity
- **Medium-term:** extension of symptom-free intervals
- **Long-term:** complete recovery

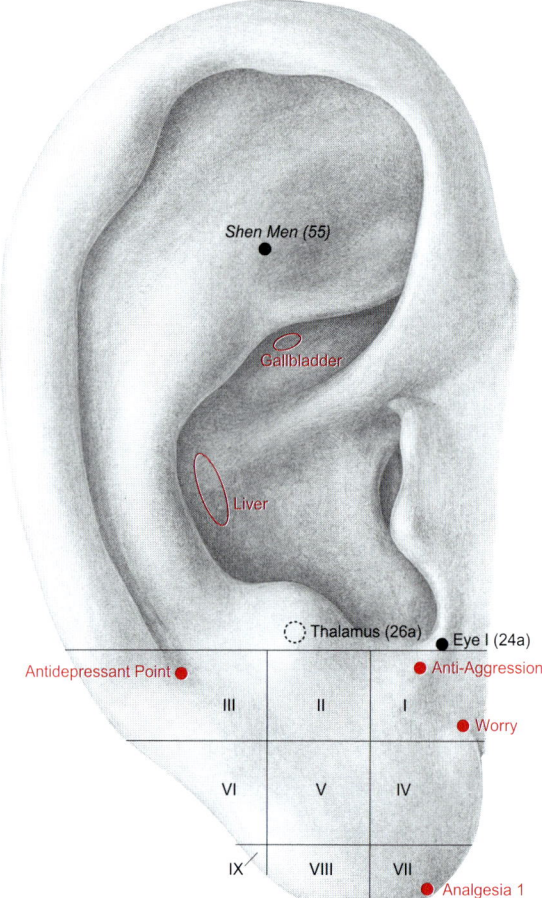

Fig. 7.4-4

7.4.4 'Gallbladder Migraine'

Description

- Attacks often triggered by stress and emotions (corresponding to Liver/Gallbladder according to TCM), often one-sided retro-orbital pain
- Accompanying symptoms: in particular sensitivity to light, visual disturbances, nausea and vomiting
- Triggered/exacerbated by: stimulating substances such as alcohol or coffee
- Occurs particularly during the early hours of the morning
- Duration: several hours

Point prescription

French points
- Analgesic point: **Analgesia 1** (› 6.7.5)
- Stabilising points: **Liver, Gallbladder** (› 6.4.1)
- Psychological points: **Antidepressant Point** (› 6.8.5), **Worry, Anti-Aggression** (› 6.8.5)

Chinese points
- Stabilising point: **Eye I (24a)** (› 6.3.4)
- Analgesic points: *Shen Men* **(55)** (› 6.7.2), **Thalamus (26a)** (› 6.7.4)

Treatment Intervals

- Depending on the frequency of the attacks initially every 2–7 days, later twice monthly until symptoms have subsided completely

Treatment Course and Prognosis

The longer the duration of the disorder, the longer treatments will be necessary; the first treatment course generally takes approximately 6 months. Especially at the start of the therapy patient compliance is crucial: triggers, such as stress, should be avoided!

- **Short-term:** reduction of analgesic medication due to decreased pain intensity
- **Mid-term:** longer symptom-free intervals
- **Long-term:** complete recovery

7.5 Neuralgias

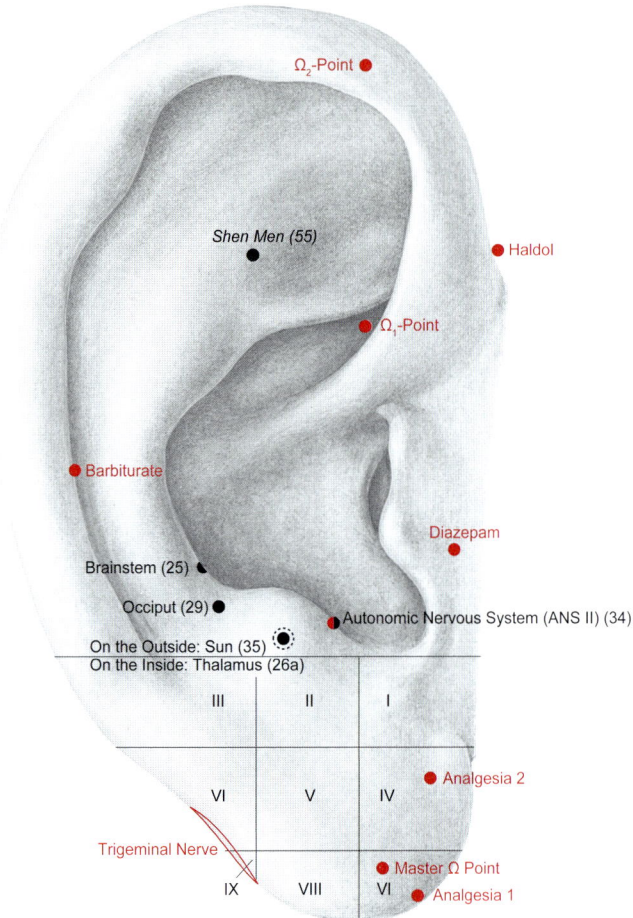

Fig. 7.5-1

7.5.1 Trigeminal Neuralgia

Description

- Recurrent paroxysmal pain affecting the area supplied by the trigeminal nerve, lasting seconds to minutes
- Typically affects women during the second half of their lives
- Causes: idiopathic; eye or dental disorders, sinusitis; mechanic nerve damage (e.g. due to tumours or fractures); in conjunction with vascular disorders, metabolic disorders, infections, intoxication, or multiple sclerosis
- Triggers: touching certain areas of the skin (trigger zones), changes in temperature, etc.

Point Prescription

French points

- Local point: **Trigeminal Nerve** (› 6.3.4)
- Analgesic points: **Analgesia 1** and **Analgesia 2** (› 6.7.5)
- Psychological points: **Diazepam** (› 6.7.3), **Barbiturate** (› 6.7.1), **Haldol** (› 6.8.6), **Omega Axis** (› 6.12.1)

Chinese points

- Analgesic points: **Sun (35), Occiput (29), ANS II (34)** (› 6.7.4), *Shen Men* **(55)** (› 6.7.2), **Brainstem (25)** (› 6.10.4), **Thalamus (26a)** (› 6.7.4)

Treatment Intervals

- For daily pain attacks: initially once daily until pain-free intervals last several days and/ or the pain intensity has diminished, then once weekly until symptoms have subsided completely

Treatment Course and Prognosis

The longer the duration of the disorder, the longer the treatment course required. Often there is:

- within days: reduction of analgesic medication due to decreased pain intensity
- within weeks: symptom-free periods for several days or even a week
- within months: no more recurrences

7.5.2 Toothache

Description

Toothache always requires a referral to the dentist. However, reducing tooth ache with auricular acupuncture is certainly indicated in the following cases:

- For acute toothache: 'first aid'-acupuncture until the patient can be seen by a dentist
- As adjuvant therapy during ongoing dental treatments to shorten their duration
- For chronic pain conditions when there is no further improvement with dental treatments

Diagnosis and treatment by a dentist is essential and cannot be replaced by auricular acupuncture. However, acupuncture as adjuvant therapy can significantly reduce the intensity of the pain.

Point prescription

French points

- Local points: depending on the affected tooth/teeth: **Upper Jaw** or **Lower Jaw** (› 6.3.4)
- Analgesic points: **Analgesia 1** and **Analgesia 2** (› 6.7.5)
- Relaxing points: **Diazepam** (› 6.7.3), **Barbiturate** (› 6.7.1)

Chinese points

- Local points: **Tooth (1), Tooth (7), Upper Jaw (5), Lower Jaw (6)** (› 6.3.4), **Larynx and Tooth (27)** (› 6.3.3)
- Analgesic points: **Tooth Pain (26), Occiput (29)** (› 6.7.4), **Thalamus (26a)** (› 6.7.4)

Treatment Intervals

- **Acute symptoms:** in addition to dental treatment initially once daily until symptoms have reduced significantly
- Then once weekly until symptoms have subsided completely

Treatment Course and Prognosis

- **Acute pain:** reduction of both the duration and pain intensity after dental treatment
- **Chronic pain** (despite dental treatments): reduction of the pain intensity within one week, completely symptom-free within months

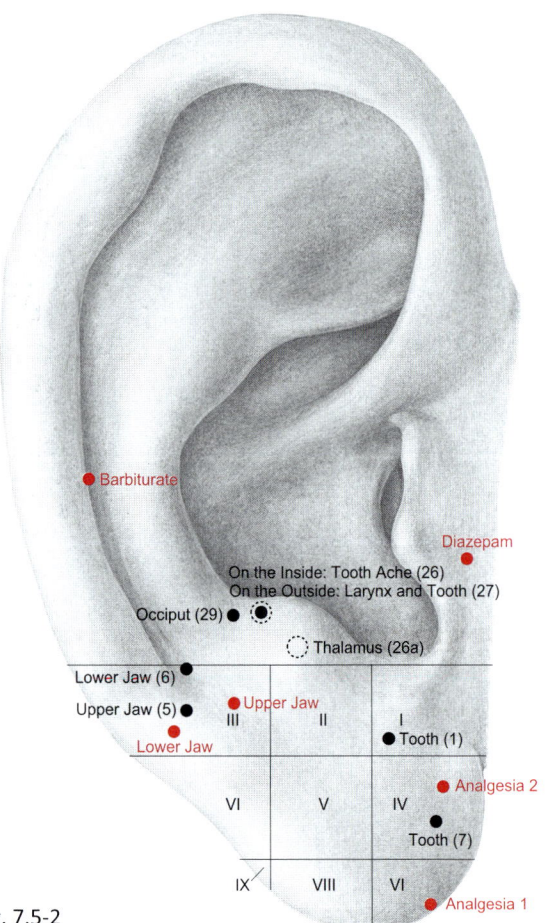

Fig. 7.5-2

8 Further Indications

8.1 Cardiovascular Disorders

8.1.1 Hypertension

- Blood pressure of > 140/90 mmHg with repeated measurements
- Predisposing factors: overweight, alcohol, psycho-emotional strain or stress
- Classification according to aetiology:
  - primary (essential) hypertension: cause unknown
  - secondary hypertension: caused by another disorder or medication/alcohol abuse (e.g. endocrine, renal, or pulmonary hypertension)
- Complications: arteriosclerosis, heart insufficiency, cerebral haemorrhage, dizziness, visual disturbances, clouding of consciousness
- **Caution:** Secondary hypertension should be excluded by conventional medicine prior to treatments since it rarely responds to auricular acupuncture. For secondary hypertension it is necessary to treat the underlying disorder, surgery may be required.

Point Prescription

French points
- Local points: **Heart II** (› 6.4.2), **Renin-Angiotensin Point** (› 6.6.3), **Neural Adrenal Cortex Point** (› 6.9.2), **Vagus Nerve** (› 6.10.7) on the anterior ear; **Heart** (› 6.11.3) on the posterior ear

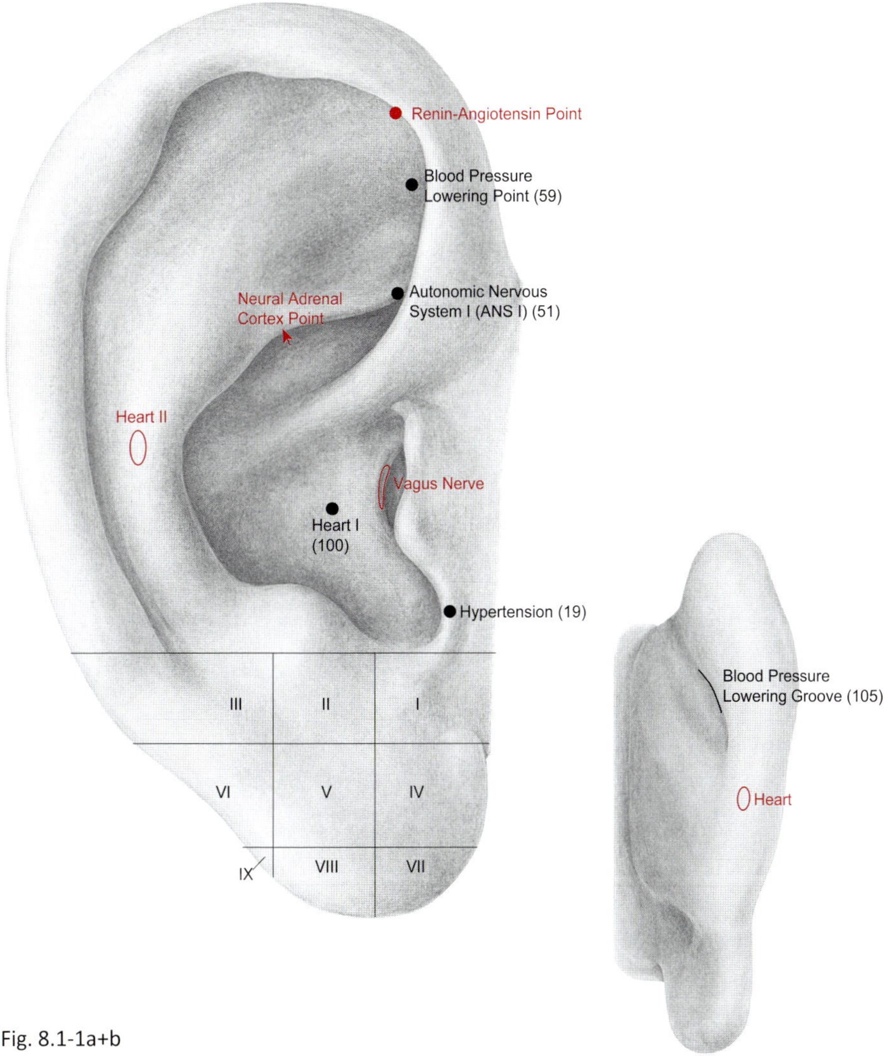

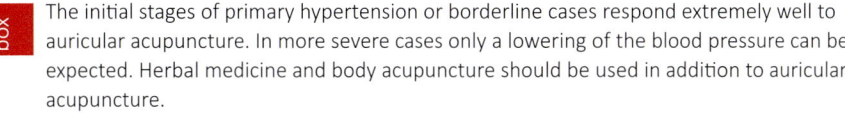

Renin-Angiotensin Point

Blood Pressure
Lowering Point (59)

Autonomic Nervous
System I (ANS I) (51)

Neural Adrenal
Cortex Point

Heart II

Vagus Nerve

Heart I
(100)

Hypertension (19)

III   II   I

VI   V   IV

IX   VIII   VII

Blood Pressure
Lowering Groove (105)

Heart

Fig. 8.1-1a+b

Chinese points

- Local points: **Heart I (100)** (› 6.4.1), **Hypertension (19)** (› 6.4.5), **Blood Pressure Lowering Point (59)** (› 6.4.7) on the anterior ear; **Blood Pressure Lowering Groove (105)** (› 6.11.3) on the posterior ear
- Stabilising point: **ANS I (51)** (› 6.6.5)

> **box** The initial stages of primary hypertension or borderline cases respond extremely well to auricular acupuncture. In more severe cases only a lowering of the blood pressure can be expected. Herbal medicine and body acupuncture should be used in addition to auricular acupuncture.

Treatment Intervals

- Initially twice weekly with daily blood pressure measurements
- Blood pressure within the normal range: treatment intervals can be extended to once weekly; with consistently normal readings twice monthly
- Consistently normal readings for over 2 months: no further treatments necessary
- Continuous reduction of blood pressure but without reaching normal values: 1-2 treatments per month accompanied by conventional therapy (medication)

Treatment Course and Prognosis

This depends on the duration and severity of the disorder as well as existing risk factors:

- **Mild hypertension:** with patient compliance (weight loss, stress reduction) approximately 6 months until symptoms disappear
- **Moderate to severe hypertension:** if there is no reduction in blood pressure within 3 months, the combination with Chinese herbal medicine (and possibly body acupuncture) or conventional therapy will be necessary

- Acupuncture has a harmonising and energetically balancing effect and therefore also supports the reduction of risk factors (e.g. alcohol, stress).

8.1.2 Coronary Heart Disease

Description

- Impaired myocardial circulation, generally caused by degenerative changes (obstruction or stenosis) of the coronary vessels
- Recurrent feelings of pressure or pain in the chest, worse with exertion, e.g. angina pectoris (› 8.1.3); may also be completely asymptomatic

Point Prescription

French points

- Local points: **Heart II** (› 6.4.2), β-**Receptor** (› 6.7.1) on the anterior ear; **Heart** (› 6.11.3) on the posterior ear
- Stabilising point: **Point Zero** (› 6.10.3)

Chinese points

- Local point: **Heart I (100)** (› 6.4.1)
- Stabilising point: **ANS I (51)** (› 6.6.5)

A thorough conventional investigation is necessary for assessing coronary stenoses and associated risks. Unstable angina pectoris (› 8.1.3) in the context of coronary heart disease is an absolute indication for admission to hospital.

Treatment Intervals

- With pain (› 8.1.3, angina pectoris): twice weekly
- Following heart surgery: 2–3 times weekly in addition to conventional therapy

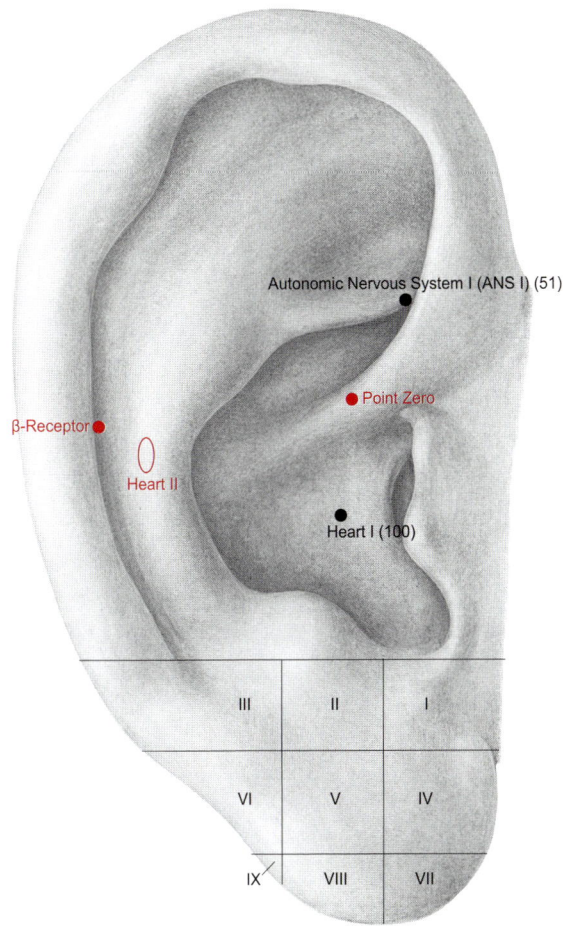

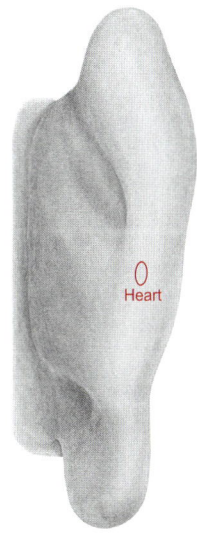

Fig. 8.1-2a+b

- Absence of symptoms: twice monthly as preventative measure for progressive arteriosclerosis

> Auricular acupuncture can alleviate or prevent pain associated with coronary heart disease. However, it cannot improve arteriosclerosis or myocardial blood supply. The combination with conventional medication (e.g. nitroglycerin spray) is often necessary.

Treatment Course and Prognosis

- **Short-term:** pain reduction
- **Medium-term:** no cure possible but the progression can be slowed down

> box
> - Reducing existing risk factors (e.g. obesity, high cholesterol, stress, nicotine abuse) is necessary for a positive treatment outcome.
> - Acupuncture harmonises the body's energetic balance and is emotionally stabilising. It also supports patient compliance (› 8.8, Treatment of Addiction)

8.1.3 Angina Pectoris

Description

- Thoracic pain lasting from seconds up to several minutes; often underlying coronary heart disease (› 8.1.2); less commonly caused by coronary spasms (Prinzmetal's or variant angina) or Roemheld syndrome (› 8.1.4, cardiac symptoms associated with meal times)
- Forms:
  - stable angina: recurrent thoracic pain, e.g. with stress or physical exertion; nitro-positive
  - unstable angina: first episode of thoracic pain or thoracic pain during rest; nitro-negative

Point Prescription

French points

- Local points: **Heart II** (› 6.4.2), **Cardiac Plexus** (› 6.10.1), β-**Receptor** (› 6.7.1) on the anterior ear; **Heart** (› 6.11.3) on the posterior ear
- Stabilising point: **Point Zero** (› 6.10.3)

Chinese points

- Local point: **Heart I (100)** (› 6.4.1),
- Stabilising points: **ANS I (51)** (› 6.6.5), *Shen Men* **(55)** (› 6.7.2)

> box
> Before starting treatments a thorough conventional diagnosis is necessary to exclude the possibility of coronary stenoses and to assess the risk of a myocardial infarction. Patients with unstable angina pectoris have to be admitted to hospital.

Treatment Intervals

- With pain: initially twice weekly, followed by longer intervals depending on the duration of symptom-free periods
- Postoperative treatments: 2–3 times weekly to support the recovery process

> box
> For Prinzmetal's angina a complete recovery is possible.

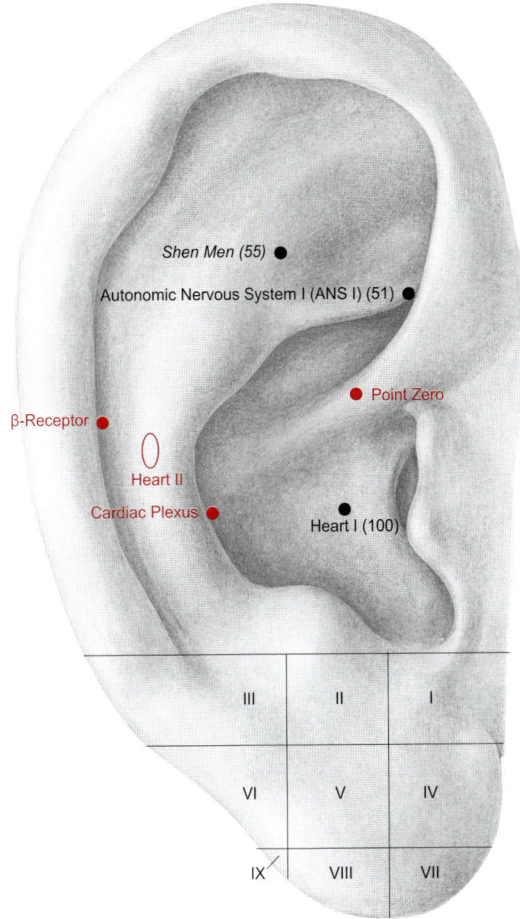

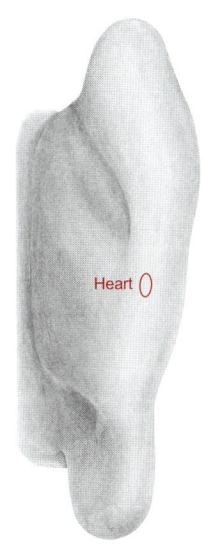

Fig. 8.1-3a+b

Treatment Course and Prognosis

Depending on the type of angina and the extent of the coronary heart disease:

- Prinzmetal's angina and stable angina pectoris **without stenoses:** the majority of cases will be pain-free within 3 months
- **Existing stenoses:** the progression can be slowed down; monthly treatments required during symptom-free intervals

Reducing existing risk factors (e.g. obesity, high cholesterol, stress, nicotine abuse) is necessary for a good treatment outcome. Acupuncture harmonises the body's energetic balance and is emotionally stabilising. It also supports patient compliance (› 8.8, Addictions)

8.1.4 Roemheld Syndrome

Description

- Cardiac arrhythmias and angina-like symptoms in conjunction with meals; possible mechanism: abdominal bloating resulting in pressure on or even displacement of the heart
- Recurrent episodes, possibly in conjunction with epigastric pain
- Affects mostly males

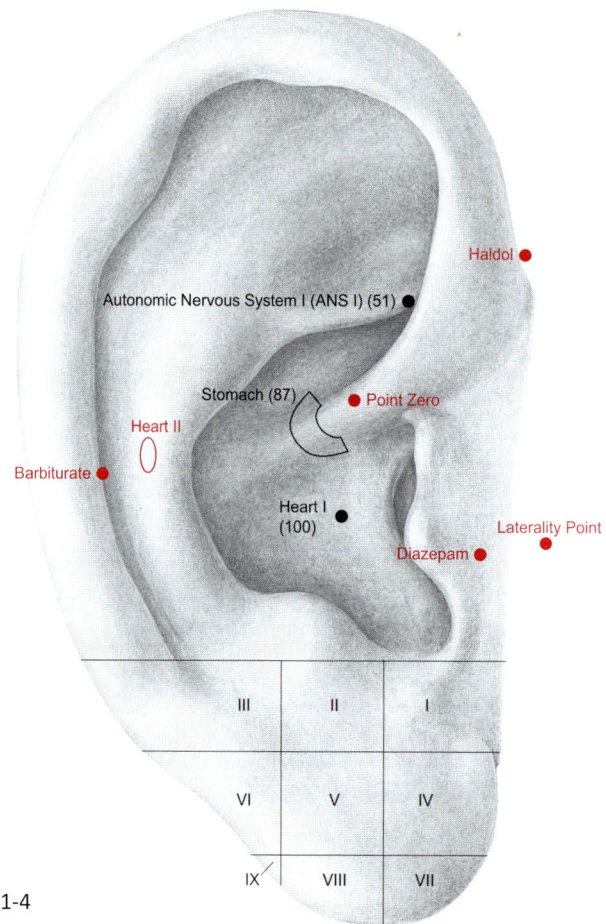

Fig. 8.1-4

Point Prescription

French points

- Local point: **Heart II** (› 6.4.2)
- Stabilising points: **Point Zero** (› 6.10.3), **Laterality Point** (› 6.8.6)
- Psychological points: **Barbiturate** (› 6.7.1), **Haldol** (› 6.8.6), **Diazepam** (› 6.7.3)

Chinese points

- Local points: **Stomach (87)**, **Heart I (100)** (› 6.4.1)
- Stabilising point: **ANS I (51)** (› 6.6.5)

Treatment Intervals

- Daily symptoms: 2–3 times weekly until symptoms have improved, then once weekly until symptoms have disappeared
- Occasional symptoms: once weekly until symptoms have disappeared

Treatment Course and Prognosis

- Recent onset: generally approximately 3–4 weeks for sustained symptomatic relief
- **Chronic stage** (> 4 weeks): approximately 3 months for a sustained relief from symptoms

 Relaxation is important as stress exacerbates symptoms.

8.1.5 Cardiac Arrhythmias

Description

Differentiation according to
- Pathogenesis: impulse-generation or impulse-conduction disorder
- Frequency: bradycardia or tachycardia
- Location: ventricular or supraventricular arrhythmias

Causes:
- Irritations or pathological changes of the coronary conduction system (coronary heart disease, myocarditis)
- Dysregulation of the autonomic nervous system
  - trigger: psycho-emotional stress
  - recurrent or continuous forms

 Before treating with auricular acupuncture, cardiac arrhythmias have to be thoroughly investigated and diagnosed by conventional medicine since some forms are life-threatening (e.g. interference dissociation, atrial flutter, or ventricular tachycardia) and have to be treated accordingly.

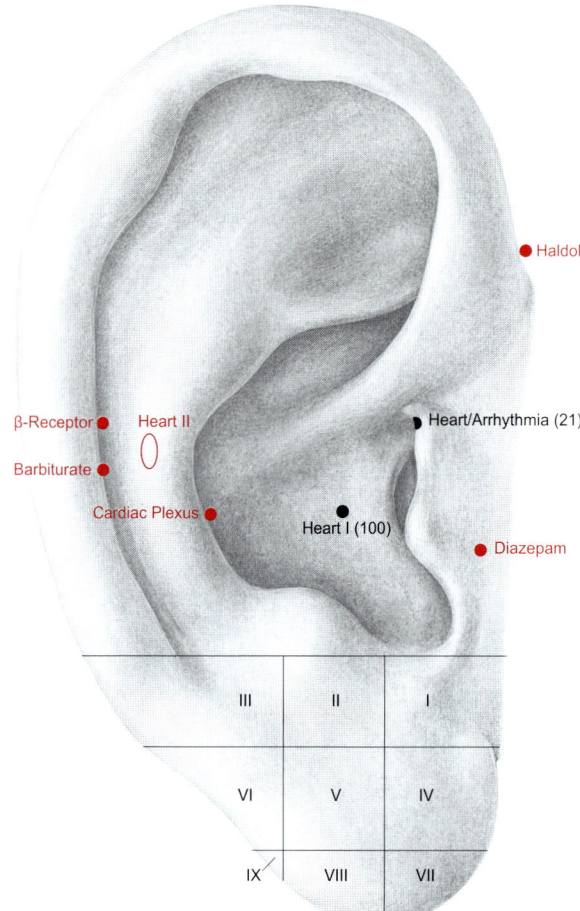

β-Receptor ●

Heart II

Barbiturate ●

Cardiac Plexus ●

Haldol ●

Heart/Arrhythmia (21)

Heart I (100)

Diazepam

III | II | I

VI | V | IV

IX | VIII | VII

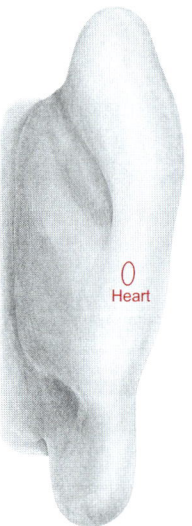

Heart

Fig. 8.1-5a+b

Point Prescription

French points
- Local points: **Heart II** (› 6.4.2), β-**Receptor** (› 6.7.1), **Cardiac Plexus** (› 6.10.1) on the anterior ear; **Heart** (› 6.11.3) on the posterior ear
- Psychological points: **Barbiturate** (› 6.7.1), **Haldol** (› 6.8.6), **Diazepam** (› 6.7.3)

Chinese points
- Local points: **Heart I (100)** (› 6.4.1), **Heart/Arrhythmia (21)** (› 6.4.5)

- Complete recovery is possible for cardiac arrhythmias triggered by the sympathetic nervous system.
- For cardiac arrhythmias caused by pathological changes, only an improvement of symptoms can be expected, particularly in advanced stages; in these cases auricular acupuncture can provide support as an adjuvant therapy to conventional treatments.

Treatment Intervals
- Daily cardiac arrhythmias: initially 2–3 times weekly until symptoms improve, then once weekly until symptoms have disappeared
- Occasional cardiac arrhythmias: once weekly until symptoms have disappeared

Treatment Course and Prognosis
- Recent onset cardiac arrhythmias: generally approximately 3–4 weeks for a sustained relief from symptoms
- Chronic arrhythmias (> 4 weeks): provided the conduction system is not irreversibly damaged (e.g. following a myocardial infarction) approximately 3 months until symptoms subside completely

8.1.6 Palpitations

Description
- The sensation of one's own heartbeat; perceived as uncomfortable or even threatening
- Causes:
  - generally psychogenic causes: emotional dysbalance, anxiety attacks; differential diagnosis: cardiac neurosis (› 8.13.3)
  - less commonly organic causes: e.g. heart disorders, hormonal disorders, anaemia

Organic causes have to be excluded before treating with auricular acupuncture (referral to a cardiac consultant!).

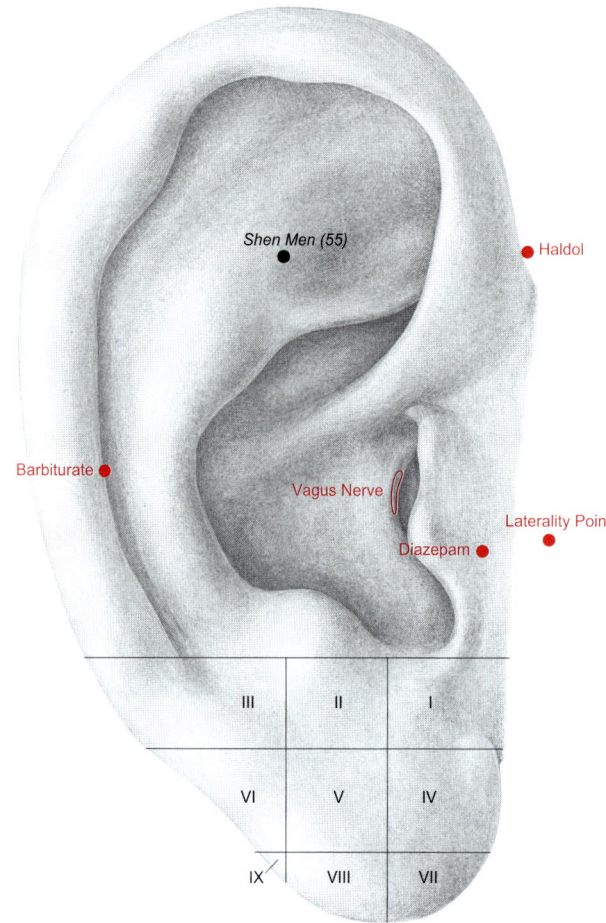

Shen Men (55)

Haldol

Barbiturate

Vagus Nerve

Laterality Point

Diazepam

III   II   I

VI   V   IV

IX   VIII   VII

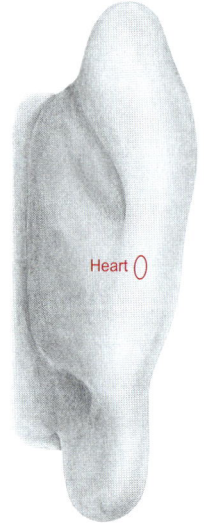

Heart

Fig. 8.1-6a+b

Point Prescription

French points

- Local points: **Vagus Nerve** (> 6.10.7) on the anterior ear; **Heart** (> 6.11.3) on the posterior ear
- Psychological points: **Barbiturate** (> 6.7.1), **Haldol** (> 6.8.6), **Diazepam** (> 6.7.3)
- Stabilising point: **Laterality Point** (> 6.8.6)

Chinese points

- Stabilising point: *Shen Men* **(55)** (> 6.7.2)

Treatment Intervals

- Palpitations on a daily basis: initially 2–3 times weekly until symptoms become milder, then once weekly until symptoms disappear
- Sporadic palpitations: once weekly until symptoms disappear

Treatment Course and Prognosis

- **Recent onset:** approximately 3–4 weeks for a sustained relief from symptoms
- **Chronic disorder** (> 4 weeks): approximately 3 months until symptoms disappear

8.2 Respiratory Disorders

8.2.1 Bronchial Asthma

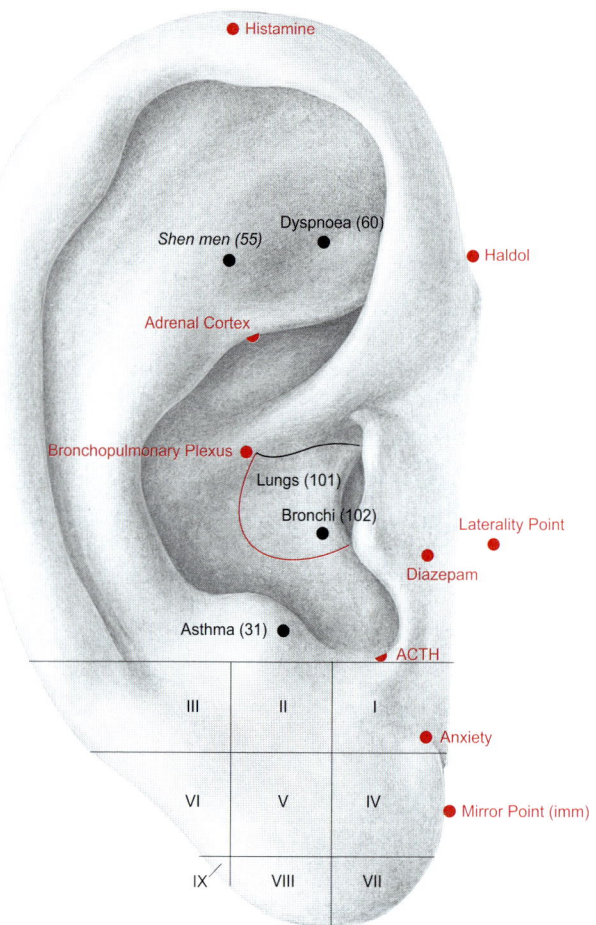

- Histamine
- Dyspnoea (60)
- Shen men (55)
- Haldol
- Adrenal Cortex
- Bronchopulmonary Plexus
- Lungs (101)
- Bronchi (102)
- Laterality Point
- Diazepam
- Asthma (31)
- ACTH

III   II   I

- Anxiety

VI   V   IV

- Mirror Point (imm)

IX   VIII   VII

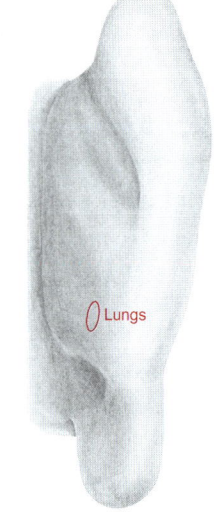

Lungs

Fig. 8.2-1a+b

Description

- Mainly paroxysmal attacks due to a complete or only partially reversible bronchial constriction with an underlying hyperreactive bronchial system
- Trigger: various exogenous or endogenous stimuli, e.g. allergens, chemical and physical inhalation irritants
- The psychological component plays an important role

Point Prescription

The point prescription is determined by RAC-palpation (› 3.1.4) rather than the specific form of asthma. The treatment protocol can be used for acute cases as well as during remission.

French points

- Local point: **Lung** (› 6.11.3) on the posterior ear
- Stabilising points: **Laterality Point** (› 6.8.6), **Bronchopulmonary Plexus** (› 6.10.1)
- Psychological points: **Anxiety** (› 6.8.5), **Haldol** (› 6.8.6), **Diazepam** (› 6.7.3)
- Antiallergic points: **Histamine** (› 6.6.4), **ACTH** (› 6.6.6), **Adrenal Cortex** (› 6.6.1) or **Immune Axis** (› 6.12.3)

Chinese points

- Local points: **Lung (101), Bronchi (102)** (› 6.4.1), **Dyspnoea (60)** (› 6.4.7), **Asthma (31)** (› 6.4.6)
- Stabilising point: *Shen Men (55)* (› 6.7.2)

 Patients with acute asthma have to be carefully monitored. If there is no treatment response within 30 minutes the patient must take medication. Acute severe asthma initially requires drug therapy.

Treatment Intervals

- Daily asthma attacks: once daily or every other day
- Several asthma attacks per week: 2–3 times weekly
- Milder forms: once weekly until symptoms have disappeared

Treatment Course and Prognosis

- For recent onset bronchial or allergic asthma: approximately 3 months of treatments until symptoms disappear
- For severe chronic bronchial asthma, possibly accompanied by emphysema: approximately 6 months until there is a significant improvement; sustained treatment results require monthly treatments for up to 2 years

- It is perfectly possible to cure predominantly allergic forms of asthma.
- If there is a strong psychological component or for longstanding cases it is generally possible to reduce at least any asthma medication and to discontinue steroidal medication.

8.2.2 Bronchitis

Description

Inflammation of the bronchial mucosa of mainly the larger bronchi, accompanied by cough and expectoration of phlegm

- Acute bronchitis: caused mostly by viral infections
- Chronic bronchitis: episodes of cough and expectoration of phlegm for at least 3 months and within 2 consecutive years
  - primary cause: nicotine abuse, air pollution, or infections
  - secondary to bronchial asthma, emphysema, lung fibrosis, tuberculosis etc.
- Chronic bronchitis in conjunction with chronic obstructive pulmonary disorder (COPD)

Point Prescription

The point prescription is determined by RAC-palpation (› 3.1.4), not the type of bronchitis.

French points

- Stabilising points: **Laterality Point** (› 6.8.6), **Bronchopulmonary Plexus** (› 6.10.1), **Point Zero** (› 6.10.3)
- Defense against infection: **Infection Axis** (› 6.12.4)

Chinese points

- Local points: **Dyspnoea (60)** (› 6.4.7), **Lung (101)**, **Bronchi (102)** (› 6.4.1)

Treatment Intervals

- **Acute bronchitis:**
  - Initially every 2–3 days until both cough and phlegm have decreased
  - Then once weekly until symptoms have disappeared
- **Chronic bronchitis:**
  - initially twice weekly
  - once the cough and phlegm subside (after approximately 4 weeks) once weekly
- **Chronic bronchitis with chronic obstructive pulmonary disorder (COPD):**
  - initially once weekly until shortness of breath has improved and there is less phlegm, then 1–twice/month

Treatment Course and Prognosis

- **Acute bronchitis:** approximately 2–4 weeks until symptoms disappear
- **Chronic bronchitis:** approximately 6 months, minor residual complaints may persist
- **Chronic bronchitis with chronic obstructive pulmonary disorder (COPD):** a complete cure is not possible due to damage to the lung tissue; shortness of breath will improve with long-term treatments only.

 If there is nicotine abuse auricular acupuncture will not result in any significant improvement. It is essential that this is explained to the patient. Stopping smoking is a requirement for achieving any therapeutic results.

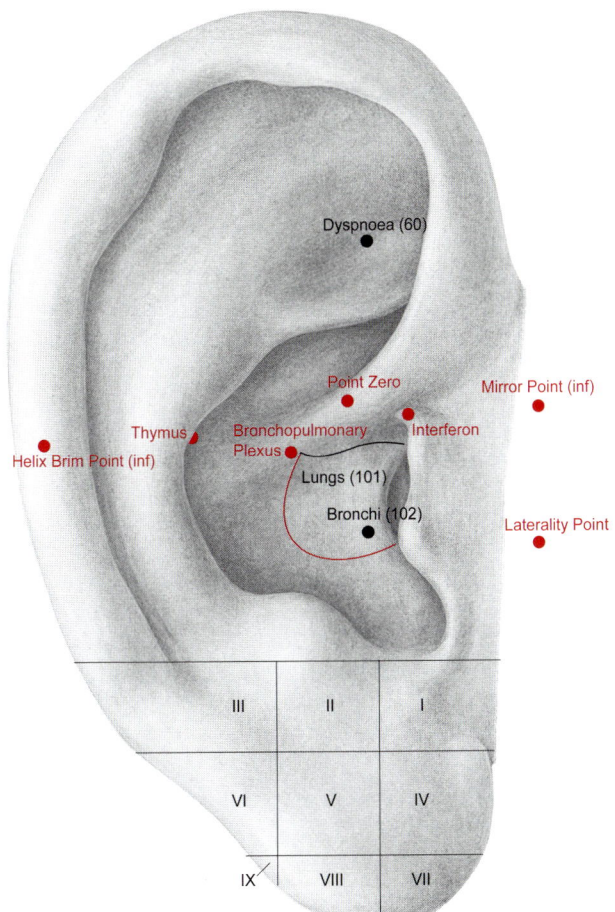

Dyspnoea (60)

Point Zero

Mirror Point (inf)

Thymus
Helix Brim Point (inf)

Bronchopulmonary
Plexus

Interferon

Lungs (101)

Bronchi (102)

Laterality Point

III II I

VI V IV

IX VIII VII

Fig. 8.2-2

8.2.3 Bronchopulmonary Infection

Description

- Respiratory infection, mainly of viral, less commonly of bacterial origin
- Symptoms vary according to organ involvement:
  - nose and paranasal sinuses: head cold (blocked nose), possibly headache
  - throat/pharynx: sore throat, loss of voice
  - lungs: cough, dry or with phlegm

Point Prescription

The point prescription depends on the organs involved and RAC-palpation (› 3.1.4).

French points

- Local points: possibly **Nose**, **Nasal Mucosa** (› 6.3.4)
- Stabilising points: **Laterality Point** (› 6.8.6), **Bronchopulmonary Plexus** (6.10.1), **Point Zero** (› 6.10.3)
- Defense against infection: **Thymus** (› 6.6.1), **Interferon** (› 6.7.3), **Infection Axis** (› 6.12.4)

Chinese points

- Local points: **Thorax (42)** (› 6.4.4), **Lung (101)**, **Bronchi (102)** (› 6.4.1), **Dyspnoea (60)** (› 6.4.7), possibly **Larynx and Tooth (27)** (› 6.3.3), **Palate (2)**, **Floor of the Mouth (3)** (› 6.3.4)

Treatment Intervals

- **Acute stage:** initially once daily or every other day, then 2–3 times weekly until symptoms have disappeared
- Start of treatments **after the acute stage:** 2–3 times weekly until symptoms have disappeared

- Acupuncture can significantly accelerate the healing process of a viral infection.
- If the patient shows signs of pneumonia (findings include crackles and an aggravation of breath sounds) he/she should be referred to a consultant.
- Auricular acupuncture can be continued while the patient is taking antibiotics (improvement of pulmonary symptoms, fewer side effects).

Treatment Course and Prognosis

- Generally symptoms disappear after one or a few days depending on the severity and the extent of organ involvement.
- With a weak constitution or a persistent infection it may take 2–4 weeks until symptoms disappear.

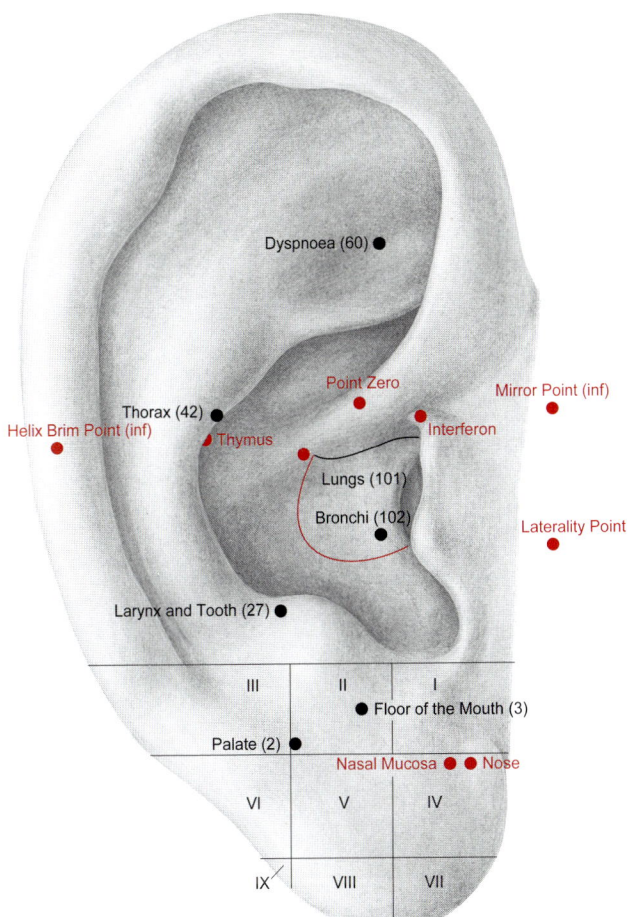

Dyspnoea (60)

Point Zero

Mirror Point (inf)

Thorax (42)

Helix Brim Point (inf)

Thymus

Interferon

Lungs (101)

Bronchi (102)

Laterality Point

Larynx and Tooth (27)

III   II   I

Floor of the Mouth (3)

Palate (2)

Nasal Mucosa ● ● Nose

VI   V   IV

IX   VIII   VII

Fig. 8.2-3

8.2.4 Sinusitis

Description

- Inflammation of the paranasal sinuses; often following acute rhinitis with difficulty breathing due to nasal blockage, or in conjunction with a bronchopulmonary infection (› 8.2.3)
- May become chronic, often with an allergic component; typical symptoms include: fatigue, headache, general malaise, impaired performance, recurrent post-nasal drip perceived as unpleasant
- Chronic cases often act as an interference field (› 5.7)

> **box** Sometimes patients with chronic sinusitis have become so used to the condition that they don't even mention it as part of their medical history. However, since chronic sinusitis can act as an interference field it can trigger or exacerbate disorders that are not as such associated with it. It is therefore essential that the treatment of chronic sinusitis is always included in the treatment approach.

Point Prescription

French points

- Local points: **Nose**, **Nasal Mucosa** (› 6.3.4), **Maxillary Sinus**, **Frontal Sinus**, **Ethmoidal Sinus**, **Sphenoidal Sinus** (listed according to decreasing frequency of occurrence) (› 6.3.3)
- Defense against infection: **Thymus** (› 6.6.1), **Interferon** (› 6.7.3), **Infection Axis** (› 6.12.4)
- Stabilising points: **Point Zero** (› 6.10.3), **Laterality Point** (› 6.8.6)

Chinese points

- Local points: **External Nose (14)**, **Internal Nose (16)** (› 6.3.2), *Shen Men* **(55)** (› 6.7.2)

Treatment Intervals

- **Acute stage:** twice weekly
- As nasal breathing becomes easier: once weekly to twice monthly until symptoms have disappeared

Treatment Course and Prognosis

- Treatment results can vary greatly; nasal breathing often eases straight away
- Symptoms generally disappear within a few weeks to several months

> **box** Nasal polyps are no contraindication for auricular acupuncture and may even diminish during the treatment course. Scheduled surgery can sometimes be avoided.

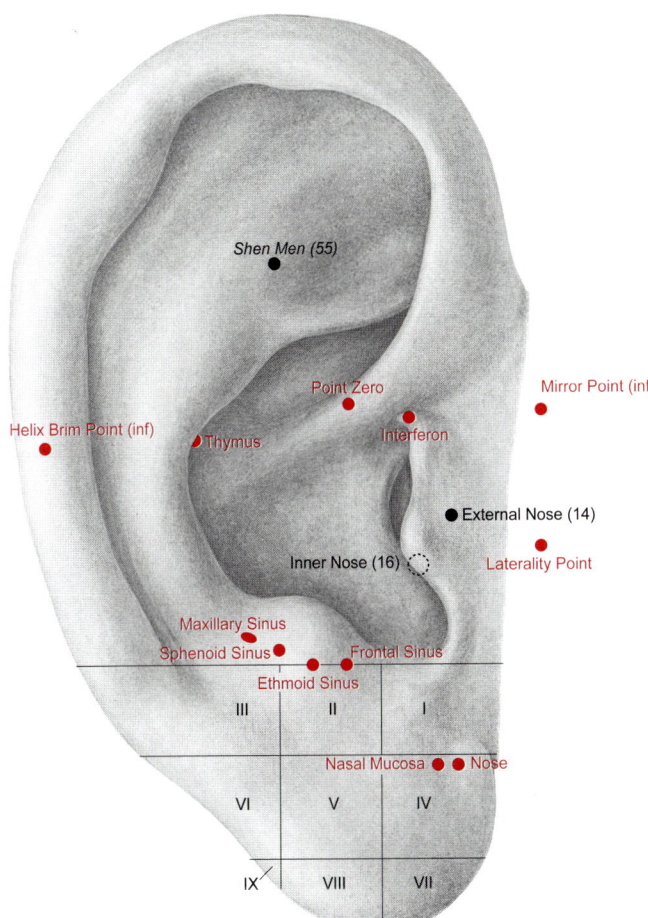

Shen Men (55)

Point Zero

Mirror Point (inf)

Helix Brim Point (inf)

Thymus

Interferon

External Nose (14)

Inner Nose (16)

Laterality Point

Maxillary Sinus

Sphenoid Sinus

Frontal Sinus

Ethmoid Sinus

III

II

I

Nasal Mucosa

Nose

VI

V

IV

IX

VIII

VII

Fig. 8.2-4

8.2.5 Tonsillitis

Description

- Bacterial or viral inflammation of the pharyngeal and palatine tonsils with difficulty swallowing
- Typically red and swollen tonsils
- Often chronically recurrent
- Both chronic tonsillitis as well as tonsillectomy scars can act as an interference field (› 5.7).

Point Prescription

French points

- Local point: **Tonsil** (› 6.3.4)
- Defense against infection: **Thymus** (› 6.6.1), **Interferon** (› 6.7.3), **Infection Axis** (› 6.12.4)

Chinese points

- Local points: **Tonsil I (73)**, **Tonsil II (74)**, **Tonsil III (75)** (› 6.3.1) and **Tonsil IV (10)** (› 6.3.4), **Throat (41)** (› 6.4.4), **Larynx/Pharynx (15)** (› 6.4.5)

- To eliminate the possibility of a streptococcal colonization the patient should be referred for a throat swab. In the meantime auricular acupuncture can be continued as adjuvant therapy (to speed up the healing process and alleviate the side effects of antibiotics).
- Peritonsillar abscesses (unilateral redness and protrusion of the affected palatine arch, high fever) have to be treated surgically. However, whether surgery is indeed necessary should be considered very carefully since tonsillectomy scars can act as interference fields (› 5.7.1).

Treatment Intervals

- **Acute tonsillitis:** initially once daily or every other day until redness and difficulty swallowing has significantly reduced, then 1–2 times weekly until symptoms have disappeared
- **Chronic recurrent tonsillitis:** 1–2 times weekly until symptoms have disappeared
- **Tonsillectomy scar as interference field**: treatment of the scar as projected onto the ear should be included in the treatment during remission of the primary illness

Even for chronic recurrent tonsillitis auricular acupuncture can achieve a permanent relief from symptoms!

Treatment Course and Prognosis

- **Acute tonsillitis:** generally 2–3 weeks until symptoms disappear
- **Chronic recurrent tonsillitis:** mostly 2–6 weeks until symptoms disappear

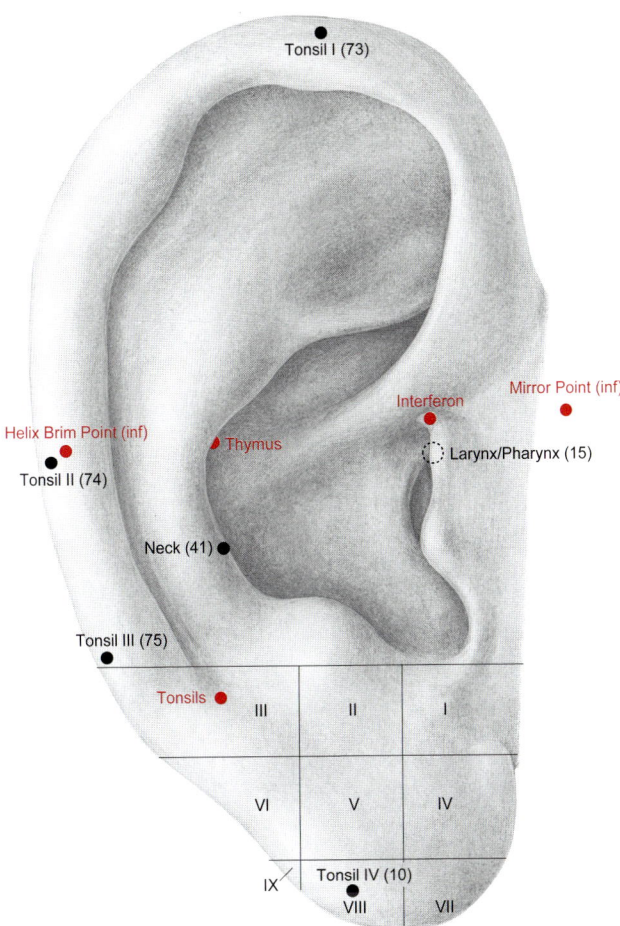

Tonsil I (73)

Mirror Point (inf)

Interferon

Helix Brim Point (inf)

Larynx/Pharynx (15)

Thymus

Tonsil II (74)

Neck (41)

Tonsil III (75)

Tonsils

III

II

I

VI

V

IV

IX

Tonsil IV (10)

VIII

VII

Fig. 8.2-5

8.2.6 Parotitis

Description

- Acute or chronic recurrent inflammation of the parotid gland with painful swelling and reddening
- Causes:
  - viral infectious disease (mumps)
  - bacterial infection, e.g. due to a weakened immune system after severe surgery
  - secondary to the blockage of the submandibular duct caused by salivary gland stones (very rare)

Point Prescription

The various forms of parotitis can be treated with the same protocol. In cases of a blocked duct, points relating to the immune system can be omitted. The point description is determined by RAC-palpation (› 3.1.4).

French points

- Local point: **Parotid Gland** (› 6.3.4)
- Immunostimulant points: **Thymus** (› 6.6.1), **Interferon** (› 6.7.3), **Infection Axis** (› 6.12.4)

Chinese points

- Local points: **Parotid Gland (30)** (› 6.3.3), **Cheek (11)** (› 6.3.4)

 Abscesses require surgical intervention and possibly treatment with antibiotics. In the rare case of a blocked duct due to a stone this has to be removed by a specialist consultant.

Treatment Intervals

- **Acute parotitis:** initially once daily or every other day until both pain and swelling have significantly diminished; then 1–2 times weekly until symptoms have disappeared
- **Chronic recurrent parotitis:** 1–2 times weekly until symptoms have disappeared

Treatment Course and Prognosis

- **Acute parotitis:** generally 2–3 weeks until symptoms disappear; acupuncture can alleviate the course of viral parotitis (mumps) and shorten it to just a few days
- **Chronic recurrent parotitis:** usually 2–3 months until symptoms disappear
- **Reactive parotitis due to a stone:** following the removal of the stone one acupuncture treatment should be sufficient for symptoms to subside

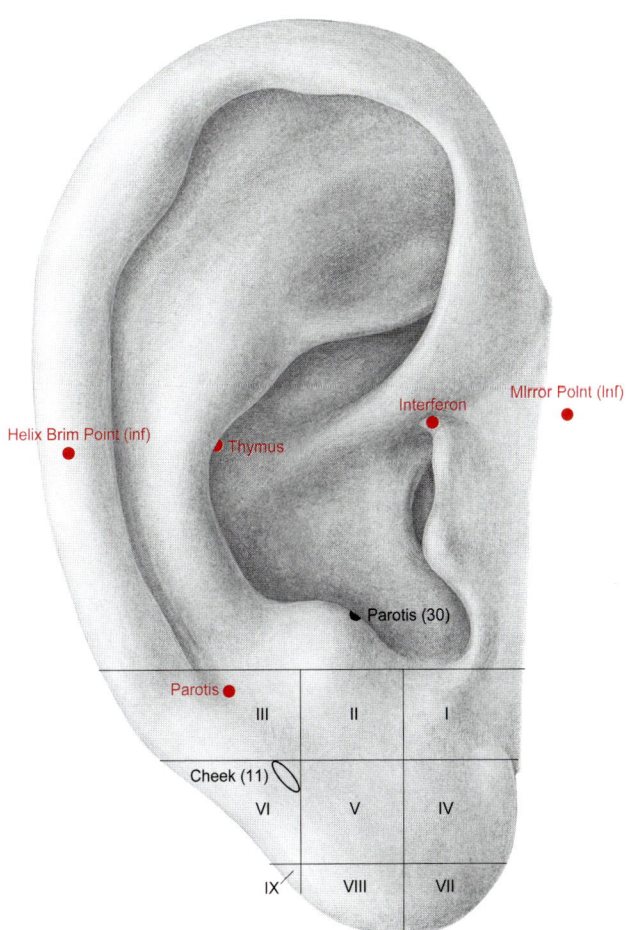

Helix Brim Point (inf)
Thymus
Interferon
Mirror Point (inf)
Parotis (30)
Parotis
III
II
I
Cheek (11)
VI
V
IV
IX
VIII
VII

Fig. 8.2-6

8.3 Gastrointestinal Disorders

8.3.1 Nausea

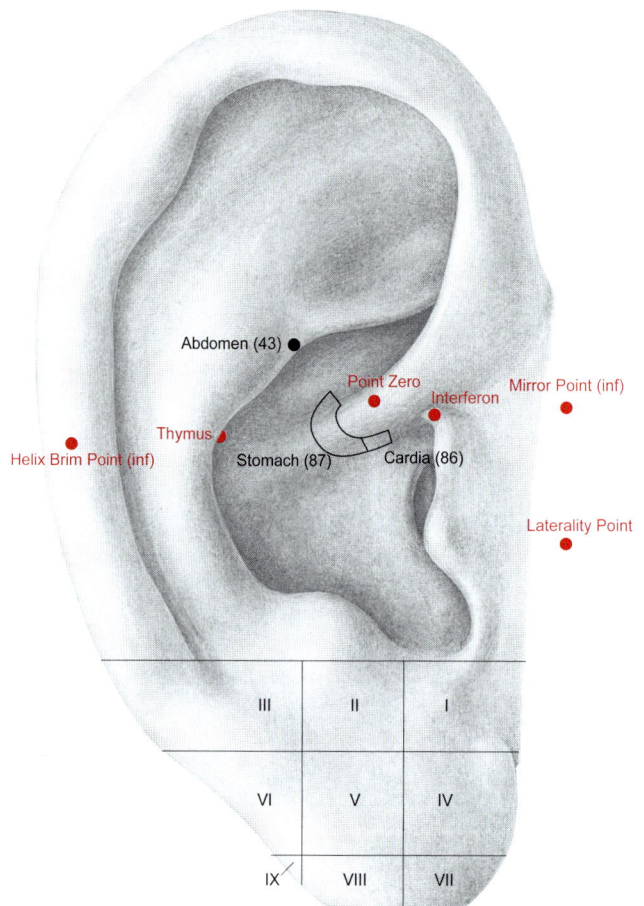

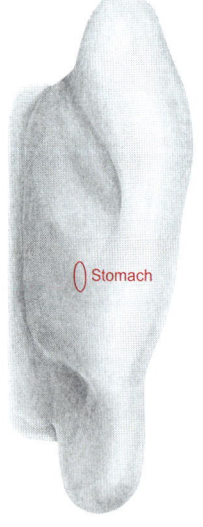

Fig. 8.3-1a+b

Description

- Acute nausea, in conjunction with e.g.
  - gastrointestinal infections
  - migraines
  - travel sickness
- Chronic nausea, with e.g.
  - severe illnesses such as tumours or after chemotherapy
  - disturbed balance (e.g. Menière's disease)

Point Prescription

French points

- Local point: **Stomach** (› 6.11.3) on the posterior ear
- Stabilising points: **Point Zero** (› 6.10.3), **Laterality Point** (› 6.8.6)
- Immunostimulant points: **Thymus** (› 6.6.1), **Interferon** (› 6.7.3), **Infection Axis** (› 6.4.1)

Chinese points

- Local points: **Stomach (87)** (› 6.4.1), **Cardia (86)** (› 6.4.1), **Abdomen (43)** (› 6.4.4)

 For recurrent nausea organic causes have to be ruled out (e.g. a tumour requires surgery).

Treatment Intervals

- **Acute nausea:** once daily or every other day
- **Chronic nausea**, also nausea due to chemotherapy: 2–3 times weekly

Treatment Course and Prognosis

- **Acute nausea:** generally symptoms disappear after one or a few days
- **Chronic nausea:** 2–4 weeks until symptoms disappear
- **Nausea with an underlying malignancy or with chemotherapy:** generally significant improvement after a few days

8.3.2 Gastritis

Description

- Inflammation of the mucosa of the stomach, often accompanied by recurrent epigastric pain; acute and chronic forms
- Causes include: infection with helicobacter pylori, alcohol, NSAIDs, biliary reflux, excess stomach acid, autoimmune processes
- Triggered/exacerbated by: nicotine, caffeine, stress
- Complications: ulcer (› 8.3.3)

Point Prescription

French points

- Local point: **Neural Stomach Point** (› 6.9.2)
- Defense against infection: **Thymus** (› 6.6.1), **Interferon** (› 6.7.3), **Infection Axis** (› 6.12.4)
- Psychological points: **Haldol** (› 6.8.6), **Barbiturate** (› 6.7.1), **Diazepam** (› 6.7.3)
- Stabilising point: **Point Zero** (› 6.10.3)

Chinese points

- Local points: **Stomach (87)**, **Cardia (86)** (› 6.4.1), **Abdomen (43)** (› 6.4.4)
- Stabilising point: *Shen Men* **(55)** (› 6.7.2)

- For epigastric complaints a gastroscopy should be carried out before starting auricular acupuncture to eliminate the possibility of an ulcer or carcinoma.
- For helicobacter pylori eradication therapy is necessary (combination of antibiotics and gastric acid secretion inhibitors)

Treatment Intervals

- **Acute gastritis:** every other day until symptoms have disappeared
- **Chronic gastritis:** initially twice weekly; once symptoms start to subside or there are pain-free intervals of more than a week (after approximately 4 weeks): once weekly until there is a sustained relief from symptoms

Treatment Course and Prognosis

- **Acute gastritis:** approximately 2 weeks until symptoms disappear
- **Chronic gastritis:** approximately 6 months until symptoms disappear

- Chronic nicotine or caffeine abuse, or continued stress will prevent a complete recovery; residual symptoms will remain. Regular acupuncture (approximately once monthly) will be necessary for sustained therapeutic results.
- While chronic atrophic gastritis (a form of gastritis affecting elderly patients with atrophied gastric mucosa) generally responds to treatment, therapeutic results tend to be limited.

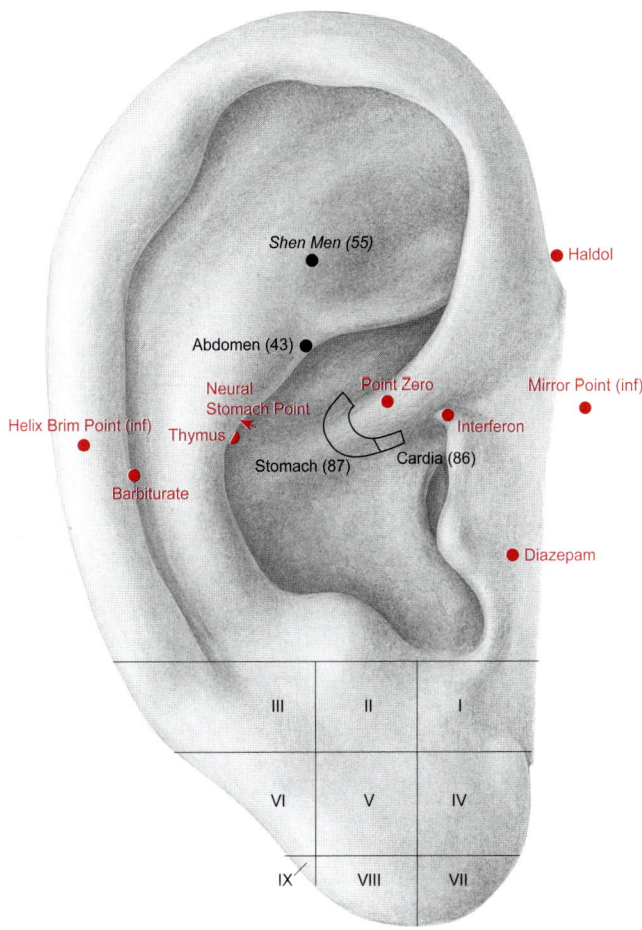

Fig. 8.3-2

8.3.3 Ventricular and Duodenal Ulcers

Description

- Mostly recurrent inflammation and ulceration of the gastric or duodenal mucosa
- Epigastric pain, especially postprandial or on an empty stomach (duodenal ulcer)
- Causes: helicobacter pylori (nearly 100 % of duodenal ulcers, approximately 80 % of ventricular ulcers), NSAIDs, acetylisalicylic acid (ASA), less frequently glucocorticoids, Zollinger-Ellison syndrome
- Exacerbating factors: nicotine, caffeine, stress

Point Prescription

French points

- Local point: **Neural Stomach Point**(› 6.9.2)
- Psychological points: **Diazepam** (› 6.7.3), **Anti-Aggression** (› 6.8.5), **Frustration** (› 6.8.3)
- Stabilising point: **Point Zero** (› 6.10.3)

Chinese points

- Local points: **Stomach (87)** (› 6.4.1), **Duodenum (88)** (› 6.4.1), **Abdomen (43)** (› 6.4.4)
- Stabilising point: *Shen Men* **(55)** (› 6.7.2), **Diaphragm (82)** (› 6.4.3)

- In cases of epigastric pain a gastroscopy should be carried out before starting treatment with auricular acupuncture to eliminate the possibility of a carcinoma.
- For severe ulcers conservative treatment with proton inhibitors (e.g. omeprazole) is the treatment of choice due to the risk of perforation.

Treatment Intervals

Severe ulcers should be treated by conventional medicine. In these cases auricular acupuncture can provide support as an adjuvant therapy to accelerate the healing process. Only mild cases should be treated with just auricular acupuncture.

- **Acute stage:** once daily or every other day
- **Chronic stage** (pain more than once monthly): 1–2 times weekly until the pain has completely subsided

> If ulcers are caused by NSAIDs or glucocorticoids, these drugs should be slowly reduced or discontinued and, if possible, replaced by auricular acupuncture. The point prescription depends on the relevant indication.

Treatment Course and Prognosis

- **Acute and chronic stage:** significant reduction of the complaint within 1–2 weeks
- Start of treatment during the **acute stage:** symptoms generally disappear within up to 4 weeks

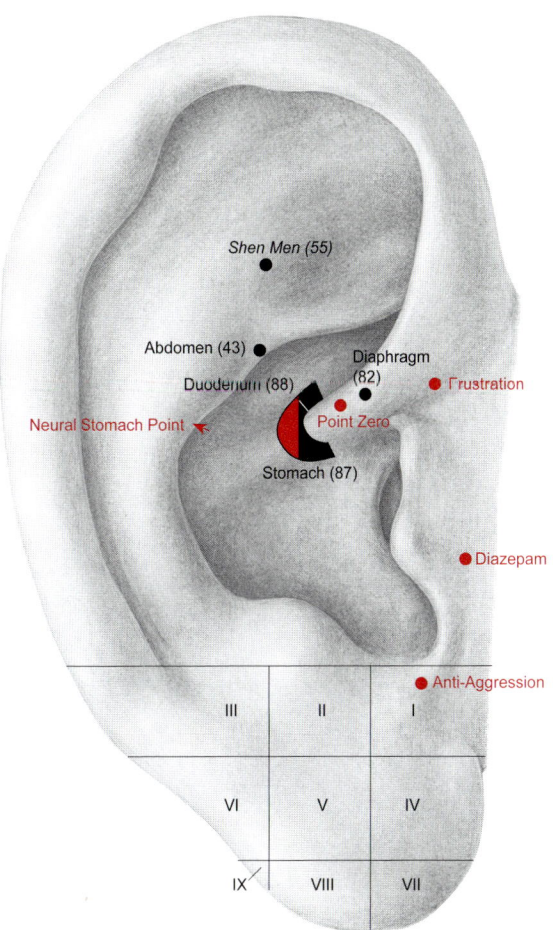

Shen Men (55)

Abdomen (43)

Duodenum (88)

Diaphragm (82)

Frustration

Point Zero

Neural Stomach Point

Stomach (87)

Diazepam

Anti-Aggression

III II I

VI V IV

IX VIII VII

Fig. 8.3-3

box

Chronic nicotine or caffeine abuse, continuous stress, or certain drugs (e.g. NSAIDs, gluco-corticoids, aspirin) can prevent the healing of an ulcer or cause it to re-occur.

8.3.4 Cholelithiasis and Cholecystitis

Description

- Cholelithiasis: gall stones; 50 % of cases are asymptomatic (incidental sonographic findings); otherwise recurrent, often diffuse epigastric pain (especially following the intake of fatty foods, alcohol, and coffee) or biliary colic
- Cholecystitis: inflammation of the gallbladder; in over 90 % of cases caused by gallstones

Point Prescription

French points

- Local points: **Gallbladder**, also **Liver** (› 6.4.1)
- Analgesic points: **Analgesia 1 and 2** (› 6.7.5)
- Defense against infection: **Thymus** (› 6.6.1), **Interferon** (› 6.7.3), **Infection Axis** (› 6.12.4)
- Relaxing points: **Diazepam** (› 6.7.3), **Haldol** (› 6.8.6)

Chinese points

- Analgesic points: **Sun (35)**, **Thalamus (26a)**, **Occiput (29)** (› 6.7.4), *Shen Men* **(55)** (› 6.7.2)

- Curative treatment with auricular acupuncture is possible only in cases of biliary sludge.
- In cases of gallstones auricular acupuncture can trigger colic. Endoscopic surgery is therefore the treatment of choice.
- Acute cholecystitis requires the immediate referral to hospital!

Treatment Intervals

- **Asymptomatic cholecystolithiasis:** no treatment required; auricular acupuncture may trigger colic
- **Biliary sludge:** once weekly until there is a complete recovery (sonographic check-ups)
- **Acute pain:** once daily until there is a sustained reduction in pain, possibly until a stone has been passed or there has been surgery

Treatment Course and Prognosis

- **Cholecystitis:** approximately 2–3 weeks until symptoms have disappeared
- **Biliary sludge:** treatments required for up to 3 months

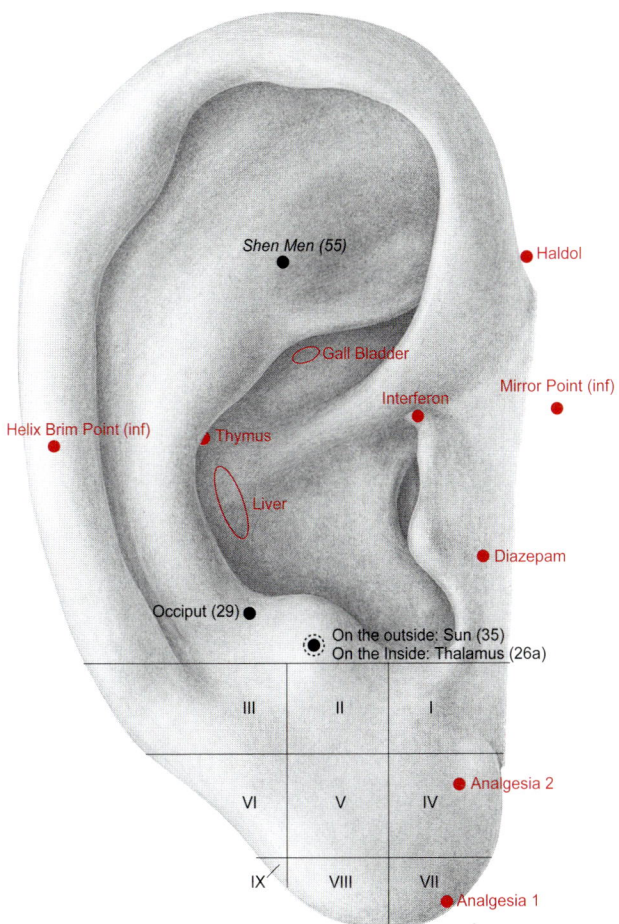

Shen Men (55)

Haldol

Gall Bladder

Interferon

Mirror Point (inf)

Helix Brim Point (inf)

Thymus

Liver

Diazepam

Occiput (29)

On the outside: Sun (35)
On the Inside: Thalamus (26a)

III II I

VI V IV Analgesia 2

IX VIII VII Analgesia 1

8.3.5 Appendicitis

Description

- Acute appendicitis:
  - pain in the right lower abdomen, often accompanied by loss of appetite, nausea, and vomiting
  - rapid onset, often within a few hours
- Chronic recurrent irritation of the appendix: episodic pain in the right lower abdomen, maybe constipation, weight loss

Point Prescription

French points

- Local point: **Caecum** (› 6.4.1)
- Analgesic points: **Analgesia 1 and 2** (› 6.7.5)
- Defense against infection: **Thymus** (› 6.6.1), **Interferon** (› 6.7.3), **Infection Axis** (› 6.12.4)

Chinese points

- Local points: **Appendix IV (90)** (› 6.4.1), **Appendix I (68)**, **Appendix II (69)**, **Appendix III (70)** (› 6.4.2)
- Analgesic points: **Sun (35)**, **Thalamus (26a)**, **Occiput (29)** (› 6.7.4)

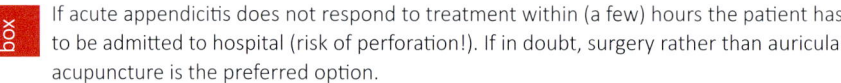

> If acute appendicitis does not respond to treatment within (a few) hours the patient has to be admitted to hospital (risk of perforation!). If in doubt, surgery rather than auricular acupuncture is the preferred option.
>
> In female patients it is sometimes possible to distinguish between oophorosalpingitis and appendicitis by RAC-palpation. However, appendicitis is often accompanied by an inflammation of the ovary and ovarian duct and vice versa. In such cases both auricular points will be active.

Treatment Intervals

- **Acute appendicitis:** surgery is the treatment of choice; attempt to treat (for a few hours): acupuncture every 1–2 hours until the pain has reduced significantly; if there is no response to the treatment, admission to hospital is necessary
- **Chronic recurrent irritation of the appendix:**
  - initially once daily until there is a significant reduction of the pain
  - then once weekly until symptoms have disappeared

Treatment Course and Prognosis

- **Acute appendicitis:** symptoms may improve within hours
- **Chronic recurrent irritation of the appendix:** generally up to 3 months until symptoms have disappeared

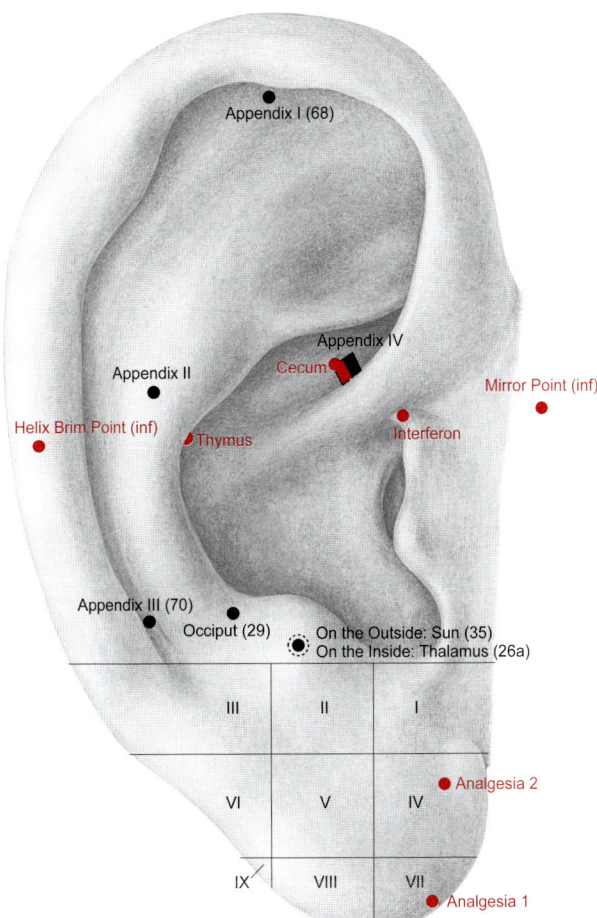

Fig. 8.3-5

8.3.6 Hepatitis

Description

- Seropositive hepatitis A:
  - transmitted by fecal-oral/oral fecal route (sexual contact, contaminated food)
  - incubation period: approximately 15–20 days
  - symptoms, course of disease: predominantly debility and general symptoms of infection; generally complete recovery, chronicity is very rare; tests will remain seropositive; vaccination possible
- Seropositive hepatitis B:
  - mostly parenteral transmission (e.g. blood transfusion, used syringes); but also oral-fecal route (sexual contact)
  - incubation period: approximately 50–180 days
  - symptoms and course of disease: during the acute stage primarily debility and unspecific symptoms of infection, only rarely jaundice; vaccination possible; can be fatal (1 %), can become chronic (cirrhosis of the liver)
- Seropositive hepatitis C:
  - mostly parenteral transmission (e.g. blood transfusion, used syringes); but also oral/fecal route (sexual contact)
  - incubation period: approximately 40–85 days
  - symptoms and course of disease: during the acute stage primarily debility and unspecific symptoms of infection, only rarely jaundice; can become chronic (cirrhosis of the liver); currently no vaccination available

Point Prescription

The same treatment protocol applies to all forms of hepatitis. For aggressive cases of hepatitis B and C TCM is a beneficial complementary therapy

French points

- Local point: **Liver** (› 6.4.1)
- Defense against infection: **Thymus** (› 6.6.1), **Interferon** (› 6.7.3), **Infection Axis** (› 6.12.4)
- Stabilising points: **Point Zero** (› 6.10.3), **Laterality Point** (› 6.8.6)

Chinese points

- Local points: **Hepatitis Point (61)** (› 6.4.7), **Liver I (76)**, **Liver II (77)** (› 6.4.3), **Liver (97)** (› 6.4.1)

> **box** Acupuncture can boost the immune response but it has no effect on the infectivity. Patient education is therefore crucial (e.g. transmission through sexual intercourse!).

Treatment Intervals

- **Hepatitis A, B and C**, acute stage: 2–3 times weekly until symptoms have disappeared
- **Hepatitis B and C**, chronic stage: 2–4 times monthly, generally for several years

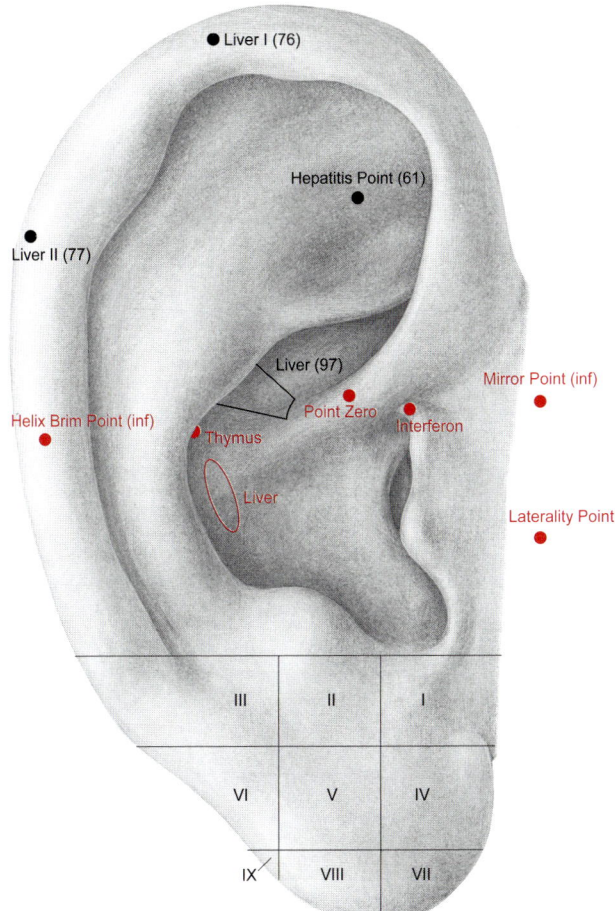

Fig. 8.3-6

Treatment Course and Prognosis

- **Acute stage** (duration approximately 2–4 weeks): the course of the disease can be shortened, especially with hepatitis A; for hepatitis B acupuncture reduces the risk of chronicity
- **Chronic stage** (hepatitis B and C):
  - development of cirrhosis of the liver can be slowed down
  - general malaise (fatigue, weakness) generally disappears

8.3.7 Meteorism

Description

- Accumulation of air or gas in the intestines or the abdominal cavity, possibly accompanied by diffuse abdominal pain
- Often occurs together with functional dyspepsia or other nervous disorders such as aerophagia
- Trigger: foods that cause bloating (e.g. cabbage), food intolerances, stress, candidiasis

> **box** Patients with severe gastrointestinal disorders such as tumours (e.g. colon carcinoma) have to be referred to a consultant for a thorough diagnosis and possibly undergo surgery before starting treatment with acupuncture.

Point Prescription

Regardless of the cause the following points should be treated based on RAC-palpation (› 3.1.4):

French points
- Local points: **Rectum** (› 6.4.1) on the anterior ear; **Point Zero Retro** (› 6.11.4) on the posterior ear
- Stabilising points: **Point Zero** (› 6.10.3), **Laterality Point** (› 6.8.6)
- Psychological points: **Barbiturate** (› 6.7.1), **Haldol** (› 6.8.6), **Diazepam** (› 6.7.3)

Chinese points
- Local points: **Colon (91)** (› 6.4.1), maybe **Stomach (87)** (› 6.4.1)
- Stabilising point: **ANS I (51)** (› 6.6.5)

> **box** Auricular acupuncture may resolve candidiasis without the requirement for systemic treatment (such as nystatin). Assumed mechanism: strengthening the immune system allows the intestinal flora to regenerate so that candida overgrowth will subside.

Treatment Intervals

- Daily meteorism: 2–3 times weekly until symptoms improve, then once weekly until symptoms have disappeared
- Sporadic meteorism: once weekly until symptoms have disappeared

Treatment Course and Prognosis

- Recent onset **acute meteorism:** usually about 3–4 weeks for a sustained relieve from symptoms
- **Chronic meteorism** (> 4 weeks): approximately 3 months for a sustained relieve from symptoms

> **box** Learning relaxation techniques such as *Qi* Gong, Yoga, or autogenic training can accelerate the treatment results.

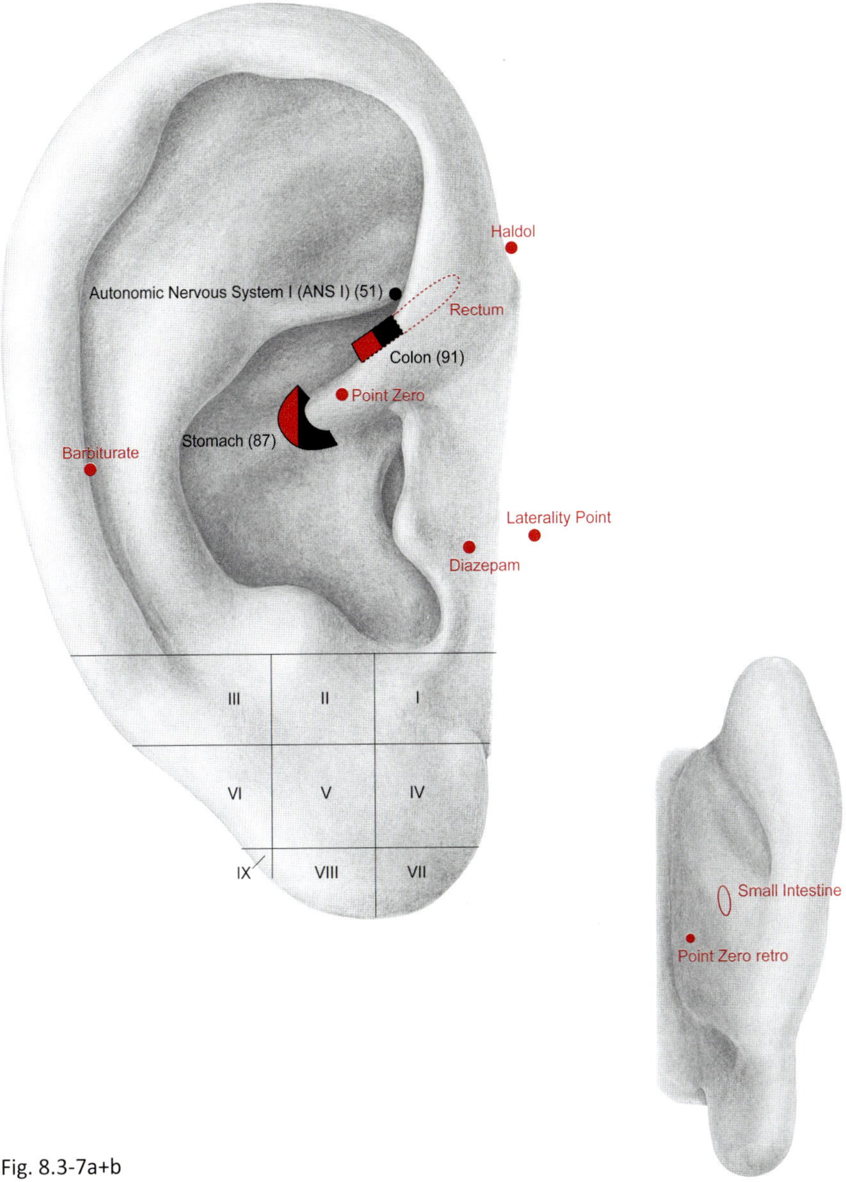

Haldol

Autonomic Nervous System I (ANS I) (51)

Rectum

Colon (91)

Point Zero

Stomach (87)

Barbiturate

Laterality Point

Diazepam

III | II | I

VI | V | IV

IX | VIII | VII

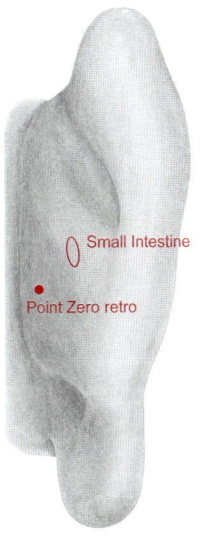

Small Intestine

Point Zero retro

Fig. 8.3-7a+b

8.3.8 Constipation

Description

- Increased intervals between bowel movements (varies from person to person, approximately > 3 days) combined with hard stools
- Often chronic, habitual constipation; possibly as accompanying symptom of other disorders or a side effect of certain drugs
- Constipation often leads to laxative abuse which in turn exacerbates the constipation (vicious circle)
- Contributing factors: a diet low in fibre, lack of exercise, too little fluid intake

> **box** Stenosing processes (e.g. as a result of tumours) have to be ruled out before starting treatments with auricular acupuncture.

Point Prescription

French points

- Local points: **Colon**, **Rectum** (› 6.4.1) on the posterior ear
- Stabilising points: **Point Zero** (› 6.10.3), **Laterality Point** (› 6.8.6)
- Psychological points: **Barbiturate** (› 6.7.1), **Haldol** (› 6.8.6), **Diazepam** (› 6.7.3)

Chinese points

- Local point: **Colon (91)** (› 6.4.1)
- Stabilising points: *San Jiao* **(104)** (› 6.10.1), **ANS I (51)** (› 6.6.5)

Treatment Intervals

- Initially (for approximately 4 weeks) 2–3 times weekly
- Then once weekly (if constipation persists)

Treatment Course and Prognosis

- **Short-term constipation** (up to a few months): usually approximately 4 weeks until symptoms disappear
- **Chronic constipation** (for several months and up to several years, sometimes for decades): approximately 3–6 months until symptoms disappear

> **box** Patient compliance is essential for good treatment results. Sufficient intake of fibres and fluids is essential, laxatives should be discontinued. Long-standing laxative abuse can damage the intestines to such an extent that a complete recovery is no longer possible.

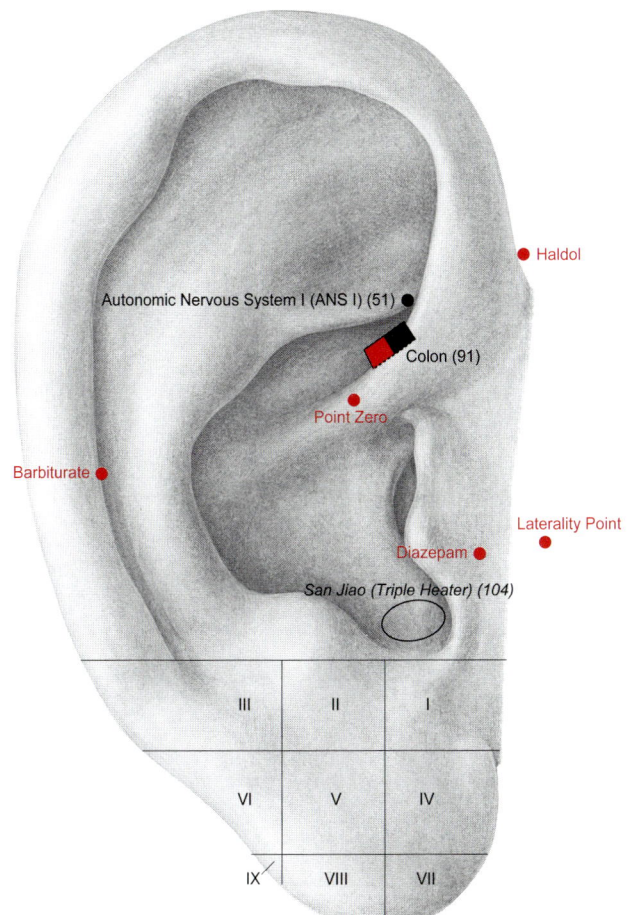

Haldol

Autonomic Nervous System I (ANS I) (51)

Colon (91)

Point Zero

Barbiturate

Laterality Point

Diazepam

San Jiao (Triple Heater) (104)

III   II   I

VI   V   IV

IX   VIII   VII

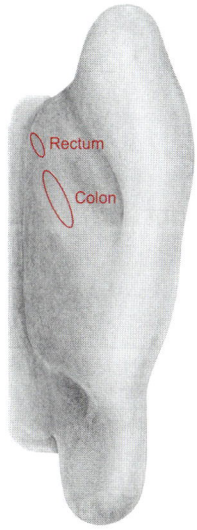

Rectum

Colon

Fig. 8.3-8a+b

8.3.9 Diarrhoea

Description

- More than three bowel movements with unformed stools per day
- Causes:
  - gastrointestinal infections (e.g. salmonella, shigella, enterotoxic strains of E. coli)
  - food allergies or intolerances (e.g. dairy)
  - side effects of drugs, e.g. antibiotics, NSAIDs, digitalis, stomach medication)
  - stress or other psychological strain (especially in emotionally unstable patients)
  - chronic inflammatory intestinal disorders, e.g. ulcerative colitis (› 8.3.10), Crohn's disease (› 8.3.11)

Point Prescription

French points

- Local point: **Rectum** (› 6.4.1)
- Stabilising points: **Point Zero** (› 6.10.3), **Laterality Point** (› 6.8.6)
- Psychological points: **Barbiturate** (› 6.7.1), **Diazepam** (› 6.7.3)
- Defense against infection (if indicated): **Thymus** (› 6.6.1), **Interferon** (› 6.7.3), **Infection Axis** (› 6.12.4)

Chinese points

- Local points: **Colon (91)** (› 6.4.1), **Rectum (81)** (› 6.4.3)
- Stabilising points: **Shen Men (55)** (› 6.7.2), **ANS I (51)** (› 6.6.5)

> **box** Severe disorders of the gastrointestinal tract (e.g. colon carcinoma) require investigation and diagnosis by conventional medicine. Stool tests are also important for diagnosing infections (e.g. salmonella).

Treatment Intervals

- **Acute mild gastrointestinal infections:**
  - 2–3 times weekly until symptoms have disappeared
- **Acute severe gastrointestinal infections** (e.g. salmonellosis, dysentery): auricular acupuncture as adjuvant therapy with conventional treatments
  - initially 3–4 times weekly until symptoms improve
  - then once weekly until symptoms have disappeared
- **Non-infectious diarrhoea** (e.g. stress-related):
  - initially twice weekly until symptoms improve
  - then once weekly until symptoms have disappeared

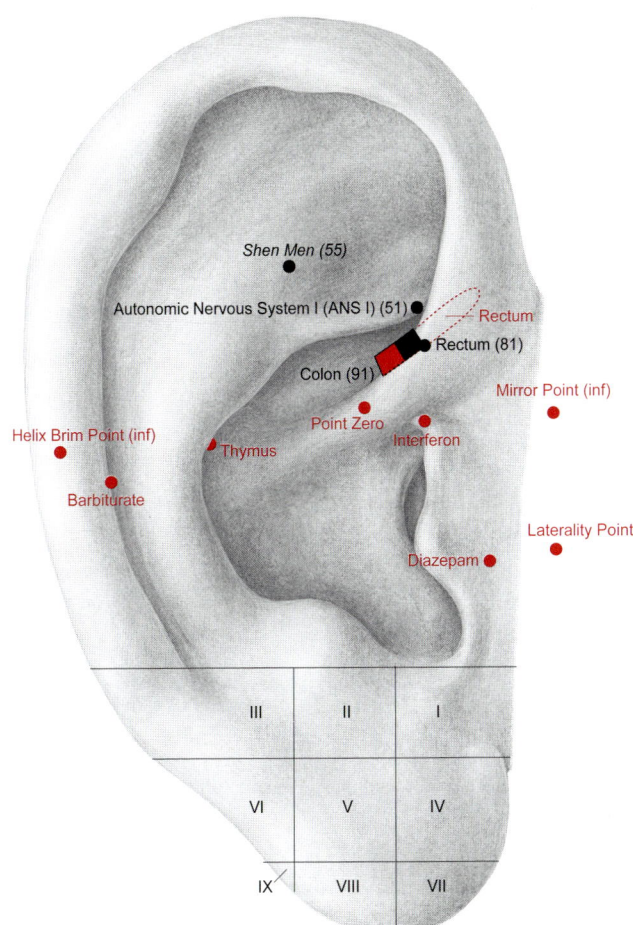

Fig. 8.3-9

Treatment Course and Prognosis

- **Acute mild gastrointestinal infection:**
  - depending on the patient's constitution 2–10 days until symptoms have disappeared
- **Acute severe gastrointestinal infection** (e.g. salmonellosis, dysentery):
  - 1–4 days until symptoms improve
  - 1–3 weeks until symptoms have disappeared
- **Non-infectious diarrhoea** (e.g. stress-related):
  - 1–2 weeks until symptoms improve
  - approximately 3 months until symptoms disappear

8.3.10 Ulcerative Colitis

Description

- Chronic inflammatory, recurrent disorder of the colon; initially affects the rectum, then spreading to more proximal areas
- Diffuse abdominal pain accompanied by diarrhoea mixed with blood and mucus
- Psychological component, e.g. stress can trigger a flare-up
- Depending on duration and extent increased risk of malignant degeneration

> **box** Patients with ulcerative colitis require regular colonoscopies due to the risk of malignant degeneration.

Point Prescription

French points

- Local point: **Rectum** (› 6.4.1)
- Stabilising points: **Point Zero** (› 6.10.3), **Laterality Point** (› 6.8.6)
- Psychological points: **Barbiturate** (› 6.7.1), **Diazepam** (› 6.7.3), **Omega Axis** (› 6.12.1)
- Immunostimulant points: **Immune Axis** (› 6.12.3), **ACTH** (› 6.6.6), **Adrenal Cortex** (› 6.6.1)

Chinese points

- Local points: **Colon (91)** (› 6.4.1), **Rectum (81)** (› 6.4.3)
- Stabilising points: ***Shen Men* (55)** (› 6.7.2), **ANS I (51)** (› 6.6.5)

Treatment Intervals

- **Acute episode:** once daily or every other day until symptoms improve; once there are pain-free intervals of > 1 week (after approximately 4 weeks) once weekly until there is a sustained relief from symptoms
- **Preventative treatments** during symptom-free intervals: approximately once monthly for about 6 months

Treatment Course and Prognosis

- During acute episodes: depending on the severity 4–8 weeks until diarrhoea has subsided
- Longer symptom-free intervals after approximately 6 months
- Lasting relief from symptoms possible after several years

> **box** Auricular acupuncture has a psychologically stabilising effect and supports the immune system. Both these components are important for the successful treatment of ulcerative colitis.

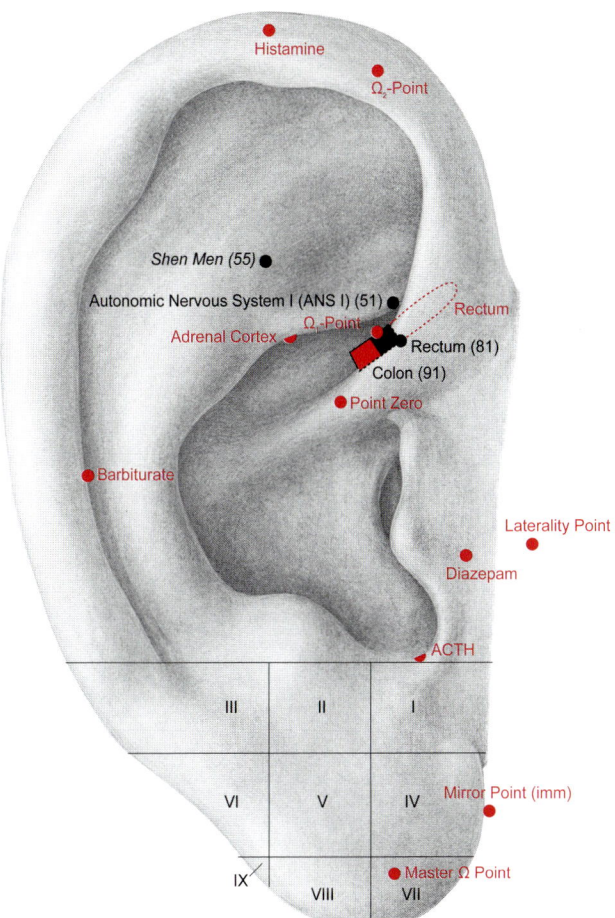

Fig. 8.3-10

8.3.11 Crohn's Disease

Description

- Chronic inflammatory, granulomatous disease, affecting particularly the terminal ileum (in 40 % of cases only the ileum) and the colon
- Colicky abdominal pain with diarrhoea (only rarely mixed with blood)
- Exacerbating factor: psychological stress
- Complications: ulcerations and fistulas, stenosis, ileus

Point Prescription

French points

- Local point: **Cecum** (› 6.4.1)
- Stabilising points: **Point Zero** (› 6.10.3), **Laterality Point** (› 6.8.6)
- Psychological points: **Barbiturate** (› 6.7.1), **Diazepam** (› 6.7.3), **Omega Axis** (› 6.12.1)
- Immunostimulant points: **Immune Axis** (› 6.12.3), **ACTH** (› 6.6.6), **Adrenal Cortex** (› 6.6.1)

Chinese points

- Local points: **Duodenum (88)**, **Small Intestine (89)**, **Colon (91)** (› 6.4.1),
- Stabilising points: *Shen Men* **(55)** (› 6.7.2), **ANS I (51)** (› 6.6.5)

Treatment Intervals

- **Acute episode:** every 2 days until the diarrhoea has stopped, then once weekly until there is sustained relief from symptoms
- **Prophylaxis** (during symptom-free intervals): approximately once monthly until there is a sustained remission for > 6 months

Treatment Course and Prognosis

- Acute relapse: 2–4 weeks until diarrhoea stops
- Prolonged symptom-free intervals after 3–6 months (depending on the severity of the disease)
- Sustained relief from symptoms is possible after several years, provided there are no late effects (e.g. fistulas)

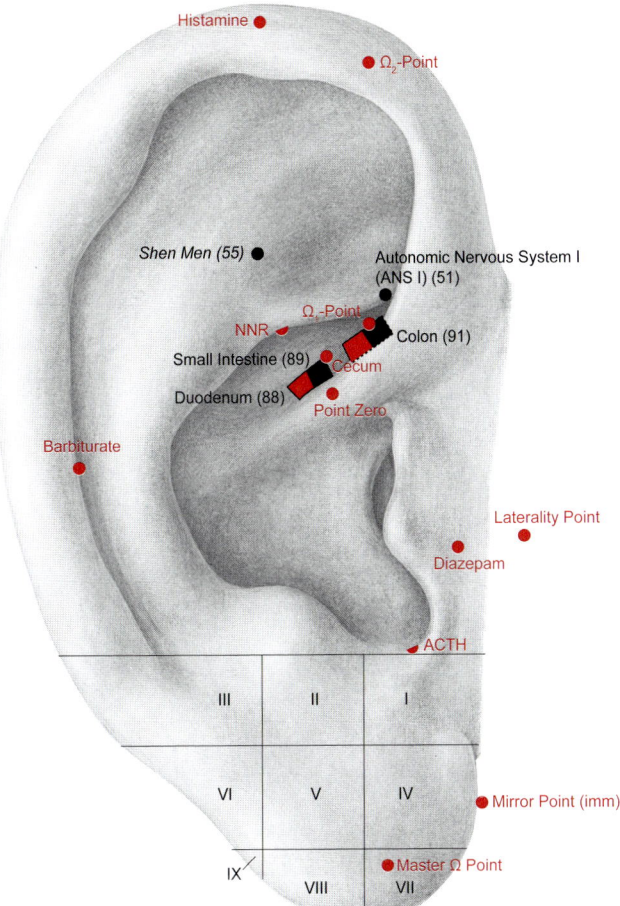

Fig. 8.3-11

8.3.12 Haemorrhoids

Description

- Dilation of the rectal venous plexus
  - Grade 1: slight haemorrhoidal protrusion into the anal canal
  - Grade 2: prolapse upon straining followed by spontaneous reposition
  - Grade 3: prolapse requiring manual reposition
  - Grade 4: prolapse which cannot be repositioned manually
- Itching, stools covered by bright blood
- Possibly pain with defecation

> **box** Anal bleeding requires investigation by rectoscopy to eliminate the possibility of a tumour.

Point Prescription

French points

- Local point: **Haemorrhoids** (› 6.4.1)
- Stabilising point: **Point Zero** (› 6.10.3)
- Analgesic points (if indicated): **Analgesia 1 and 2** (› 6.7.5)

Chinese points

- Local point: **Rectum (81)** (› 6.4.3)
- Stabilising point: *Shen Men* **(55)** (› 6.7.2)
- Analgesic point (if indicated): **Thalamus (26a)** (› 6.7.4)

> **box** Auricular acupuncture is suitable for the treatment of grade 1 and 2 haemorrhoids. Grade 3 and 4 haemorrhoids generally require surgical intervention; auricular acupuncture can accelerate the post-operative healing process.

Treatment Intervals

- Pain and bleeding (grade 1 and 2): once daily or every other day until the pain has subsided
- Grade 3 and 4: short-term as pain-relief prior to surgery; after surgery twice weekly until symptoms have disappeared
- Chronic recurrent haemorrhoids (grades 1 or 2): once weekly

Treatment Course and Prognosis

- **Grades 1 and 2:** reduction of haemorrhoids and symptomatic relief depend on the duration of the disorder but generally within 1–3 months
- **Grades 3 and 4,** post-operative acupuncture: following surgery, symptoms generally subside within 2 weeks

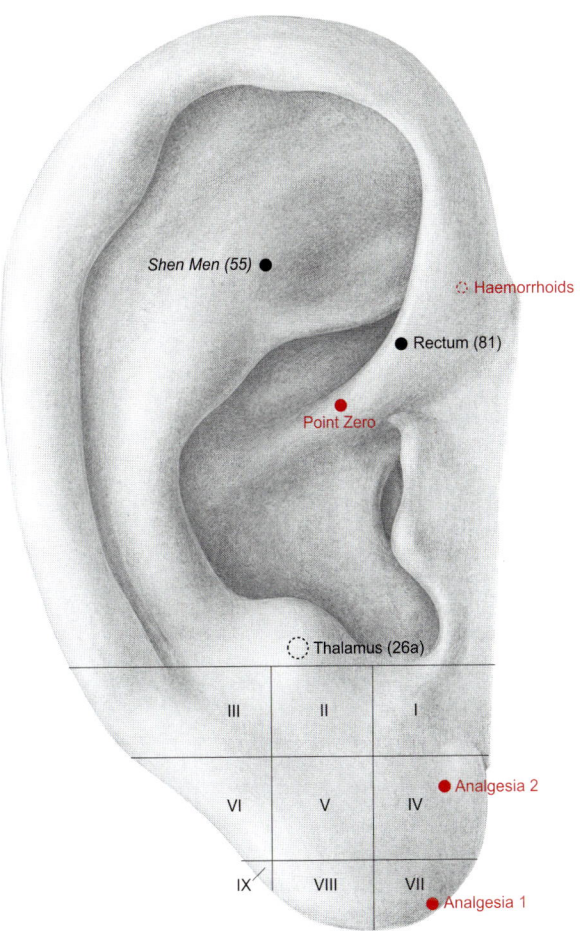

Shen Men (55)

Haemorrhoids

Rectum (81)

Point Zero

Thalamus (26a)

III II I

Analgesia 2

VI V IV

IX VIII VII

Analgesia 1

8.4 Urogenital Disorders

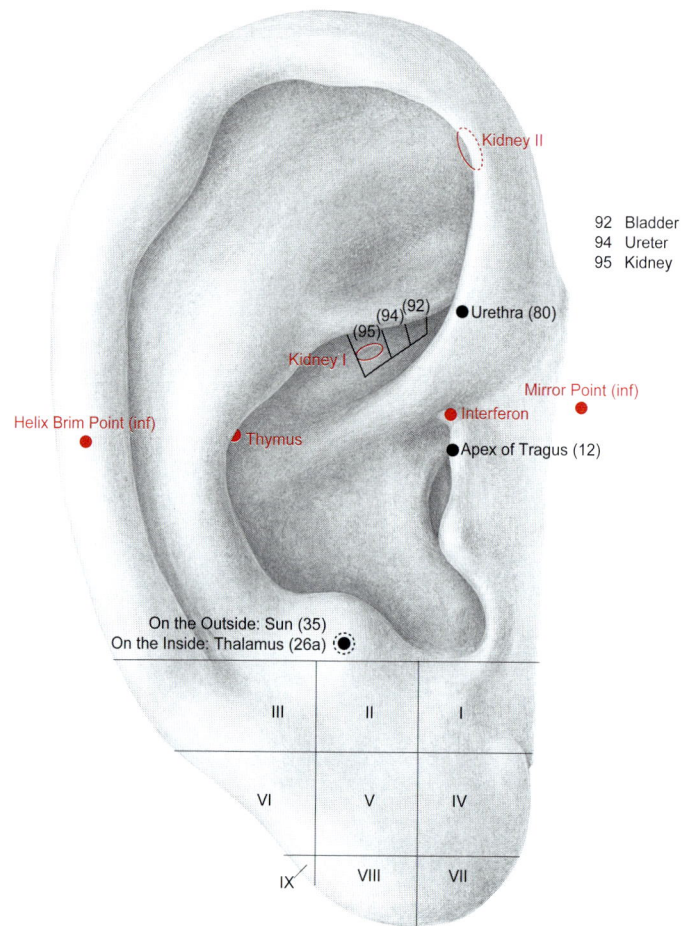

92 Bladder
94 Ureter
95 Kidney

Fig. 8.4-1

8.4.1 Urinary Tract Infection

Description

- Inflammatory disorder of the lower (bladder, urethra) and/or upper (renal pelvis) urinary tract, mostly bacterial infection; typically accompanied by dysuria but can be asymptomatic
- Trigger: exposure to cold (weather, cold seats, cold sweat), swimming pools, sexual intercourse
- More prevalent in women; in men often in conjunction with organic disorders of the urogenital system (e.g. prostrate adenoma)

Children, men, pregnant women as well as women with chronic recurrent urogenital infections should be thoroughly investigated by conventional medicine prior to auricular acupuncture.

Point Prescription

French points

- Local points: **Kidney I** (› 6.5.1), **Kidney II** (› 6.5.4)
- Defense against infection: **Infection Axis** (› 6.12.4), **Interferon** (› 6.7.3), **Thymus** (› 6.6.1)

Chinese points

- Local points: **Bladder (92)** (› 6.5.1), **Urethra (80)** (› 6.5.2), **Ureter (94)** (› 6.5.1), **Kidney (95)** (› 6.5.1)
- Analgesic points (if indicated): **Apex of Tragus (12)** (› 6.7.3), **Thalamus (26a)** (› 6.7.4)

 The patient should be advised to drink sufficient fluids (about 3 litres daily!).

Treatment Intervals

- **Acute urinary tract infection:** 2–3 times weekly until symptoms have disappeared
- **Chronic recurrent urinary tract infection:** once weekly until symptoms have disappeared (approximately 3–4 weeks)

Treatment Course and Prognosis

- **Acute urinary tract infection:** 1–2 weeks until symptoms have disappeared; auricular acupuncture shortens the course of the disease, antibiotics can generally be avoided
- **Chronic recurrent urinary tract infection:** depending on the duration of the disorder 1–3 months until symptoms disappear

8.4.2 Urinary Incontinence

Description

- Involuntary passing of urine, especially in women
- Four main forms:
  - Stress incontinence: increased pressure in the pelvic cavity leads to passing of urine
  - Overflow incontinence: urinary dribbling, e.g. with obstructions (such as prostate hyperplasia
  - Reflex incontinence: neurogenic bladder disorder, e.g. with paraplegic syndrome
  - Urge-incontinence: irresistible urge to urinate with involuntary loss of urine, e.g. with urinary tract infections

Point Prescription

French points

- Local point: **Bladder** (› 6.11.3) on the posterior ear
- Stabilising points: **Laterality Point** (› 6.8.6), **Point Zero** (› 6.10.3)

Chinese points

- Local point: **Bladder (92)** (› 6.5.1),
- Stabilising point: **Branching Point (83)** (› 6.10.1)

Treatment Intervals

- **Stress incontinence:** once weekly until there is sustained relief from symptoms
- **Reflex incontinence** without irreversible nerve damage:
  - recent onset: 2–3 times weekly
  - chronic disorder (> 4 weeks): initially once weekly until symptoms have improved significantly; then twice monthly until symptoms have disappeared

Treatment Course and Prognosis

- **Stress incontinence:**
  - symptoms often disappear within 3 months
  - no results with acupuncture: surgery may be necessary
- **Reflex incontinence** without irreversible nerve damage:
  - improvement within 4–8 weeks
  - complete recovery possible within 6 months; whether this can be achieved depends on the cause

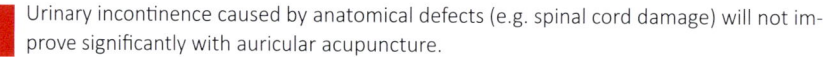

Urinary incontinence caused by anatomical defects (e.g. spinal cord damage) will not improve significantly with auricular acupuncture.

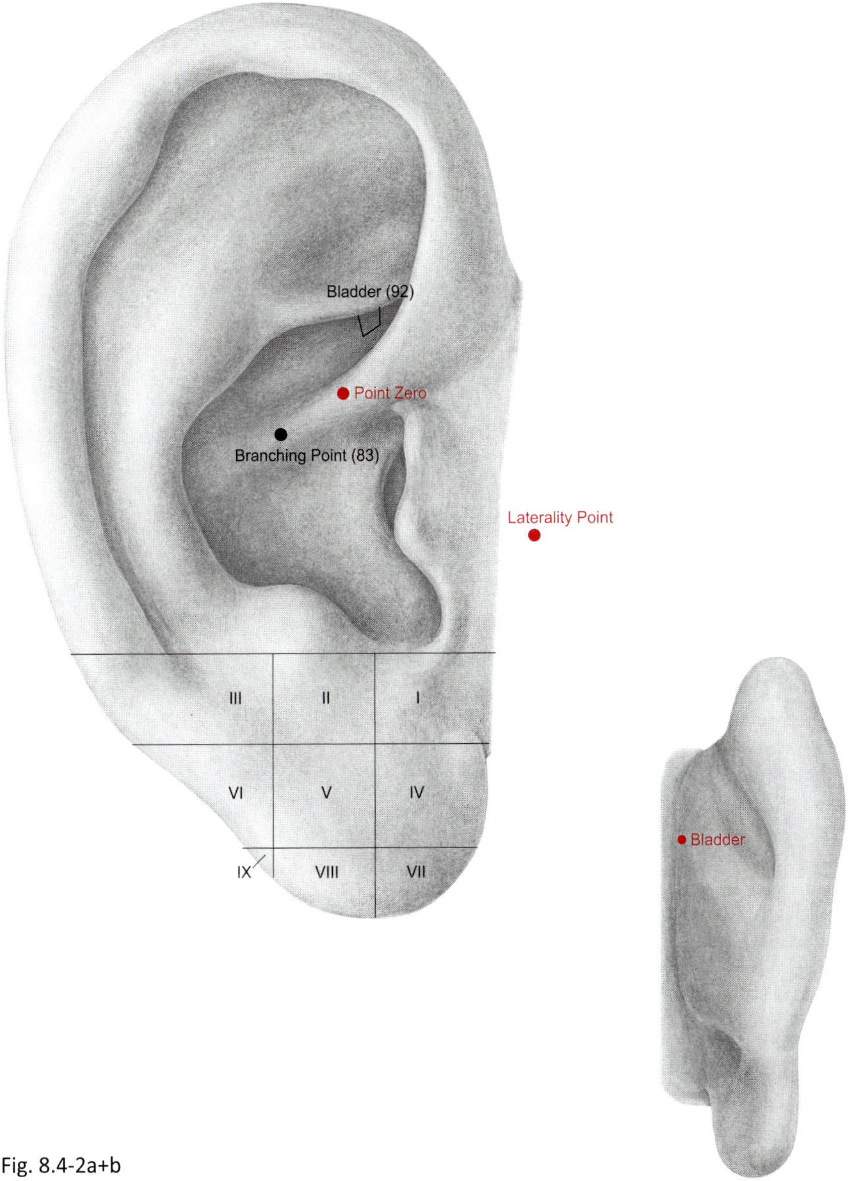

Bladder (92)

● Point Zero

● Branching Point (83)

Laterality Point
●

III | II | I

VI | V | IV

IX | VIII | VII

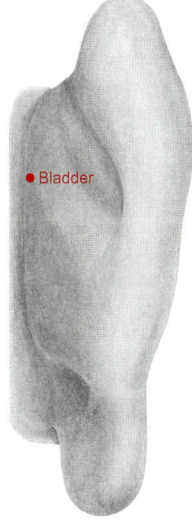

● Bladder

Fig. 8.4-2a+b

8.4.3 Urinary Retention

Description

- After urinating some residual urine remains in the bladder; frequent urination with a small amount
- Causes:
  - surgery, e.g. for urinary incontinence or in the genital area
  - prostate adenoma, sclerosis of the sphincter, urethral stricture
  - neurogenic bladder
  - side effects of medication (e.g. antihistamines, anticholinergics)
  - psychological causes

> **box** It is essential to investigate the cause of the urinary retention with conventional medicine before starting acupuncture treatments. Anatomical damage (such as scar formation, sclerosis of the bladder sphincter, prostate adenoma, or tumours) requires conventional treatments.

Point Prescription

French points

- Local point: **Bladder** (› 6.11.3) on the posterior ear
- Stabilising points: **Laterality Point** (› 6.8.6), **Point Zero** (› 6.10.3)
- Psychological points: **Diazepam** (› 6.7.3), **Barbiturate** (› 6.7.1), **Haldol** (› 6.8.6), **Omega Axis** (› 6.12.1)

Chinese points

- Local point: **Bladder (92)** (› 6.5.1)
- Stabilising point: **Branching Point (83)** (› 6.10.1)

Treatment Intervals

- Once weekly until symptoms have disappeared

Treatment Course and Prognosis

- **Residual urine due to a neurogenic bladder:**
  - depending on the cause symptoms disappear within 3–6 months
  - if symptoms do not disappear within one year, results beyond an improvement of symptoms is not to be expected
- **Residual urine due to medication side effects:**
  - improvement of symptoms within 2–4 weeks
  - for a sustained relief of symptoms it is generally necessary to discontinue medication
- **Residual urine due to psychological causes:**
  - improvement of symptoms within 1–3 months
  - sustained relief of symptoms generally within 3–6 months

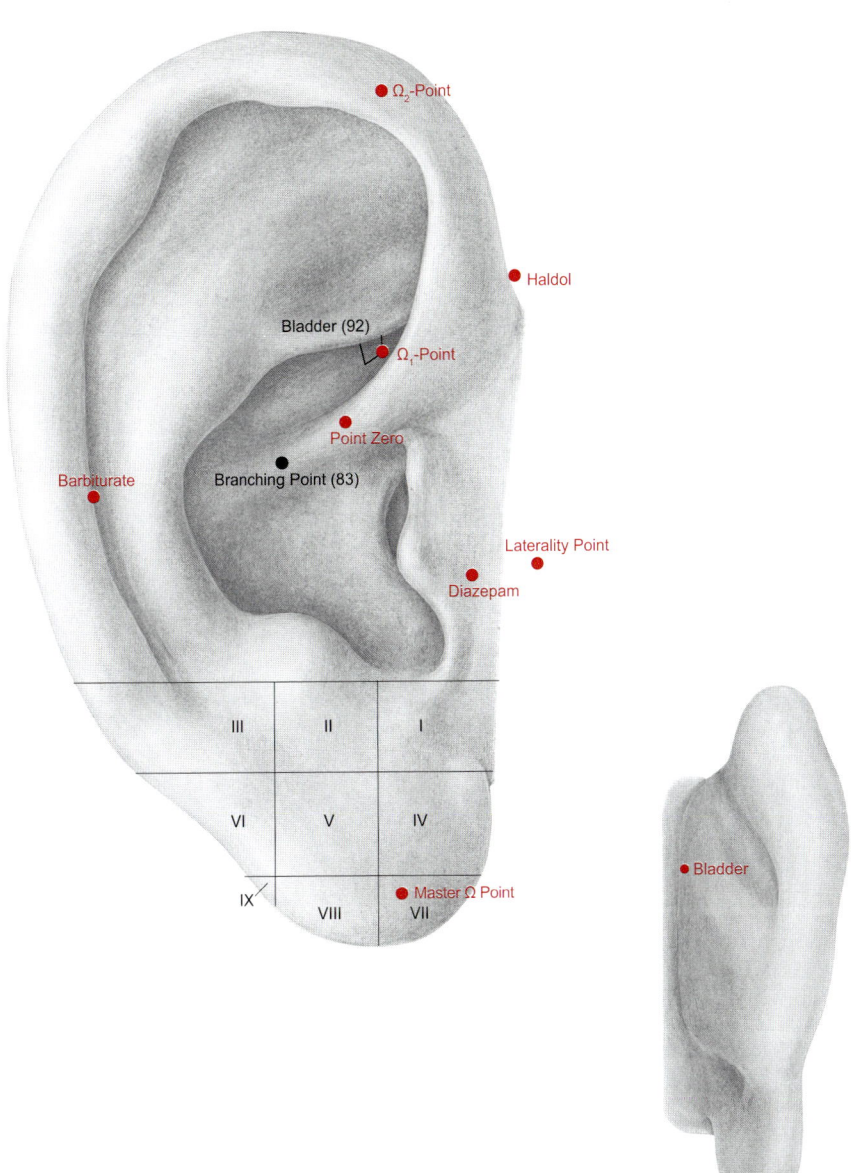

Ω$_2$-Point

Haldol

Bladder (92)

Ω$_1$-Point

Point Zero

Barbiturate

Branching Point (83)

Laterality Point

Diazepam

III   II   I

VI   V   IV

IX

VIII   VII

Master Ω Point

Bladder

Fig. 8.4-3a+b

8.4.4 Nephrolithiasis

Description

- Recurrent formation of stones of varying sizes and composition in the kidneys, the renal pelvis, and the urinary tract
- Chronic kidney stones: often asymptomatic; larger stones can cause dull recurrent pain in the lumbar area or along the course of the ureters (due to their size larger stones cannot move and become stuck)
- Mobilisation (or passing) of stones: acute colicky abdominal pain along the course of the ureters; depending on the location of the stone the pain may radiate to the lumbar region, groin, or genital area; microhematuria, gross hematuria
- Exacerbating factors:
  - protein-rich foods; increased fluid loss (hot and arid climate, insufficient fluid intake)
  - endocrine disorders affecting calcium metabolism, e.g. hyperparathyrodism
  - disorders affecting uric acid metabolism

Point Prescription

The point prescription is determined by RAC-palpation (› 3.1.4):

French points

- Local points: **Kidney I** (› 6.5.1), **Kidney II** (› 6.5.4)
- Relaxing points: **Diazepam** (› 6.7.3), **Barbiturate** (› 6.7.1)

Chinese points

- Local points: **Kidney (95)**, **Ureter (94)** (› 6.5.1)
- Analgesic point: **Thalamus (26a)** (› 6.7.4)

 Acupuncture is contraindicated if a stone cannot be passed naturally (risk of complications with larger concrements). Such cases require therapy with cystoscopy or shock wave lithotripsy.

Treatment Intervals

- **Acute colic:** once or twice daily until passing of the stone
- **During pain-free remission:** 3 times weekly until passing of the stone; **Caution:** acupuncture can trigger acute colic
- Acupuncture as adjuvant therapy with conventional therapy (e.g. lithotripsy): twice weekly until stone fragments have been passed, or post-operatively to accelerate the healing process

- During an acute colic conventional spasmolytic medication is the treatment of choice (e.g. analgesics).
- Once the acute colic has subsided auricular acupuncture can promote the passage of the stone.
- Sufficient fluid intake is crucial.

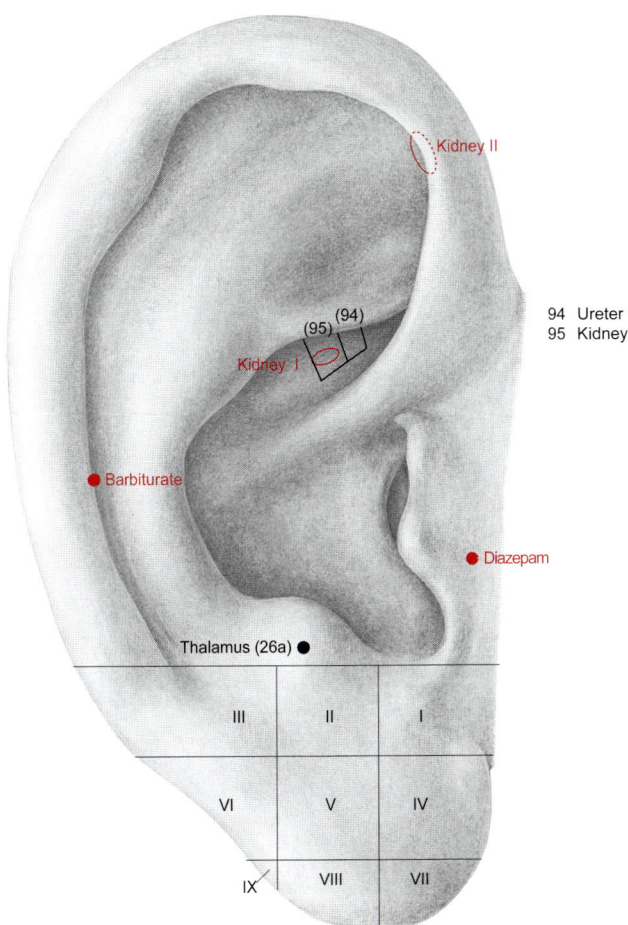

Kidney II

(94)
(95)

Kidney I

94 Ureter
95 Kidney

Barbiturate

Diazepam

Thalamus (26a)

III	II	I
VI	V	IV
IX	VIII	VII

Fig. 8.4-4

Treatment Course and Prognosis

- **Acute colic:** symptoms usually subside after one to several days, especially with smaller concrements
- **Prophylaxis** following stone removal: 3 months for a sustained relief from symptoms

box

Prophylaxis and curative therapy with auricular acupuncture is possible only after resolving the underlying disorder (e.g. hyperparathyroidism). Otherwise, auricular acupuncture can provide symptomatic relief during pain attacks.

8.4.5 Prostatic Hyperplasia (Prostate Adenoma)

Description

- Benign enlargement of the prostate; occurs in 60 % of males over the age of 50
- Symptoms: delayed urinary stream, weak stream; possibly urinary frequency, dysuria, and nocturia; in advanced stages incomplete voiding

> **box** Before starting acupuncture treatments urological diagnostic tests should be carried out to exclude the possibility of a prostate carcinoma.

Point Prescription

French points
- Local points: **Prostate** (› 6.5.2) on the anterior ear; possibly **Bladder** (› 6.11.3) on the posterior ear
- Stabilising point: **Point Zero** (› 6.10.3)

Chinese points
- Local points: **Prostate (93)** (› 6.5.1), possibly **Bladder (92)** (› 6.5.1)

Treatment Intervals

- Initially once weekly until urinary difficulties have improved (after approximately 4 weeks)
- Then 2–3 times monthly until there is no further improvement

Treatment Course and Prognosis

- Improvement of dysuria and nocturia after approximately 1–3 months due to changes in the blood flow to the adenoma.
- Only a limited reduction of prostate hyperplasia is possible

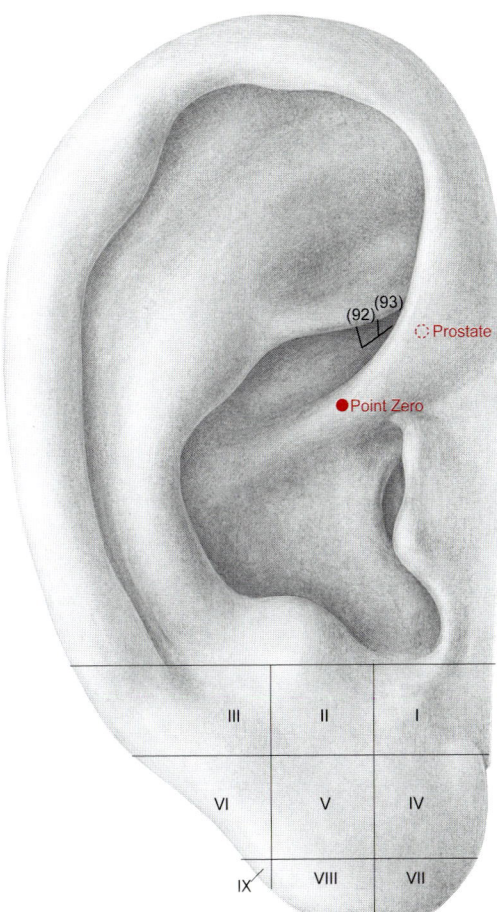

(92) (93)
◌ Prostate

● Point Zero

92 Bladder
93 Prostate

● Bladder

III | II | I
VI | V | IV
IX | VIII | VII

Fig. 8.4-5a+b

8.4.6 Sexual and Erectile Dysfunction

Description

- Forms: erectile dysfunction, ejaculatory dysfunction (e.g. premature ejaculation; male infertility due to low sperm count (oligospermia) or absence of sperm (azoospermia)
- Causes:
  - psychological, e.g. stress, excessive strain, exhaustion
  - organic, e.g. Peyronie's disease, hydrocoele, hernia, foreskin anomalies; diabetes mellitus, obesity, Graves' disease; history of pelvic or spinal surgery
  - toxicological, e.g. alcohol/drug abuse, certain medications (β-blockers, psychopharmacological drugs)

> **box** Before starting treatment with acupuncture possible organic causes of the sexual dysfunction should be investigated and treated if necessary (surgery?).

Point Prescription

French points
- Hormonal point: **Testes/Ovaries** (› 6.5.2)
- Stabilising points: **Point Bosch** (› 6.5.2), **Laterality Point** (› 6.8.6)
- Psychological points: **Haldol** (› 6.8.6), **Frustration** (› 6.8.3), **Omega Axis** (› 6.12.1)

Chinese points
- Local points: **Testes (32)** (› 6.5.3), **External Genitalia (79)** (› 6.5.2), **Ovaries (23)** (› 6.5.1)

Treatment Intervals

- Initially once weekly for approximately 4 weeks
- Then 2–3 times monthly

Treatment Course and Prognosis

- **Psychological causes:** depending on the duration of the disorder approximately 3–6 months until satisfactory sexual intercourse is possible or the sperm count is increasing
- **Toxicological causes:** curative treatments are possible only if the noxious agent can be eliminated or the relevant medication is replaced; otherwise continued supportive treatments will be necessary
- **Organic causes:** successful treatment of the sexual dysfunction is possible if the underlying disorder is resolved
- **In all cases:** if there is no response to auricular acupuncture (possibly complemented by body acupuncture and Chinese herbal medicine) for > 6 months no further improvement can be expected with acupuncture

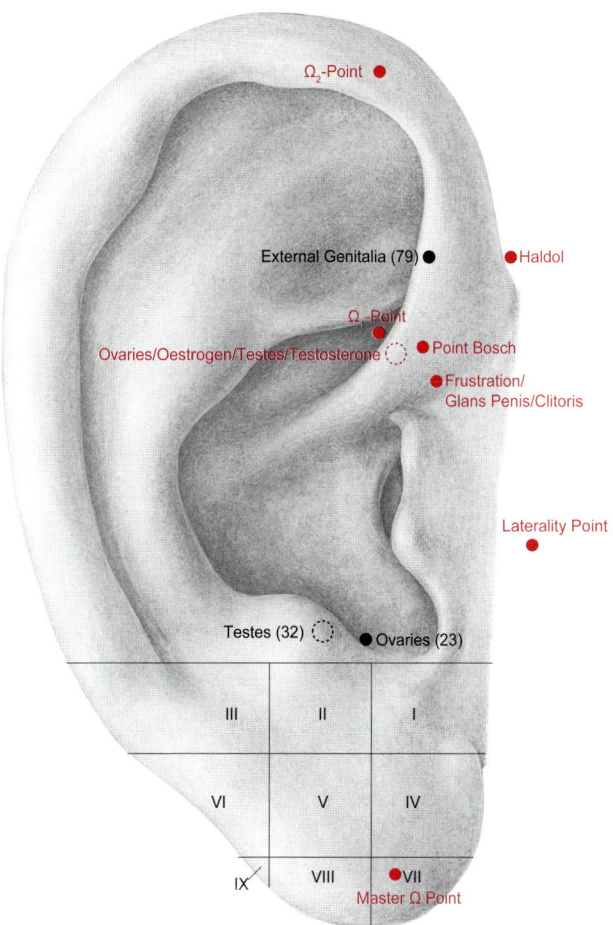

Ω_2-Point ●

External Genitalia (79) ●   ● Haldol

Ω_1-Point ●

Ovaries/Oestrogen/Testes/Testosterone ⭘ ● Point Bosch

● Frustration/
Glans Penis/Clitoris

Laterality Point
●

Testes (32) ⭘   ● Ovaries (23)

III	II	I
VI	V	IV
IX	VIII	●VII

Master Ω Point

Fig. 8.4-6

8.4.7 Enuresis

Description

- Unintentional passing of urine after the age of 4
- Generally during the night only (nocturnal enuresis), only rarely during the day; in 25 % of cases enuresis both during the day and night
- causes:
  - often psychological strain, e.g. neglect or withdrawal of affection
  - organic causes: e.g. cystitis, spina bifida, or malformation of the urogenital system

Point Prescription

French points

- Local point: **Bladder** (› 6.11.3) on the posterior ear
- Stabilising points: **Laterality Point** (› 6.8.6), **Point Zero** (› 6.10.3)
- Psychological points: **Omega Axis** (› 6.12.1), **Antidepressant Axis** (› 6.12.6), **Haldol** (› 6.8.6), **Anti-Aggression** (› 6.8.5)

Chinese points

- Local point: **Bladder (92)** (› 6.5.1)
- Stabilising point: **Branching Point (83)** (› 6.10.1)

> **box** For enuresis due to organic causes (e. g. urinary tract infections [› 8.4.1]) acupuncture treatments have to be modified accordingly. This could be a combination of acupuncture and conservative or surgical treatments (in cases of malformation of the urogenital system) or exclusively conventional treatments.

Treatment Intervals

- Initially once weekly until wetting has significantly reduced; the best time for acupuncture/laser treatments is the early evening (› 4.2)
- Then twice monthly until symptoms have disappeared

> **box** Children should be treated with a laser (› 4.2), not with needles.

Treatment Course and Prognosis

- Enuresis due to psychological causes: generally 3–6 months until symptoms disappear
- Both diagnosis and treatment should focus on the psychosocial component (› 8.15.2)

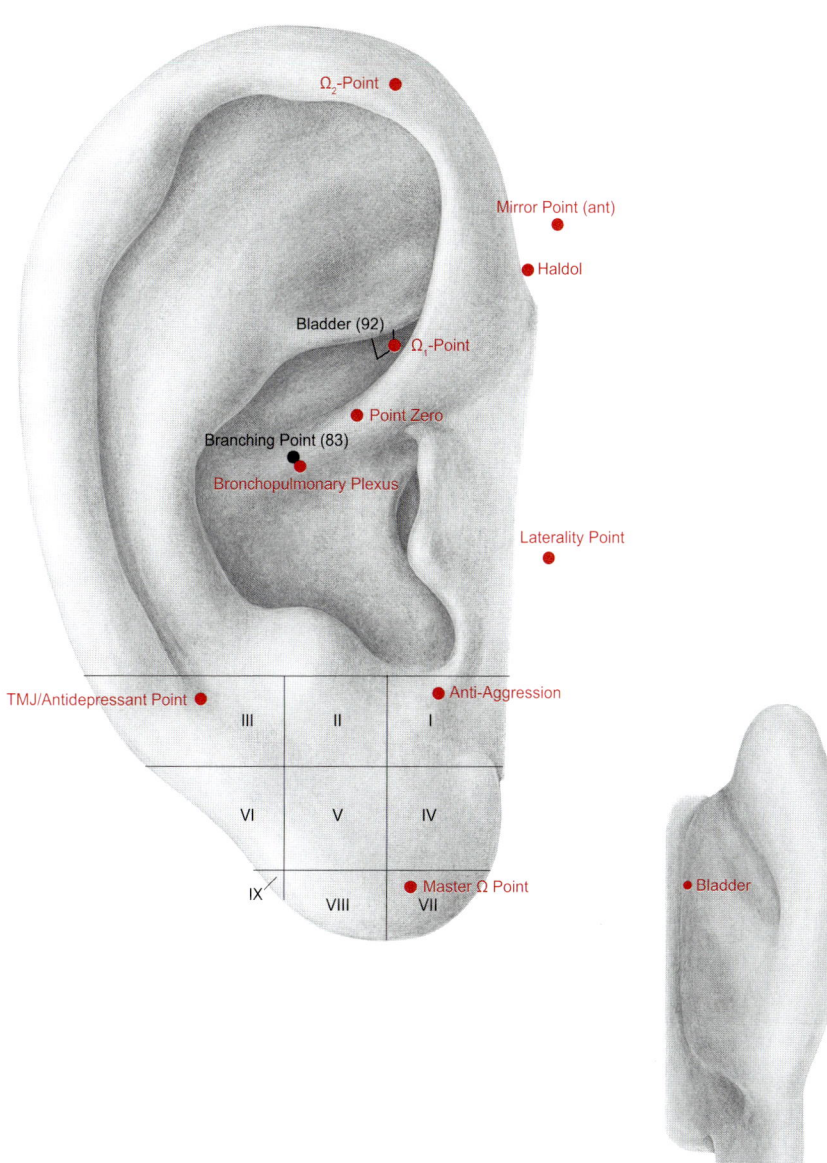

Ω_2-Point

Mirror Point (ant)

Haldol

Bladder (92)
Ω_1-Point

Point Zero

Branching Point (83)

Bronchopulmonary Plexus

Laterality Point

TMJ/Antidepressant Point

Anti-Aggression

III   II   I

VI   V   IV

IX

VIII   VII

Master Ω Point

Bladder

Fig. 8.4-7a+b

8.5 Skin Disorders

8.5.1 Atopic Dermatitis (Atopic Eczema)

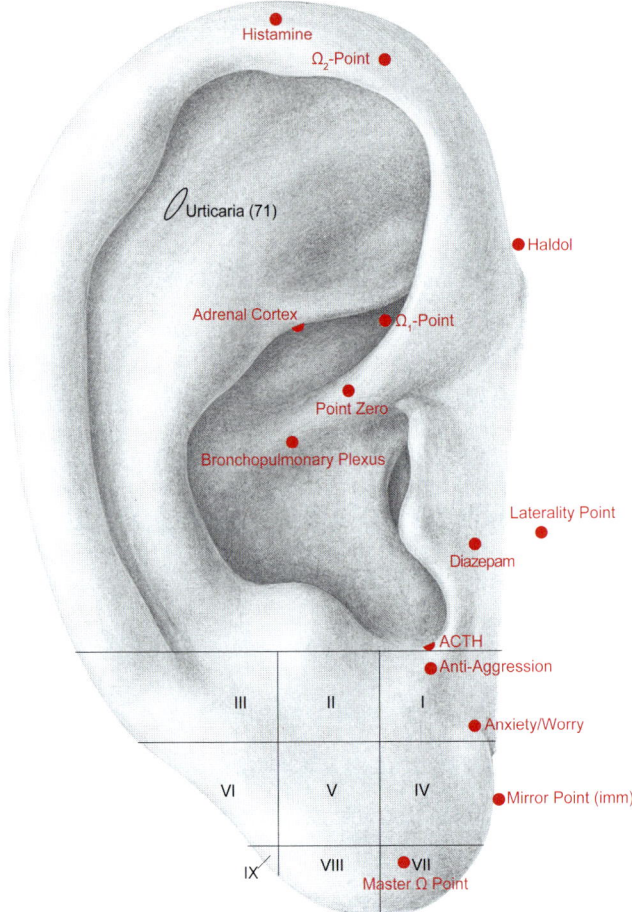

Fig. 8.5-1

Description

- Chronic or chronic recurrent itching eczema (pruritus often much worse during the night), often accompanied by other atopic disorders (also by allergic rhinitis › 8.6.1 or bronchial asthma › 8.2.1)
- Areas most affected: knee creases, elbow creases, face, neck
- Aetiology: polygenic inheritance; increased tendency to allergies; exacerbated by psychological stress and itching
- Sequelae/accompanying disorders: lichenification (coarsening of the epidermis), candidiasis, secondary pyoderma

Point Prescription

French points

- Local point: **Bronchopulmonary Plexus** (› 6.10.1)
- Immunostimulant points: **Immune Axis** (› 6.12.3), **Adrenal Cortex** (› 6.6.1), **ACTH** (› 6.6.6), **Histamine** (› 6.6.4)
- Stabilising points: **Laterality Point** (› 6.8.6), **Point Zero** (› 6.10.3)
- Psychological points: **Omega Axis** (› 6.12.1), **Anxiety, Worry** (› 6.8.5), **Haldol** (› 6.8.6), **Diazepam** (› 6.7.3), **Anti-Aggression** (› 6.8.5)

Chinese points

- Stabilising point: **Urticaria zone (71)** (› 6.10.2)

- During or after cortisone treatment the immunostimulant points should be treated very cautiously as they may trigger an initial worsening of symptoms.
- As symptoms improve to auricular acupuncture cortisone preparations can be slowly reduced.

Treatment Intervals

- **Acute episode:** 2–3 times weekly
- Once the **acute episode** has **subsided**: 2–4 times monthly

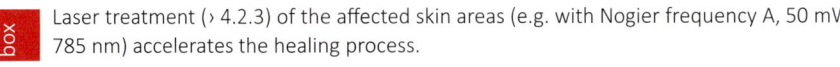

Laser treatment (› 4.2.3) of the affected skin areas (e.g. with Nogier frequency A, 50 mW, 785 nm) accelerates the healing process.

Treatment Course and Prognosis

- During acute episodes eczema and itching generally subside within a few days
- Sustained reduction of symptoms (symptoms rarely disappear completely) after approximately 1–2 years; cortisone can be discontinued in most cases

8.5.2 Psoriasis

Description

- Chronic relapsing skin disorder; often in the form of itching plaques covered by silvery white scaly skin and with sharply delineated borders
- Areas most affected: scalp, flexor side of the knees and elbows, sacrum
- Triggered/exacerbated by: psychological stress, pregnancy, infections, alcohol, certain medications (such as NSAIDs, β-Blocker)
- Accompanying symptoms: possibly joint pain (psoriatic arthritis)

Point Prescription

French points

- Local point: **Bronchopulmonary Plexus** (› 6.10.1)
- Immunostimulant points: **Immune Axis** (› 6.12.3), **Adrenal Cortex** (› 6.6.1), **ACTH** (› 6.6.6)
- Stabilising points: **Laterality Point** (› 6.8.6), **Point Zero** (› 6.10.3)
- Psychological points: **Omega Axis** (› 6.12.1), **Haldol** (› 6.8.6), **Diazepam** (› 6.7.3), **Anti-Aggression** (› 6.8.5)

Chinese points

- Stabilising point: **Urticaria Zone (71)** (› 6.10.2)
- Immunostimulant points: **Endocrine System (22)** (› 6.6.2), **Adrenal Glands (13)** (› 6.6.6), **Pituitary Gland (28)** (› 6.6.7)

- During or after cortisone treatment immunostimulant points should be treated very cautiously as they may trigger an initial worsening of symptoms.
- As symptoms continue to respond to auricular acupuncture cortisone preparations can be slowly reduced.

Treatment Intervals

- **Acute episode:** 2–3 times weekly
- Once the **acute episode** has **subsided**: 2–4 times monthly

Extensive laser treatment of the affected skin areas (e.g. with Nogier frequency A, 50 mW, 785 nm › 4.2.3) can further accelerate the healing process. Of additional benefit is the combination with Psoralen plus ultraviolet A therapy (PUVA). Cortisone, on the other hand, should be avoided.

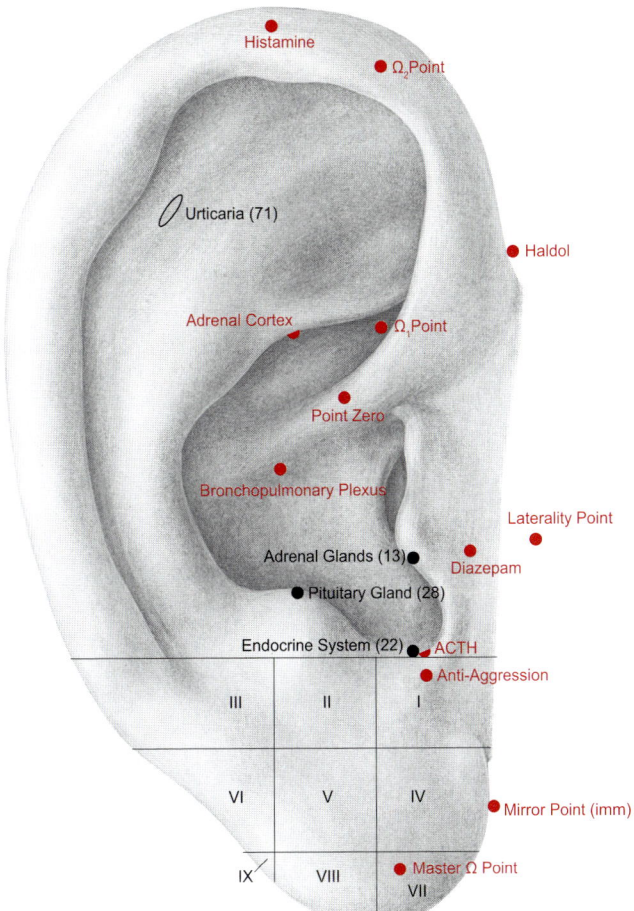

Fig. 8.5-2

Treatment Course and Prognosis

- During acute episodes plaques and itching as well as hyperkeratosis may subside within days
- With auricular acupuncture only a sustained reduction of symptoms (symptoms rarely disappear completely) can be achieved within 1–2 years; a sustained relief from symptoms can be achieved in the same period by combining auricular acupuncture with body acupuncture and Chinese herbal medicine

8.5.3 Herpes Zoster (Shingles)

Description

- Neurotropic viral infection caused by a reactivation of the varicella zoster virus; often occurs a long time after the initial infection (chickenpox)
- Generally unilateral, segmental skin rash with blisters; the rash may be preceded, accompanied, or outlasted by severe pain
- Usually affects one or more thoracic segments (the area supplied by a spinal nerve); the face (oculomotor nerve [ophthalmic zoster], facial nerve, or trigeminal nerve) is affected less commonly
- Risk of postherpetic neuralgia: pain along the affected segment persisting after the rash has healed

Point Prescription

French points

- Defense against infection: **Thymus** (› 6.6.1), **Interferon** (› 6.7.3), **Infection Axis** (› 6.12.4), **Neural Thymus Point** (› 6.9.2)
- Stabilising points: **Point Zero** (› 6.10.3), **Laterality Point** (› 6.8.6)
- Psychological points: **Diazepam** (› 6.7.3), **Barbiturate** (› 6.7.1), **Haldol** (› 6.8.6)

Chinese points

- Analgesic points: **Sun (35)** (› 6.7.4), **Thalamus (26a)** (› 6.7.4), **Occiput (29)** (› 6.7.4)
- Stabilising point: **Shen Men (55)** (› 6.7.2), **Apex of the Ear (78)** (› 6.10.3)

Treatment Intervals

- To promote healing of the rash and provide pain relief: depending on the severity of the case 2–3 times weekly
- Once both the pain and the rash have subsided: once weekly
- For neuralgias persisting for > 8 weeks: 2–3 times monthly

> **box** Extensive laser treatment of the affected skin areas (e.g. with Nogier frequency A, 50 mW, 785 nm › 4.2.3) can further accelerate the healing of the rash.

Treatment Course and Prognosis

- Depending on the patient's age and the severity of the case: 1–3 months

> **box** Auricular acupuncture can significantly shorten the duration of the disease, lower the risk of postherpetic neuralgia, and reduce the requirement for analgesic medication.

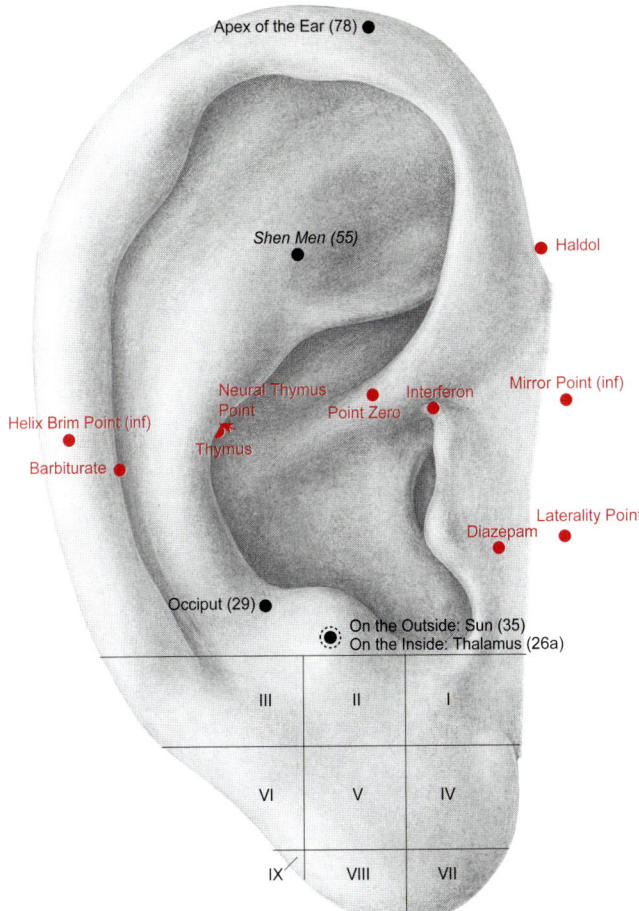

Apex of the Ear (78) ●

Shen Men (55) ●

● Haldol

Neural Thymus Point ●

Interferon ●

Point Zero ●

● Mirror Point (inf)

Helix Brim Point (inf) ●

Thymus

Barbiturate ●

Laterality Point ●

Diazepam ●

Occiput (29) ●

On the Outside: Sun (35)
On the Inside: Thalamus (26a)

III	II	I
VI	V	IV
IX	VIII	VII

Fig. 8.5-3

8.6 Allergic Diseases

8.6.1 Allergic Rhinitis (Hay Fever)

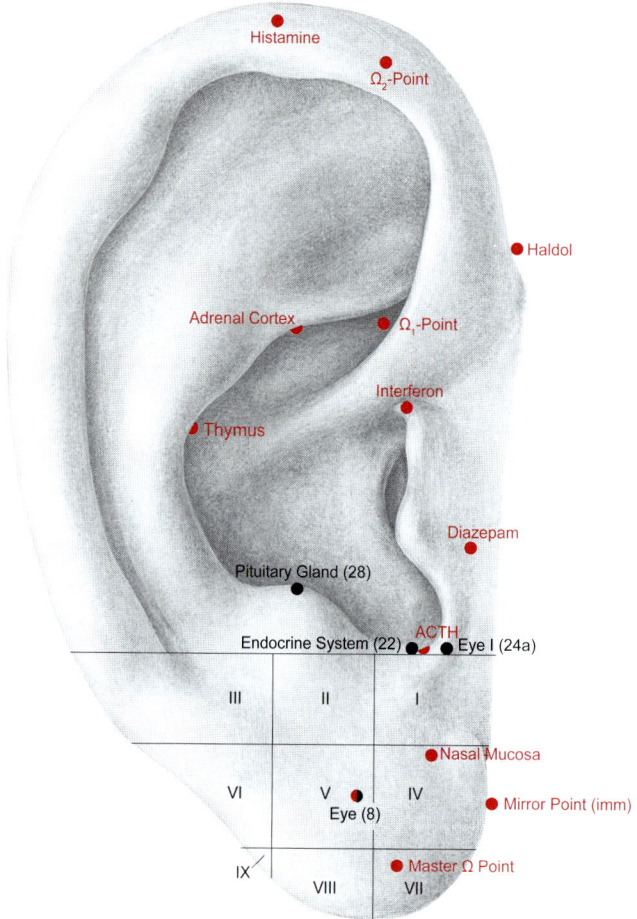

Histamine

Ω_2-Point

Haldol

Adrenal Cortex

Ω_1-Point

Interferon

Thymus

Diazepam

Pituitary Gland (28)

ACTH

Endocrine System (22)

Eye I (24a)

III   II   I

Nasal Mucosa

VI   V   IV

Eye (8)

Mirror Point (imm)

IX   Master Ω Point

VIII   VII

Fig. 8.6-1

Description

- Allergic reaction of the mucosa of the upper respiratory tract to the pollen of flowering plants and grasses; especially during high pollen count in spring and summer
- Symptoms:
  - burning or itching of the nose, eyes, and the palate
  - sneezing fits with clear discharge
  - periorbital swelling
- Atopic disorder, such as atopic dermatitis (› 8.5.1) and bronchial asthma (› 8.2.1)

Point Prescription

French points

- Local point: **Nasal Mucosa** (› 6.3.4)
- Immunostimulant points: **Interferon** (› 6.7.3), **Histamine** (› 6.6.4), **ACTH** (› 6.6.6), **Adrenal Cortex** (› 6.6.1), **Immune Axis** (› 6.12.3), **Thymus** (› 6.6.1)
- Psychological points: **Haldol** (› 6.8.6), **Diazepam** (› 6.7.3), **Omega Axis** (› 6.12.1)

Chinese points

- Local points: **Eye (8)** (› 6.3.4), **Eye I (24a)** (› 6.3.4)
- Immunostimulant points: **Endocrine System (22)** (› 6.6.2), **Pituitary Gland (28)** (› 6.6.7)

Treatment Intervals

- **Prophylaxis:** once weekly for 6 weeks; start of prophylactic treatments 2–3 weeks prior to the expected onset of the hay fever
- Treatment start during the **acute stage:** initially 2–3 times weekly; once symptoms begin to subside 2–4 times monthly until symptoms have disappeared

Treatment Course and Prognosis

- Successful prophylaxis with auricular acupuncture possible
- Treatment start during the acute stage: generally 2–4 weeks until symptoms disappear
- Generally 1–3 months (depending on the severity) for a sustained relief from symptoms

> box
>
> Hay fever and chronic sinusitis frequently occur together. Nasal congestion may therefore persist, especially in the mornings, even after successfully resolving the allergic rhinitis. In such cases it is important to treat the sinusitis (› 8.2.4) first.

8.6.2 Urticaria (Hives)

Description

- Inflammatory reaction of the skin to an allergen with varying forms of rashes and itching:
  - locally: e.g. contact allergy
  - generalised: caused by an endogenous trigger, e.g. allergy to medication
- The trigger often remains unknown, even with allergy testing.

Point Prescription

French points

- Local point: **Bronchopulmonary Plexus** (› 6.10.1)
- Immunostimulant points: **Immune Axis** (› 6.12.3), **Adrenal Cortex** (› 6.6.1), **ACTH** (› 6.6.6), **Histamine** (› 6.6.4)
- Stabilising points: **Laterality Point** (› 6.8.6), **Point Zero** (› 6.10.3)
- Psychological points: **Omega Axis** (› 6.12.1), **Haldol** (› 6.8.6), **Diazepam** (› 6.7.3), **Anti-Aggression** (› 6.8.5)

Chinese points

- Stabilising points: **Urticaria Zone (71)** (› 6.10.2), *Shen Men* **(55)** (› 6.7.2)

 During or after cortisone treatment the immune points should be treated very cautiously as they may trigger an initial worsening of symptoms.

Treatment Intervals

- **Acute stage:** 2–3 times weekly for approximately 1–4 weeks
- Symptoms persisting for > 4 weeks: once weekly

Treatment Course and Prognosis

- If the triggering allergen can be avoided both hives and itching will disappear within days.
- Unknown allergen: treatments required for several months until symptoms disappear; postulated mechanism: strengthening the immune system prevents the reaction to the allergen.

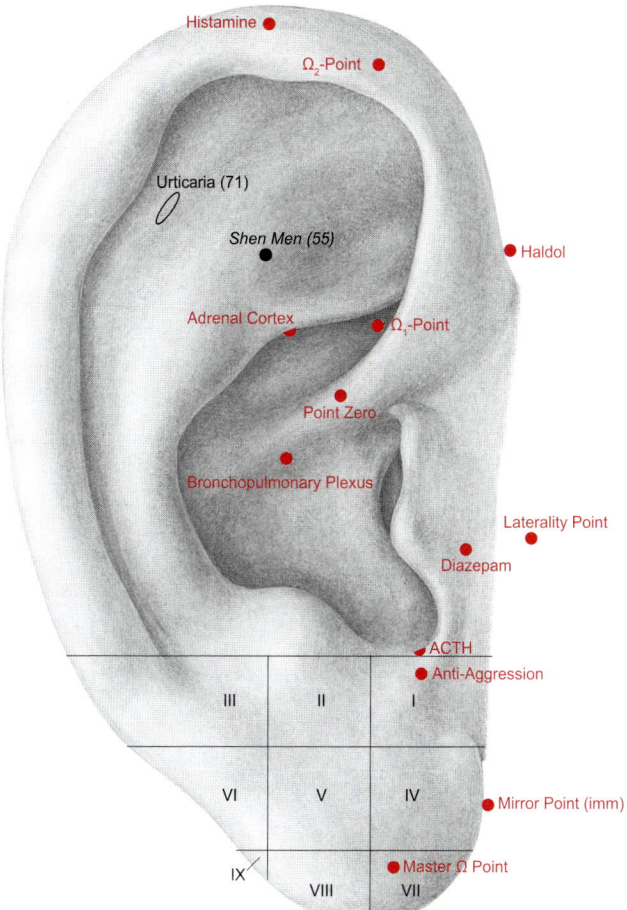

Histamine

Ω₂-Point

Urticaria (71)

Shen Men (55)

Haldol

Adrenal Cortex

Ω₁-Point

Point Zero

Bronchopulmonary Plexus

Laterality Point

Diazepam

ACTH

Anti-Aggression

III   II   I

VI   V   IV

Mirror Point (imm)

IX   VIII   VII

Master Ω Point

Fig. 8.6-2

8.6.3 Food Allergy

Description

- Immediate allergy (type I hypersensitivity) following consumption of certain foods such as cow's milk, tomatoes, citrus fruit, strawberries, nuts, fish, seafood
- Symptoms:
  - predominantly gastrointestinal reactions such as diarrhoea, bloating, abdominal pain
  - also cutaneous (hives) or respiratory reactions

Point Prescription

French points

- Immunostimulant points: **Interferon** (> 6.7.3), **Histamine** (> 6.6.4), **ACTH** (> 6.6.6), **Adrenal Cortex** (> 6.6.1), **Immune Axis** (> 6.12.3)
- Psychological points: **Haldol** (> 6.8.6), **Diazepam** (> 6.7.3), **Omega Axis** (> 6.12.1)
- Stabilising points: **Point Zero** (> 6.10.3), **Laterality Point** (> 6.8.6)

Chinese points

- Local points: **Stomach (87)**, **Small Intestine (89)**, **Colon (91)** (> 6.4.1)
- Immunostimulant points: **Endocrine System (22)** (> 6.6.2), **Pituitary Gland (28)** (> 6.6.7)

Treatment Intervals

- **Acute stage:** 2–3 times weekly
- As symptoms improve: once weekly until symptoms have disappeared

Treatment Course and Prognosis

- Treatment start during the acute stage: generally 2–4 weeks until symptoms subside; triggering foods have to be avoided initially
- Resolving the food allergy may be possible and take 2–3 months; avoiding the relevant food is then no longer necessary (probably due to the stabilisation of the immune system)

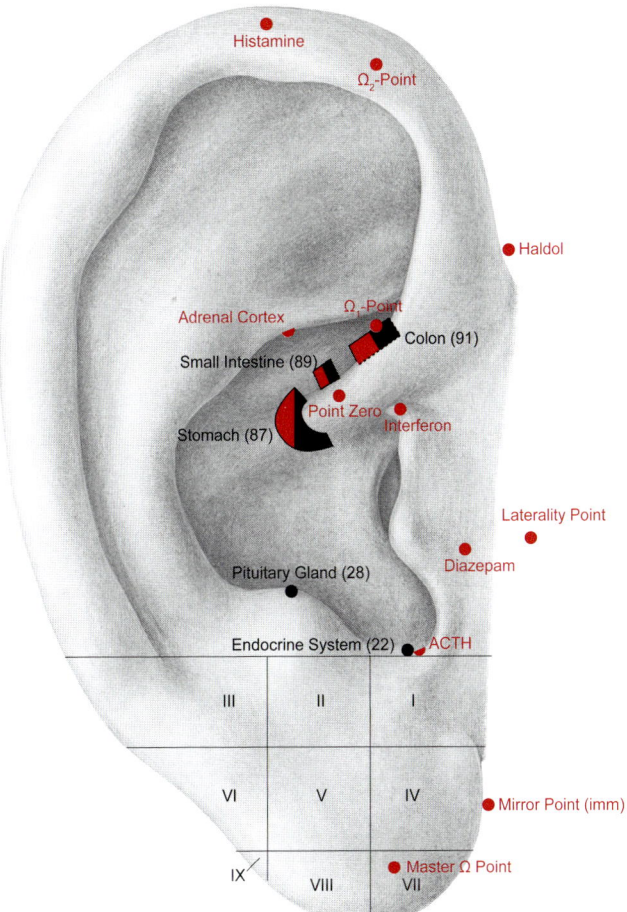

Histamine

Ω_2-Point

Haldol

Adrenal Cortex

Ω_1-Point

Colon (91)

Small Intestine (89)

Point Zero

Interferon

Stomach (87)

Laterality Point

Pituitary Gland (28)

Diazepam

Endocrine System (22)

ACTH

III

II

I

VI

V

IV

Mirror Point (imm)

IX

VIII

VII

Master Ω Point

Fig. 8.6-3

8.7 Eye Disorders

8.7.1 Macular Degeneration

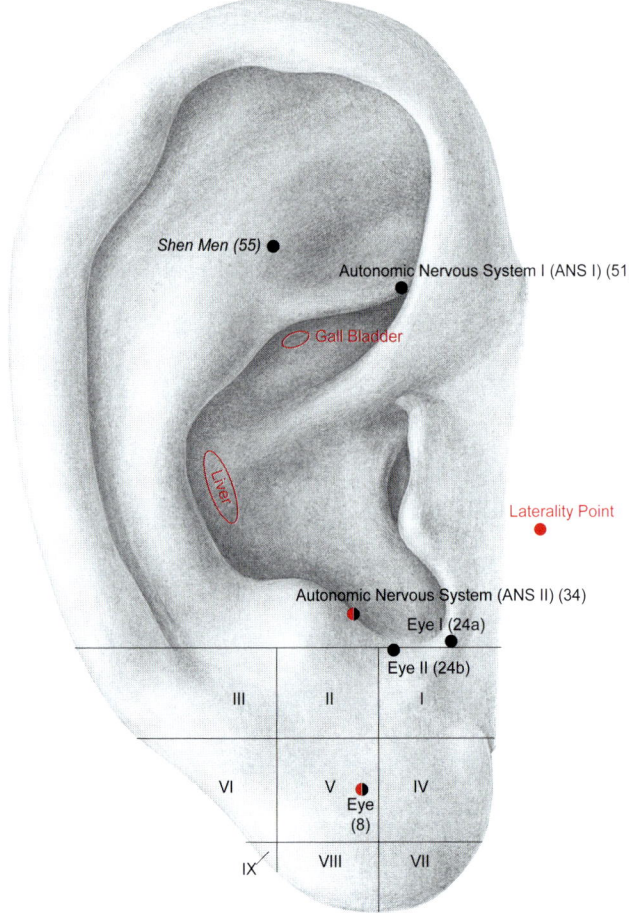

Shen Men (55)

Autonomic Nervous System I (ANS I) (51)

Gall Bladder

Liver

Laterality Point

Autonomic Nervous System (ANS II) (34)

Eye I (24a)

Eye II (24b)

III   II   I

VI   V   IV
Eye
(8)

IX   VIII   VII

Fig. 8.7-1

Description

- Progressive loss of sight
- Generally affects both eyes
- Forms: dry form with atrophy of the retinal pigment epithelium, better prognosis; wet form with serous detachment of the retina from the pigment epithelium (more severe loss of visual acuity). Either form can transform into the other.

- Causes:
  - deposits of hyaline material in the retinal pigment epithelium
  - wet form: during the final stage also subretinal neovascularization with macular scarring

Point Prescription

French points
- Local points: **Eye (8)** (› 6.3.4); **Gallbladder** (› 6.4.1), **Liver** (› 6.4.1)
- Stabilising point: **Laterality Point** (› 6.8.6)

Chinese points
- Local points: **Eye (8)**, **Eye I (24a)**, **Eye II (24b)** (› 6.3.4)
- Relaxing point: ***Shen Men* (55)** (› 6.7.2)
- Stabilising points: **ANS I (51)** (› 6.6.5), **ANS II (34)** (› 6.7.4)

Treatment Intervals

Since macular degeneration tends to progress slowly it is not possible to distinguish between acute and chronic symptoms. Once the disease has started, its chronicity is inevitable. However, its progression can be slowed down or even be arrested:

- **Initial treatment phase:** 1–2 times weekly until there is a significant subjective improvement which can be verified (in percentages) by an eye test; the extent of the improvement will depend on the previous visual impairment. Often there will be a measurable improvement of 5–15 %, probably due to the maximum stimulation of exhausted epithelial pigment cells. Damaged cells cannot regenerate.

- **Follow-up treatments:** once there is no further visual improvement 1–3 times monthly (to stabilise eyesight)

- For macular degeneration the combination of auricular and body acupuncture is highly recommended.
- The following body acupuncture points are frequently used: *Yuyao* (fish spine; in the centre of the eyebrow), GB-14, GB-1, ST-1, BL-1, LR-3, TH-3.

Treatment Course and Prognosis

- Lifelong treatments: taking a break from treatments for several months often results in a worsening of symptoms; complete remission is not possible.

8.7.2 Optic Neuritis

Description

- In children often affects both eyes, in adults mostly only one eye
- Loss of visual acuity within hours to days
- Pain on movement of the affected eye
- Central or paracentral scotoma
- Three forms can be distinguished: retrobulbar (most common form), anterior, or neuroretinitis; the first two forms often occur as precursors of multiple sclerosis but also in conjunction with collagenoses (such as lupus erythematodes), infectious diseases (e.g. Lyme disease) or vaccinations
- Causes: demyelination of the optic nerve

Point Prescription

French points

- Local points: **Eye = Eye (8)** (› 6.3.4), **Gallbladder** (› 6.4.1), **Liver** (› 6.4.1)
- Anti-inflammatory points: **Adrenal Cortex** (› 6.6.1), **ACTH** (› 6.6.6), **Immune Axis** (› 6.12.3), **Infection Axis** (› 6.12.4), **PGE$_1$/Thymus** (› 6.7.6)
- Psychological points: **Omega Axis** (› 6.12.1), **Resentment** (› 6.8.1)

Chinese points

- Local points: **Eye (8)**, **Eye I (24a)**, **Eye II (24b)** (› 6.3.4)
- Relaxing point: Shen **Men (55)** (› 6.7.2)

Treatment Intervals

- **Acute symptoms:** once daily or every 2–3 days until there is both a marked visual improvement and reduction of pain
- **Chronic symptoms:** 2–3 times weekly for approximately 4 weeks; then 1–2 times weekly until symptoms have disappeared

Treatment Course and Prognosis

- **Acute symptoms:** increasing improvement and eventually complete relief from symptoms within a few days and up to several weeks
- **Chronic symptoms:** complete remission within a few months

> **box** Following an episode of retrobulbar neuritis there is a 5-year risk of developing multiple sclerosis (› 8.11.1). The patient should be loosely monitored, recommended are early treatments with acupuncture.

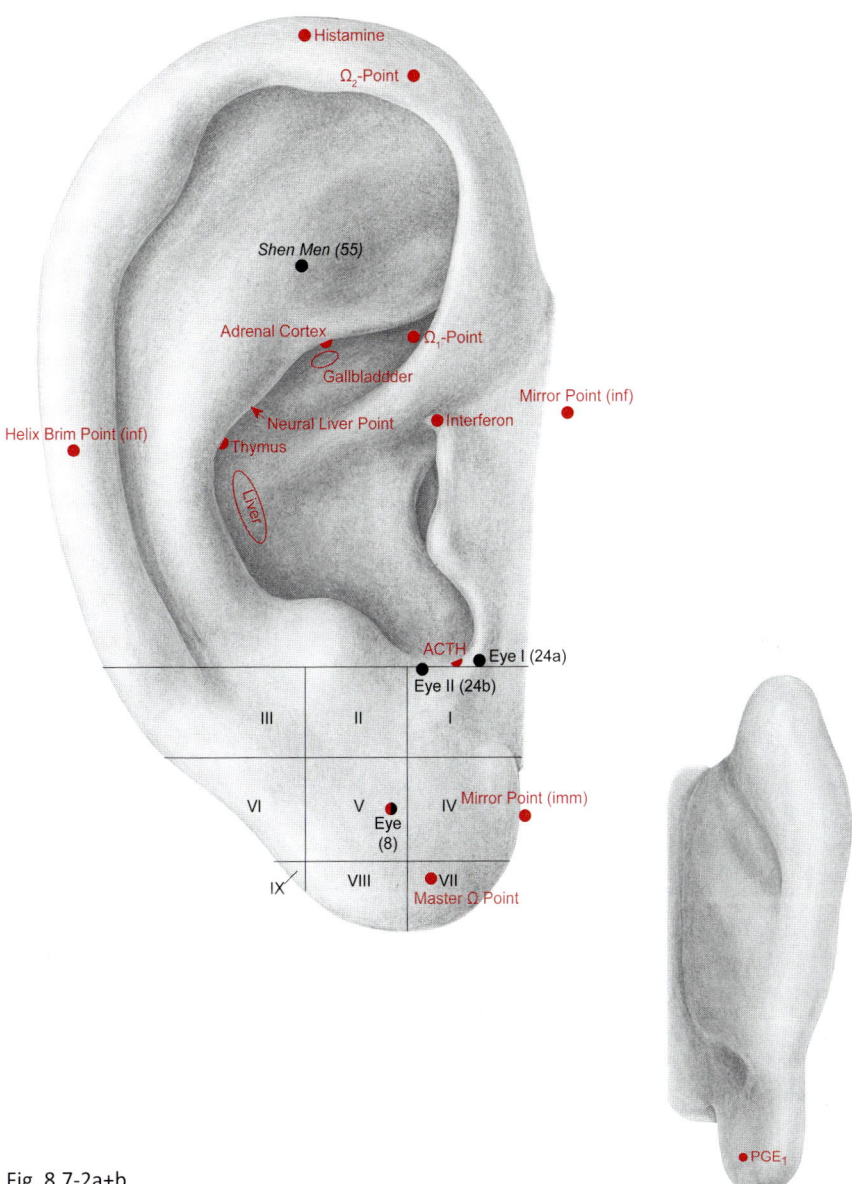

Histamine

Ω_2-Point

Shen Men (55)

Adrenal Cortex

Ω_1-Point

Gallbladder

Mirror Point (inf)

Helix Brim Point (inf)

Neural Liver Point

Interferon

Thymus

Liver

ACTH

Eye I (24a)

Eye II (24b)

III

II

I

VI

V

IV — Mirror Point (imm)

Eye (8)

IX

VIII

VII

Master Ω Point

PGE$_1$

Fig. 8.7-2a+b

8.8 Addictions

8.8.1 Nicotine Addiction

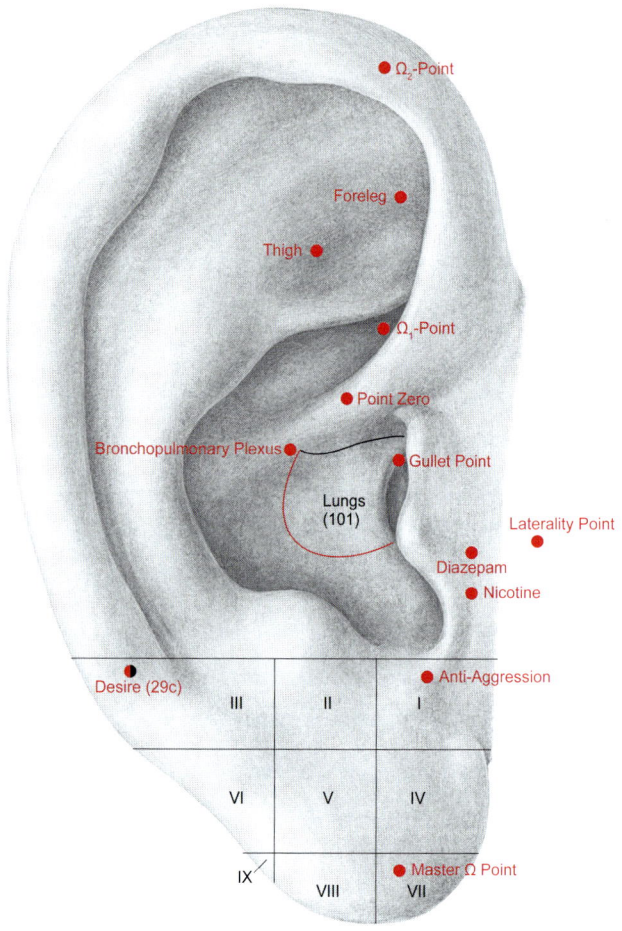

Fig. 8.8-1

Description

- Psychodynamics: oral satisfaction of needs, e.g. with stress, frustration; peer pressure
- Accompanying disorders (associated with long-term smoking) include: chronic bronchitis, peripheral arterial occlusive disease

box During nicotine withdrawal acupuncture can alleviate symptoms such as nervousness, aggression, or compensatory 'food binges'. For a successful withdrawal it is important to become aware of the habitual character of smoking, e.g. smoking when in company. The habitual nature of smoking is the most severe obstacle to treatment.

Point Prescription

Abstaining from nicotine for several days before starting treatments supports precise RAC-palpation.

French points

- Local points: **Nicotine** (› 6.8.4), **Gullet Point** (› 6.4.1)
- Psychological points: **Anti-Aggression** (› 6.8.5), **Master-Ω-Point** (› 6.8.5), **Diazepam** (› 6.7.3), **Omega Axis** (› 6.12.1)
- Stabilising points: **Point Zero** (› 6.10.3), **Laterality Point** (› 6.8.6), **Desire** (› 6.8.3)
- Points for accompanying disorders: **Bronchopulmonary Plexus** (› 6.10.1), **Lung (101)** (› 6.4.1), **Thigh**, **Foreleg** (› 6.2.3)

- 1–3 semi-permanent needles can provide additional support; of particular benefit are the points Nicotine and Gullet Point.
- The patient should be advised to repeatedly stimulate the semi-permanent needles by rotating the magnet in the guide tube (› 3.2.2), in particular if there is the urge to smoke. This can help to better cope with the craving for a cigarette.

In the beginning, acupuncture treatments can be complemented by homoeopathy, e.g. nicotinum D4 or nicotine patches.

Treatment Intervals

- **First week:** acupuncture three times weekly
- **Second week:** acupuncture twice weekly
- **As from the third week:** acupuncture once weekly until the desire to smoke has completely subsided

Treatment Course and Prognosis

- Generally 1–2 months until the patients finds it easy to cope without nicotine
- If there is no withdrawal after 2 months the prognosis is poor

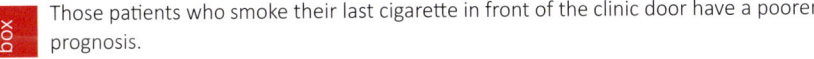

Those patients who smoke their last cigarette in front of the clinic door have a poorer prognosis.

8.8.2 Alcohol Addiction

Description

- Classification of alcohol addiction after Jellinek:
  - alpha alcoholic: no loss of control, drinking as a way to solve problems
  - beta alcoholic: habitual alcohol consumption, drinks to conform; possibly physical consequences
  - gamma alcoholic: loss of control; dependence with both physical and social consequences
  - delta alcoholic: alcoholism with dependency and inability to abstain
  - epsilon alcoholic: excessive alcohol consumption with loss of control (bingeing)
- Physical consequences include: fatty liver, cirrhosis of the liver, gastritis, pancreatitis, cardiomyopathy

Point Prescription

French points

- Local points: **Liver, Gullet Point** (› 6.4.1)
- Psychological points: **Anti-Aggression** , **Jealosy** (› 6.8.5), **Neural Liver Point** (› 6.8.1), **Diazepam** (› 6.7.3), **Haldol** (› 6.8.6), **Omega Axis** (› 6.12.1)
- Stabilising points: **Point Zero** (› 6.10.3), **Laterality Point** (› 6.8.6), **Desire** (› 6.8.3)
- Points for accompanying disorders (if indicated): e.g. **Oesophagus** (› 6.4.1)

Chinese points

- Local points: **Mouth (84)**, **Oesophagus (85)** (› 6.4.1)
- Stabilising point: **Thirst (17)** (› 6.10.5)

- As additional support 2 semi-permanent needles can be inserted, e.g. at the points Liver and Gullet Point, which can remain for up to one week. After a break of a few days new needles can be inserted.
- The patient should repeatedly stimulate the semi-permanent needles by rotating the magnet in the guide tube (› 3.2.2).

Treatment Intervals

- **First week:** 3–7 treatments to ameliorate withdrawal symptoms and to provide psychological support
- **Second week:** 2–3 treatments
- **As from the third week:** 1–2 times weekly until the patient finds it easy to abstain from alcohol

Treatment Course and Prognosis

- Generally it takes 2–3 months until patients find it easy to abstain from alcohol
- If there is no withdrawal within 6–9 months the prognosis is poor; see also drug addiction (› 8.8.3)

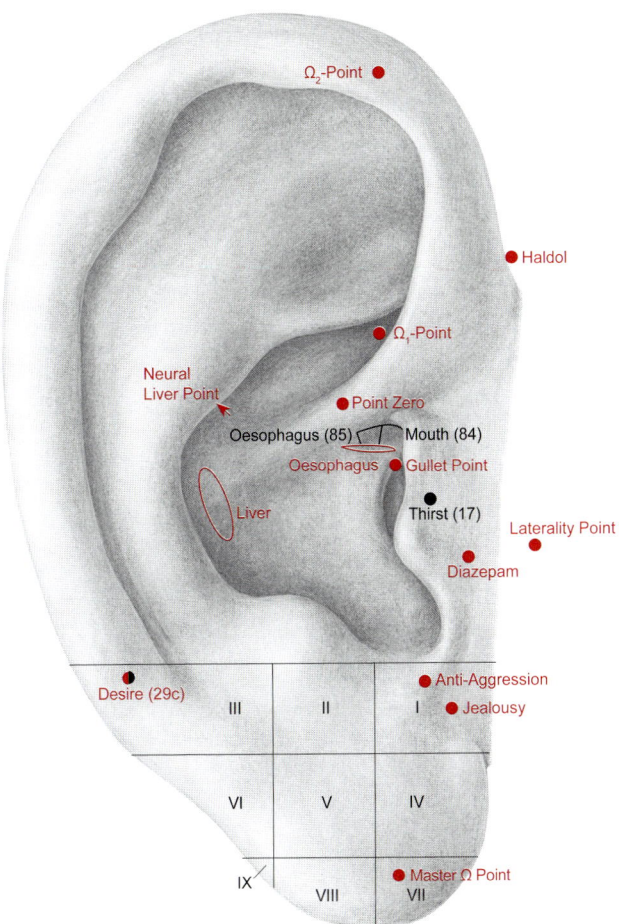

Fig. 8.8-2

- In severe cases alcohol withdrawal has to take place in a clinical setting due to the expected physical symptoms.
- Auricular acupuncture as adjuvant therapy can alleviate psychological withdrawal symptoms.

8.8.3 Drug Addiction

Description

- Depending on the drug (heroin, cocaine, hashish, LSD, ecstasy etc.) great differences regarding physical and psychological addiction
- Psychological dynamics: drug abuse often presents an escape mechanism from unresolved problems, stress, and other pressures; peer pressure may also play a role

 During the inpatient withdrawal phase auricular acupuncture is a supportive adjuvant therapy. However, it cannot provide the will necessary for withdrawal nor can it replace psychotherapeutic support.

Point Prescription

French points

- Local points: **Liver**, **Gullet Point** (› 6.4.1)
- Psychological points: **Anti-Aggression**, **Jealousy** (› 6.8.5), **Neural Liver Point** (› 6.8.1), **Diazepam** (› 6.7.3), **Haldol** (› 6.8.6), **Omega Axis** (› 6.12.1)
- Stabilising points **Point Zero** (› 6.10.3), **Laterality Point** (› 6.8.6)

Chinese points

- Local points: **Mouth** (› 6.4.1), **Oesophagus (85)** (› 6.4.1)
- **NADA** treatment protocol (**N**ational **A**cupuncture **D**etoxification **A**ssociation; USA, established in 1985): ***Shen Men* (55)** (› 6.7.2), **ANS I (51)** (› 6.6.5), **Kidney (95)** (› 6.5.1), **Liver (97)** (› 6.4.1), **Lung (101)** (› 6.4.1)

Semi-permanent needles should be added, especially at the points Liver and Gullet Point.

Treatment Intervals

- During **inpatient withdrawal phase:** initially 3–7 times weekly until the physical withdrawal process is complete; then 2–3 times weekly
- Further physical and psychological support during the **outpatient phase**: 1–2 times weekly until the patient can cope well with abstaining from the drug

Treatment Course and Prognosis

- It is impossible to provide universally applicable guidelines; the prognosis depends very much on the type of drug and patient compliance.
- A study conducted in March 1999 by Uwe Vertheim about the acupuncture project 'Palette 4' in Hamburg demonstrated a significant reduction in the consumption of cocaine and alcohol besides an improvement in general wellbeing.

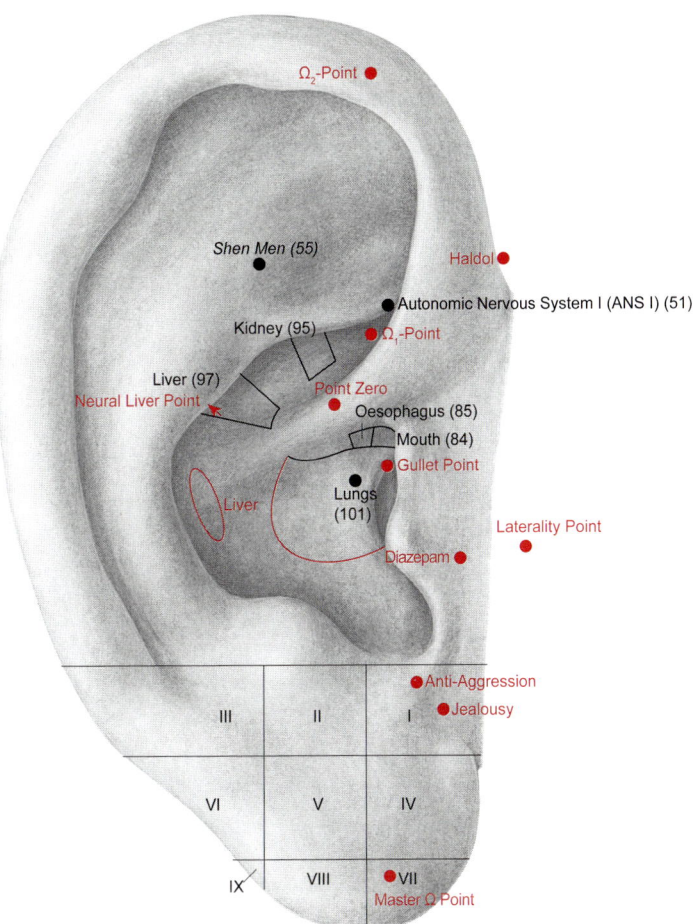

Fig. 8.8-3

8.8.4 Obesity

Description

- Obesity: a Body Mass Index (BMI) of > 30; or, after Broca, a weight 20 % higher than the standard weight (= height in centimetres minus 100)
- Overweight: A BMI of 25.0-29.9; or, after Broca, a weight 20 % higher than the standard weight (= height in centimetres minus 100)
- Psychodynamics: e.g. comfort eating (sweets etc.) to compensate for the experience of loss; comfort eating when feeling offended, upset, or anxious
- Often family history of obesity
- Possible secondary complaints include: joint problems, cardiovascular disease, dyspnoea, fatty liver, skin disorders

 Recognising underlying psychological problems and their psychogenesis is essential; in these cases behavioural therapy may be helpful. Emotional balance is a fundamental requirement for sustained weight loss. Auricular acupuncture promotes weight loss by alleviating the feeling of hunger and providing psychological support.

Point Prescription

French points
- Local points: **Gullet Point** (› 6.4.1), **Neural Stomach Point** (› 6.9.2), **Liver** (› 6.4.1)
- Psychological points: **Anti-Aggression** (› 6.8.5), **Haldol** (› 6.8.6), **Omega Axis** (› 6.12.1)
- Stabilising points: **Point Zero** (› 6.10.3), **Laterality Point** (› 6.8.6), **Desire** (› 6.8.3)

Chinese points
- Local point: **Mouth (84)** (› 6.4.1)
- Stabilising point: **Hunger (18)** (› 6.10.5)

box
- Semi-permanent needles can be added as additional support, particularly at the points Neural Stomach Point and Liver.
- Semi-permanent needles should be stimulated several times daily by rotating the magnet in the guide tube (› 3.2.2).

Treatment Intervals

- Initially once weekly until there is weight loss without much effort
- Then 2–3 times monthly until the desired weight has been reached

Treatment Course and Prognosis

- After 1–2 months the sensation of hunger should diminish, accompanied by a weight loss of approximately 1 kg/week (depending on the initial weight); treatments are necessary for up to 6 months, followed by a treatment break

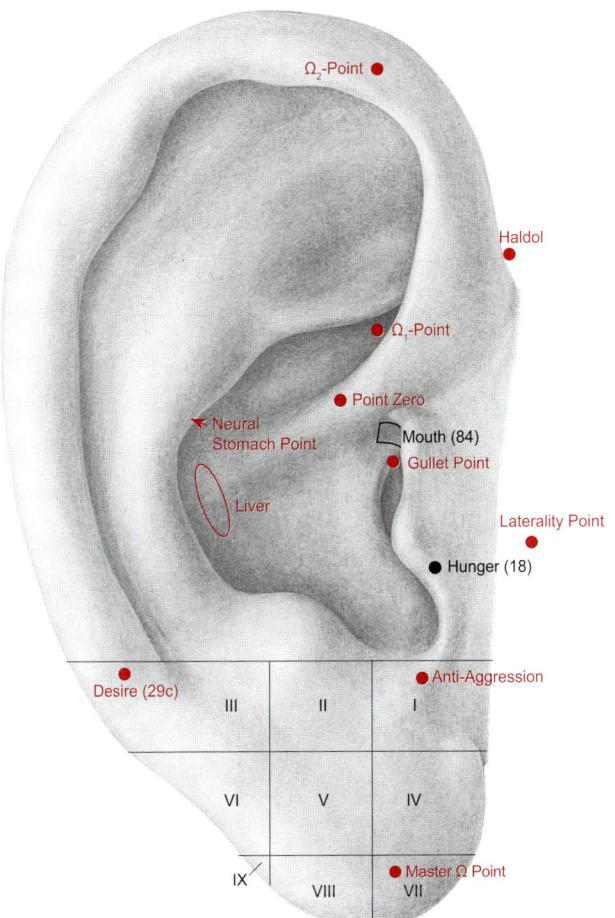

Fig. 8.8-4

8.9 Metabolic Disorders

8.9.1 Diabetes Mellitus

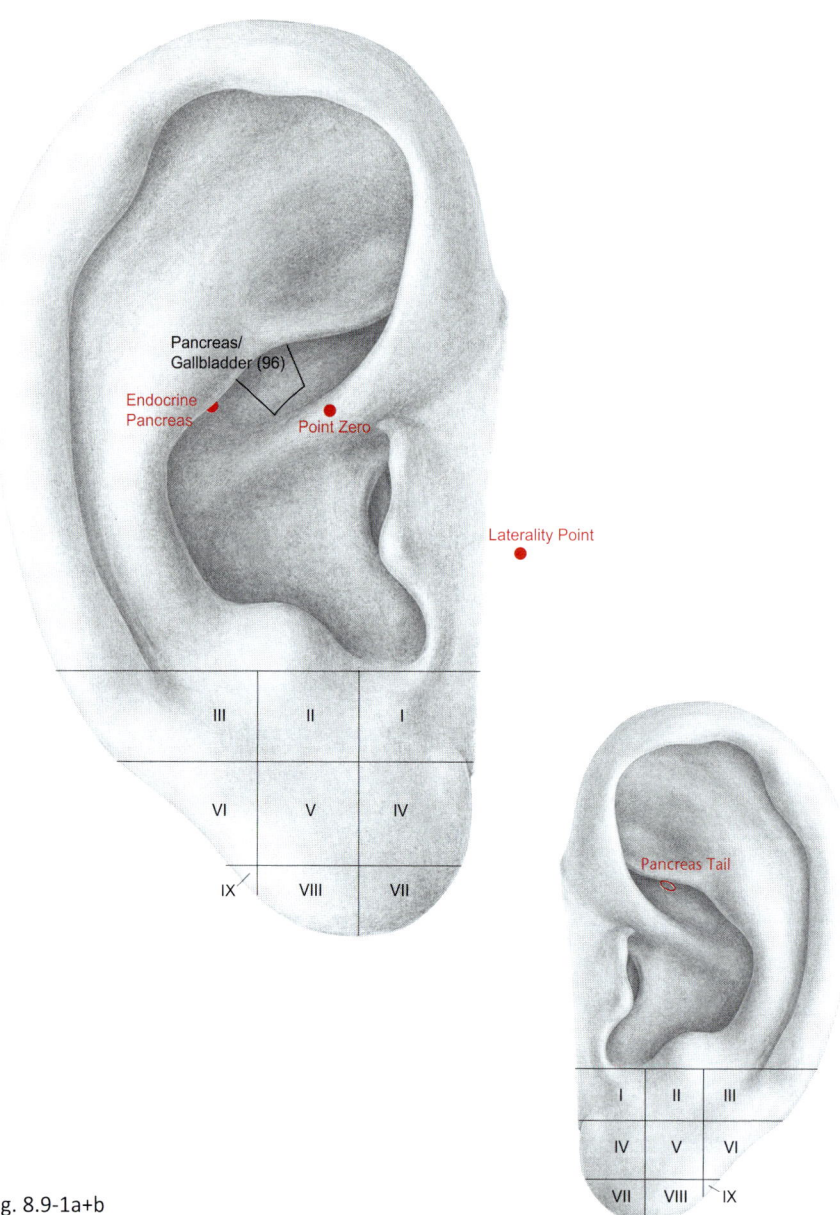

Fig. 8.9-1a+b

Description

- Glucose metabolism disorder with complete or relative lack of insulin
- Main forms:
  - Type 1 diabetes: develops during childhood or early adulthood, often progresses quickly to complete lack of insulin
  - Type 2 diabetes: formerly also known as adult-onset diabetes; the ability to synthesize insulin remains but there is relative lack of it; often occurs in conjunction with obesity
- Symptoms: during the early stages increased thirst, otherwise unspecific symptoms such as skin infections, sexual dysfunction in men, menstrual problems, fatigue
- Complications during the advanced stages include: polyneuropathy, eye disorders, kidney disorders

Point Prescription

French points
- Local points: **Pancreas Tail** (› 6.4.1), **Endocrine Pancreas** (› 6.6.1)
- Stabilising point: **Point Zero** (› 6.10.3), **Laterality Point** (› 6.8.6)
- Also see Obesity (› 8.8.4)

Chinese points
- Local point: **Pancreas/Gallbladder (96)** (› 6.4.1)

Acupuncture is only indicated for non-insulin dependent type 2 diabetes. Auricular acupuncture cannot compensate for the damaged beta cells in insulin-dependent diabetes mellitus.

Treatment Intervals

- Once weekly until oral diabetes medication can be reduced (slow reduction of diabetes medication with close monitoring of blood sugar levels [daily or every other day])
- Then 2–3 times monthly until blood sugar levels reach stable normal to borderline values
- Then approximately once monthly to keep blood sugar levels stable

Treatment Course and Prognosis

- Depending on patient compliance approximately 6 months until blood sugar levels reach stable normal to borderline values

Weight loss and a diet low in sugar improve the prognosis!

8.9.2 Hypercholesterolaemia

Description

- Elevated blood cholesterol levels (> 250 mg/dl)
- Often accompanied by obesity and diabetes mellitus (› 8.9.1)
- Exacerbated by poor diet (too much fat, eggs etc.)
- Initially asymptomatic, in advanced stages secondary vascular disorders (arteriosclerosis)

> **box**
> It is important to determine and evaluate the various lipoprotein levels (HDL, LDL, VLDL). However, elevated levels of total blood cholesterol caused by elevated HDL do not require treatment.

Point Prescription

French points
- Local point: **Liver** (› 6.4.1)
- Stabilising points: **Point Zero** (› 6.10.3), **Laterality Point** (› 6.8.6)

Chinese points
- Local point: **Liver (97)** (› 6.4.1)
- Stabilising point: *Shen Men* **(55)** (› 6.7.2)

Treatment Intervals

- Initially once weekly until cholesterol levels decrease
- Then approximately once monthly until lowered cholesterol levels are stable

Treatment Course and Prognosis

- Generally approximately 6 months until there is a significant improvement or until normal values have been reached
- If there is no improvement after 6 months further acupuncture treatments are generally not appropriate

> **box**
> A low-cholesterol diet, physical exercise, and weight loss improve the prognosis!

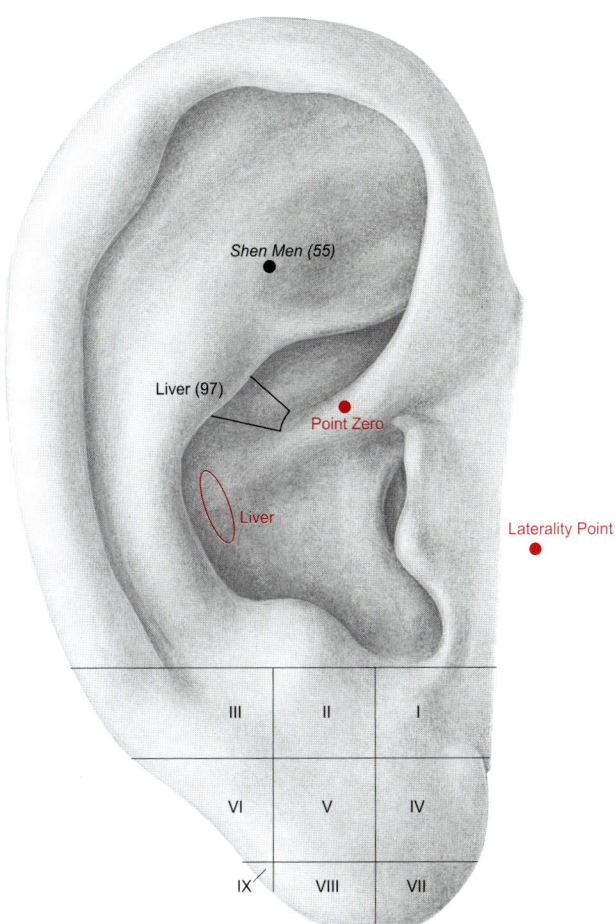

Fig. 8.9-2

8.9.3 Thyroid Disorders

Description

- Indications for auricular acupuncture:
  - nodular growth of the thyroid gland (e.g. regressive thyroid tissue, cysts)
  - hypothyroidism (e.g. Hashimoto's thyroiditis)
  - hyperthyroidism (e.g. thyroid autonomy, Graves' disease)
- Symptoms:
  - hyperthyroidism: e.g. restlessness, cardiac arrhythmias, tachycardia, hair loss
  - hypothyroidism: e.g. fatigue, weight gain
  - localised complaints owing to an enlarged thyroid gland: ranging from pressure pain on the neck to difficulty swallowing or dyspnoea

- Patients with enlarged thyroid glands have to be referred to a consultant. Approximately 2 % of 'cold' nodules are malignant.
- Patients with pronounced goitre growth accompanied by dyspnoea or difficulty swallowing have to be referred to a consultant (surgery?). A referral is also necessary for Graves' disease or autonomic thyroid adenomas that do not respond to treatments.
- Pronounced hyperthyroidism should initially be treated with conventional thyrostatic drugs. In the event of a thyrotoxic crisis (severe tachycardia, high temperature, vomiting, diarrhoea) immediate hospital admission is essential.

Point Prescription

French points

- Local points: **Thyroid Gland** (› 6.6.1), **TSH** (› 6.6.7)
- Stabilising point: **Point Zero** (› 6.10.3), **Laterality Point** (› 6.8.6), **Neural Thyroid Point** (› 6.9.2)

Chinese points

- Local point: **Thyroid Gland (45)** (› 6.6.5)

- Both hyperthyroidism and hypothyroidism can be treated with the same points.
- Acupuncture can affect both thyroid function and structure (formation of nodules, size).
- For best treatment results auricular acupuncture should be combined with body acupuncture and/or Chinese herbal medicine.

Treatment Intervals

- Initially once weekly until symptoms improve
- Then 1–2 times monthly until thyroid function is within the normal range or the struma do no longer cause any physical complaints

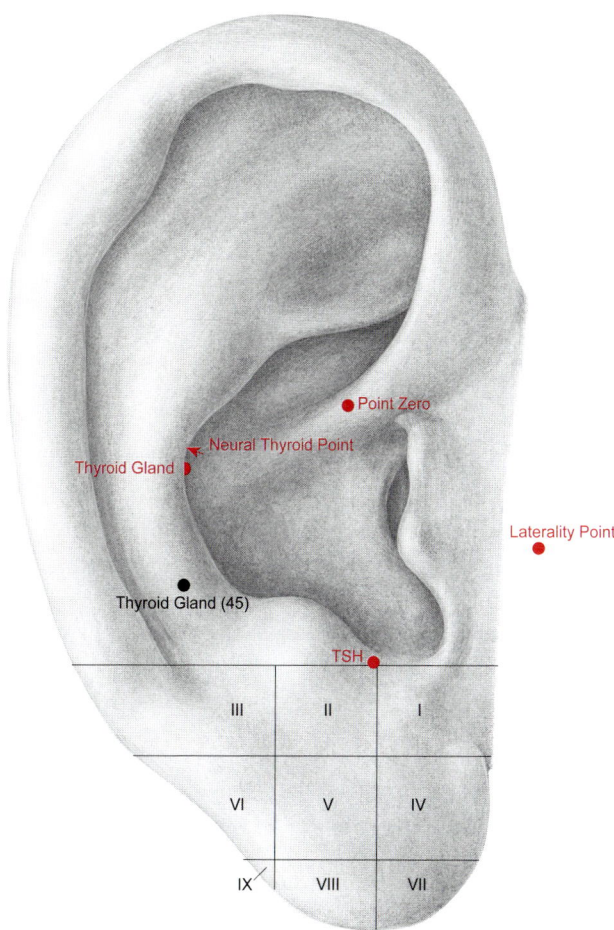

Fig. 8.9-3

Treatment Course and Prognosis

- Improvement after 1–2 months
- Complete relief from symptoms is only possible in mild cases of goitre and requires treatment for up to 6–12 months

8.9.4 Hereditary Angioedema (HAE) / Acquired Angioedema (AAE)

Description

- Recurrent swelling of the skin and mucosa, occasionally also swelling of the internal organs
- Sometimes life-threatening symptoms
- Affects approximately 0.01 % of the population, men and women are equally affected
- HAE: initial symptoms often occur during the first two decades of life
- Causes: enzyme defect: lack of C1-esterase-inhibitor (C1-INH)
  – HAE: genetic causes
  – AAE: can be drug-induced (e.g. ACE inhibitors)

Point Prescription

The same treatment protocol applies to both HAE and AAE.

French points

- Local points: **Tongue** (› 6.3.4), **Lung** (› 6.4.1), **Gullet Point** (› 6.4.1)
- Immunostimulant points: **Histamine** (› 6.6.4), **ACTH** (› 6.6.6), **Adrenal Cortex** (› 6.6.1), **Immune Axis** (› 6.12.3)
- Supporting point: **Point Zero** (› 6.10.3)
- Psychological points: **Omega Axis** (› 6.12.1), **Diazepam** (› 6.7.3), **Frustration** (› 6.8.3), **Antidepressant Point** (› 6.8.5)

Chinese points

- Local points: **Larynx and Tooth (27)** (› 6.3.3), **Tongue (4)** (› 6.3.4)
- Supporting point: **Triple Warmer (104)** (› 6.10.1)
- Immune point: **Adrenal Gland (13)** (› 6.6.6)
- Relaxing point: **Muscle Relaxation (98a)** (› 6.1.3)

Treatment Intervals

- **Acute symptoms or acute progression:** once daily until symptoms have reduced significantly, only then should antianaphylactic or immunosuppressive medication be discontinued; then once weekly until symptoms have improved or disappeared completely
- **Chronic symptoms:** approximately every 3–4 weeks as a preventative measure

Treatment Course and Prognosis

- **Acute symptoms:** generally symptoms improve within hours, complete remission within days
- **Chronic symptoms:** sustained relief from symptoms possible with regular preventative treatments, in particular for AAE

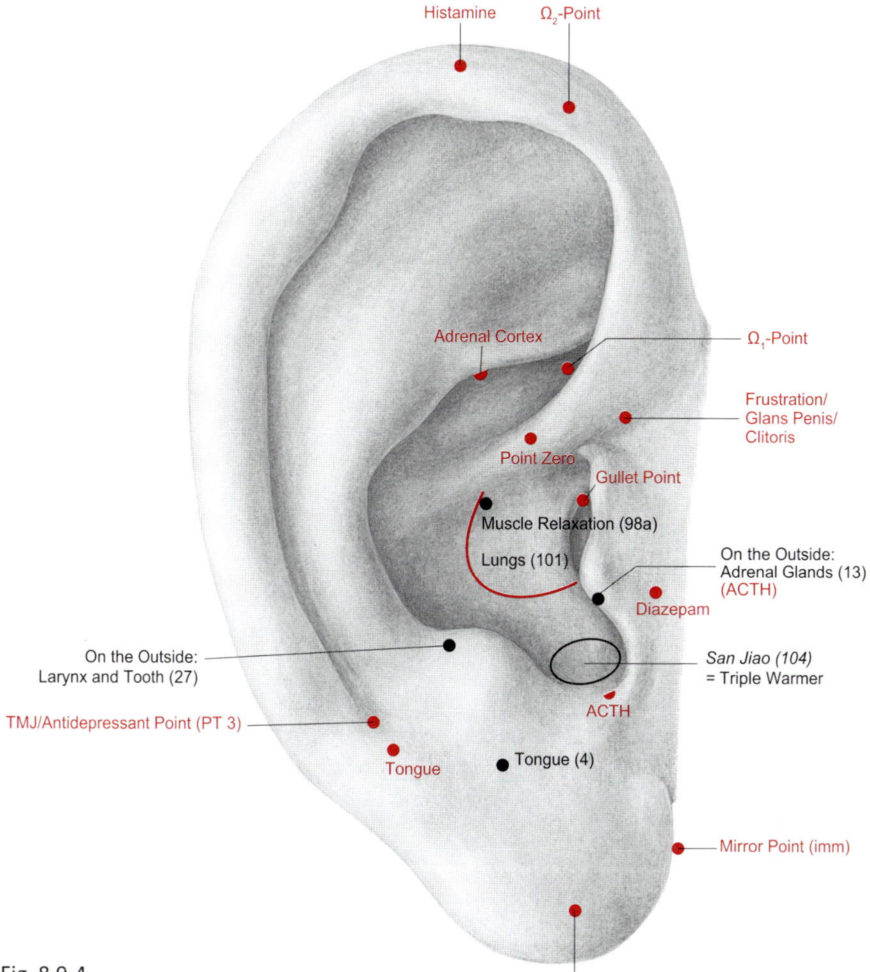

Histamine · Ω₂-Point

Adrenal Cortex · Ω₁-Point

Frustration/
Glans Penis/
Clitoris

Point Zero · Gullet Point

Muscle Relaxation (98a)

Lungs (101)

On the Outside:
Adrenal Glands (13)
(ACTH)

Diazepam

On the Outside:
Larynx and Tooth (27)

San Jiao (104)
= Triple Warmer

TMJ/Antidepressant Point (PT 3)

ACTH

Tongue (4)

Tongue

Mirror Point (imm)

Master Ω Point

Fig. 8.9-4

- Generally immunosuppressive or glucocorticoid medication does not alleviate the symptoms. However, even with auricular acupuncture treatments it may be necessary to administer C1-INH concentrate (Berinert P) intravenously or bradykinin antagonists (Icatibant) subcutaneously in acute situations.
- Androgens as long-term prevention can be substituted with acupuncture.
- The effect of acupuncture is based on strengthening the immune system (independent of the release of cortisone) and by using relaxing points.

8.10 Obstetrics and Gynaecology

8.10.1 Premenstrual Syndrome

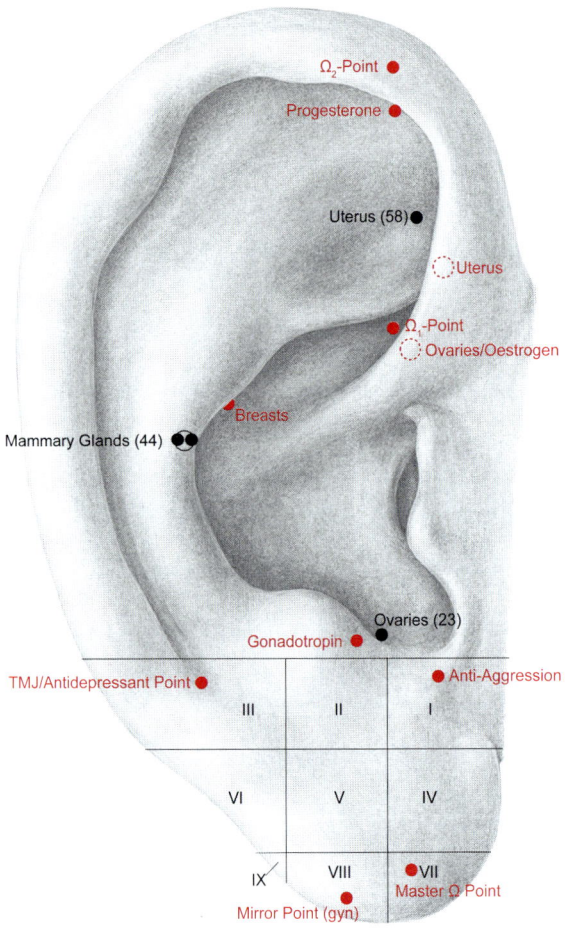

Ω_2-Point

Progesterone

Uterus (58)

Uterus

Ω_1-Point

Ovaries/Oestrogen

Breasts

Mammary Glands (44)

Ovaries (23)

Gonadotropin

TMJ/Antidepressant Point

Anti-Aggression

III II I

VI V IV

IX VIII VII

Master Ω Point

Mirror Point (gyn)

Fig. 8.10-1

Description

Occurs in the second half of the menstrual cycle, mostly several days prior to and also during menstruation; symptoms include abdominal pain, painful and distended breasts, headaches, unstable mood

Point Prescription

French points

- Local points: **Uterus** (› 6.5.2), **Breast** (› 6.6.1)
- Hormonal points: **Oestrogen** (› 6.6.4), **Progesterone** (› 6.6.3), **Gonadotropin** (› 6.6.7), **Gynaecological Axis** (› 6.12.5)
- Psychological points: **Antidepressant Point** (› 6.8.5), **Anti-Aggression** (› 6.8.5), **Omega Axis** (› 6.12.1)

Chinese points

- Local points: **Ovaries (23)** (› 6.5.1), **Uterus (58)** (› 6.5.4), **Breast (44)** (› 6.4.4)

Treatment Intervals

- **Until symptoms improve:** first acupuncture treatment approximately 4–5 days prior to the expected date of the next period; then immediately at the onset of and during the period every 2–3 days
- **Reinforcing treatments:** twice monthly until there is a sustained relief from symptoms

Treatment Course and Prognosis

- Symptoms generally improve after 1–2 menstrual cycles
- Symptoms often disappear completely after approximately 3–6 months

8.10.2 Menstrual Disorders

Description

- Various forms of menstrual disorders:
  - abnormal bleeding (hypermenorrhoea, hypomenorrhoea)
  - disorders of the cycle length (polymenorrhoea, oligomenorrhoea)
  - spotting and breakthrough bleeding
  - amenorrhoea
  - dysmenorrhoea (painful periods)
- Causes:
  - hormonal disorders
  - organic changes (e.g. uterine fibroids, endometriosis)
  - contraceptive pill (e.g. for hypomenorrhoea)
- Sometimes in combination with being underweight (› anorexia 8.13.4)

Point Prescription

French points

- Local point: **Uterus** (› 6.5.2)
- Hormonal points: **Oestrogen** (› 6.6.4), **Progesterone** (› 6.6.3), **Gonadotropin** (› 6.6.7), **Gynaecological Axis** (› 6.12.5)
- General points: **Laterality Point** (› 6.8.6), **Kidney II** (› 6.5.4)

Chinese points

- Local points: **Ovaries (23)** (› 6.5.1), **Uterus (58)** (› 6.5.4)

Treatment Intervals

- **Amenorrhoea:**
  - initially once weekly until there is a period
  - then twice monthly for two cycles for reinforcement
- **Other menstrual disorders:**
  - initially approximately twice weekly until the cycle is regular and/or the menstrual problems have resolved (after approximately 4–6 weeks)
  - then once weekly until symptoms have disappeared and there is a regular menstrual cycle
  - monthly treatments for about 3 months to obtain sustained results

Treatment Course and Prognosis

- Generally symptoms improve after 1–2 menstrual cycles
- Often symptoms disappear completely after approximately 3–6 months
- Amenorrhoea in conjunction with anorexia: it may take a year or longer until there is a period

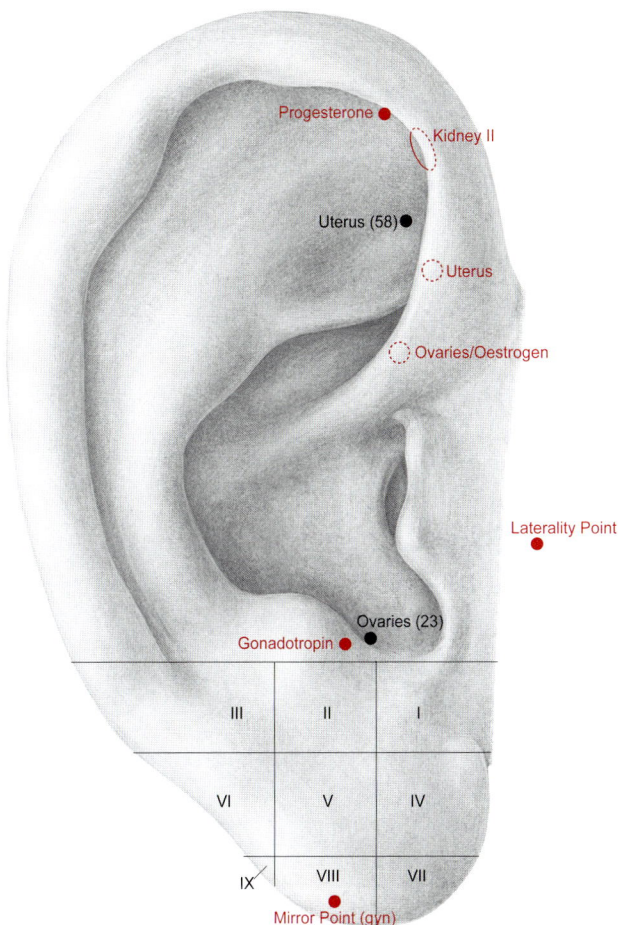

Progesterone

Kidney II

Uterus (58)

Uterus

Ovaries/Oestrogen

Laterality Point

Ovaries (23)

Gonadotropin

III   II   I

VI   V   IV

IX   VIII   VII

Mirror Point (gyn)

Fig. 8.10-2

8.10.3 Menopausal Symptoms

Description

- Symptoms caused by hormonal changes during menopause; affecting approximately 70 % of women
- Symptoms include:
  - hot flashes, sweating, dizziness, fatigue
  - mood swings, depressive mood
  - possibly organic disorders such as osteoporosis, genital atrophy

Point Prescription

French points

- Local point: **Uterus** (› 6.5.2)
- Hormonal points: **Oestrogen** (› 6.6.4), **Progesterone** (› 6.6.3), **Gonadotropin** (› 6.6.7), **Gynaecological Axis** (› 6.12.5)
- Stabilising points: **Laterality Point** (› 6.8.6), **Kidney II** (› 6.5.4)
- Psychological points: **Antidepressant Point** (› 6.8.5), **Haldol** (› 6.8.6), **Antidepressant Axis** (› 6.12.6)

Chinese points

- Local points: **Ovaries (23)** (› 6.5.1), **Uterus (58)** (› 6.5.4)

Treatment Intervals

- Once weekly until symptoms improve; existing hormone replacement medication can be discontinued at that point
- Then 2–3 times monthly until symptoms have disappeared

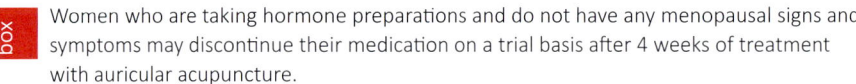

> box — Women who are taking hormone preparations and do not have any menopausal signs and symptoms may discontinue their medication on a trial basis after 4 weeks of treatment with auricular acupuncture.

Treatment Course and Prognosis

- Improvement of symptoms after 1–2 months
- Symptoms often disappear completely after 3–6 months

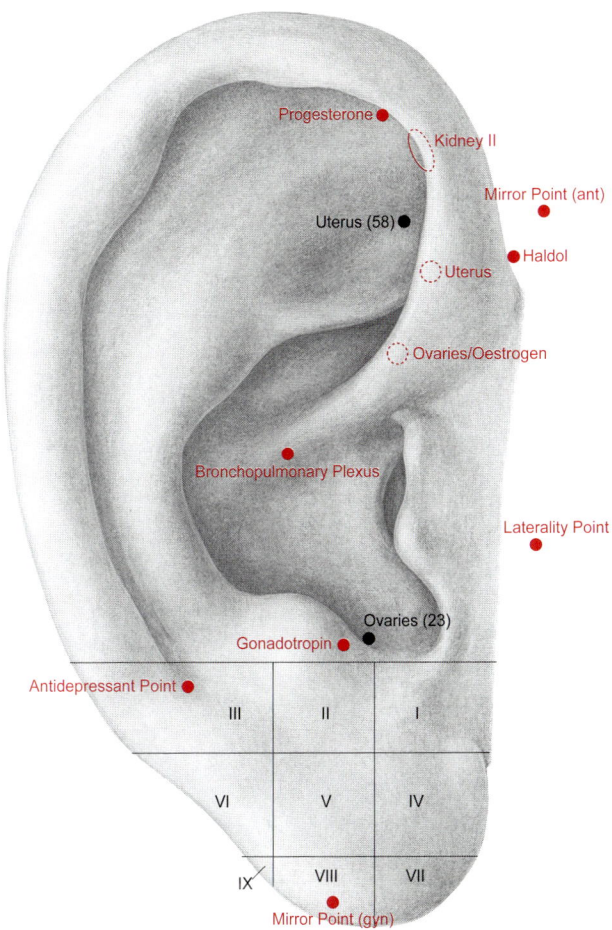

Fig. 8.10-3

8.10.4 Hyperemesis Gravidarum (Morning Sickness)

Description
- Often occurs during the first trimester of pregnancy
- Exacerbated by psychological stress
- Symptoms include:
  - nausea
  - rarely vomiting
  - aversion to certain foods

Point Prescription

French points
- Stabilising points: **Laterality Point** (› 6.8.6), **Point Zero** (› 6.10.3)
- Psychological points: **Antidepressant Point** (› 6.8.5), **Haldol** (› 6.8.6), **Antidepressant Axis** (› 6.12.6)

Chinese points
- Local point: **Stomach (87)** (› 6.4.1)
- Stabilising points: **ANS I (51)** (› 6.6.5), **ANS II (34)** (› 6.7.4)

Treatment Intervals
- 1–2 times weekly until symptoms improve

Treatment Course and Prognosis
- Symptoms generally improve after 1–2 weeks
- Symptoms often disappear completely after approximately 4 weeks

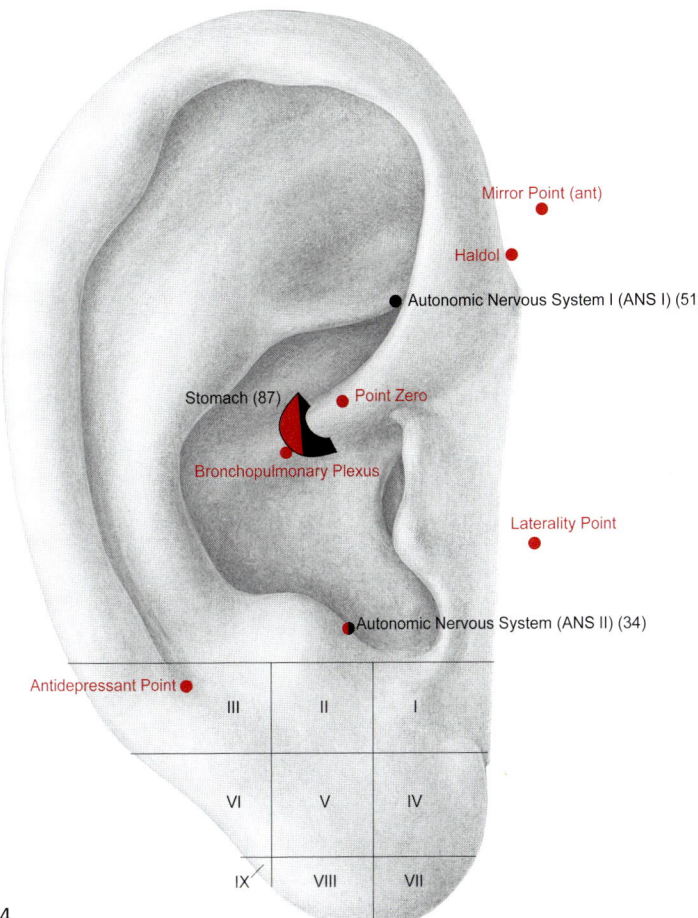

Mirror Point (ant)

Haldol

Autonomic Nervous System I (ANS I) (51)

Stomach (87)

Point Zero

Bronchopulmonary Plexus

Laterality Point

Autonomic Nervous System (ANS II) (34)

Antidepressant Point

III	II	I
VI	V	IV
IX	VIII	VII

Fig. 8.10-4

8.10.5 Fertility Disorders

Description

- Male fertility disorders:
  - low ejaculate volume: hypospermia (< 2 ml), aspermia
  - low sperm count: oligozoospermia (< 20 mio/ml), azoospermia
  - reduced sperm motility (asthenozoospermia [< 50 %], necrozoospermia)
- Female fertility disorders:
  - fallopian tube obstruction
  - dysmenorrhoea, amenorrhoea
- Causes:
  - stress, especially in men
  - recurrent urogenital tract infections (prostatitis, adnexitis)
  - eating disorders (e.g. anorexia), especially in women
  - radiation-induced damage; in men more likely to be reversible than in women since sperm, in contrast to follicles, are constantly reproduced

Point Prescription

 Gender-specific points have to be individually chosen.

French points

- Hormonal points: **Progesterone** (› 6.6.3); **Oestrogen (Ovaries)/Testosterone (Testes)** (› 6.6.4; 6.5.2), **Gynaecological Axis** (› 6.12.5)
- Energetically effective areas: **Kidney I** (› 6.5.1), **Kidney II** (› 6.5.4)
- Psychological points: **Omega Axis** (› 6.12.1), **Point Bosch** (› 6.5.2), **Frustration** (› 6.8.3)

Chinese points

- Hormonal points: **Testes (32)** (› 6.5.3), **Kidney (95)** (› 6.5.1), **Ovaries (23)** (› 6.5.1), **Endocrine System (22)** (› 6.6.2)
- Relaxing point: *Shen Men* **(55)** (› 6.7.2)

- From the view of auricular acupuncture, fertility disorders are treated the same in both men and women; the aim is to optimise the capacity of the reproductive organs and to relax the whole energetic system.
- If there are organic defects (such as incurable impotence or irreversible fallopian tube obstruction) acupuncture will not be effective!

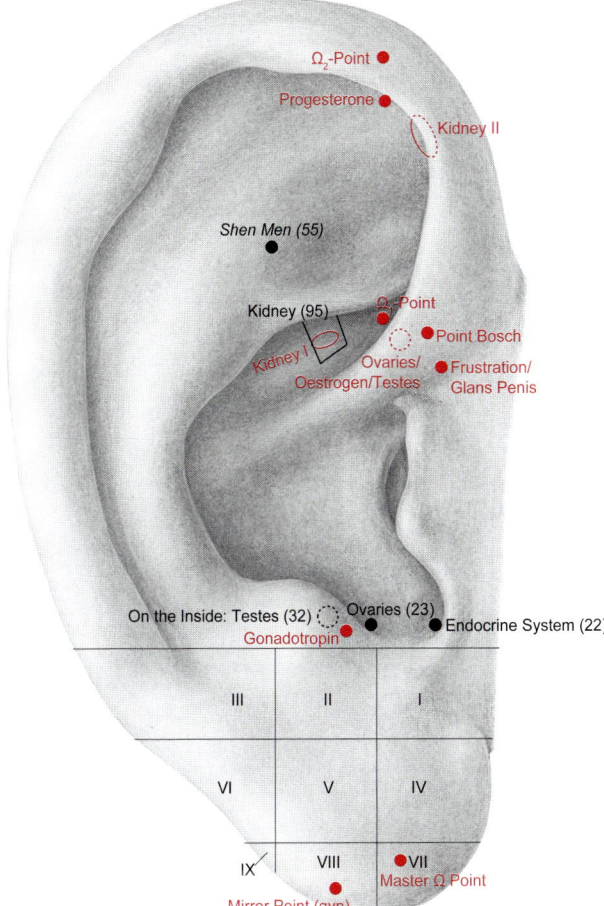

Ω_2-Point

Progesterone

Kidney II

Shen Men (55)

Kidney (95)
Ω_1-Point
Point Bosch
Kidney I
Ovaries/
Oestrogen/Testes
Frustration/
Glans Penis

On the Inside: Testes (32)
Ovaries (23)
Endocrine System (22)
Gonadotropin

III   II   I

VI   V   IV

IX   VIII   VII
Master Ω Point
Mirror Point (gyn)

Fig. 8.10-5

Treatment Intervals

- **Initial phase:** once weekly until there is significant subjective improvement of general wellbeing and a stable and positive approach to stress (approximately 4 weeks) or, in cases of amenorrhoea, until periods start
- **Follow-up treatments:** 1–3 times monthly, in women until pregnancy, in men until a semen analysis is within the normal range

Treatment Course and Prognosis

- Depending on the complexity of the disease pattern approximately 6 months to 2 years

- The points Uterus and Uterus (58) should be needled only towards the end of pregnancy for relaxation. Needling these points can trigger foetal movements.
- Hormonal points – Oestrogen, Progesterone, Gonadotropin, and Ovaries (23) – are contraindicated during pregnancy.

8.10.6 Pregnancy and Childbirth

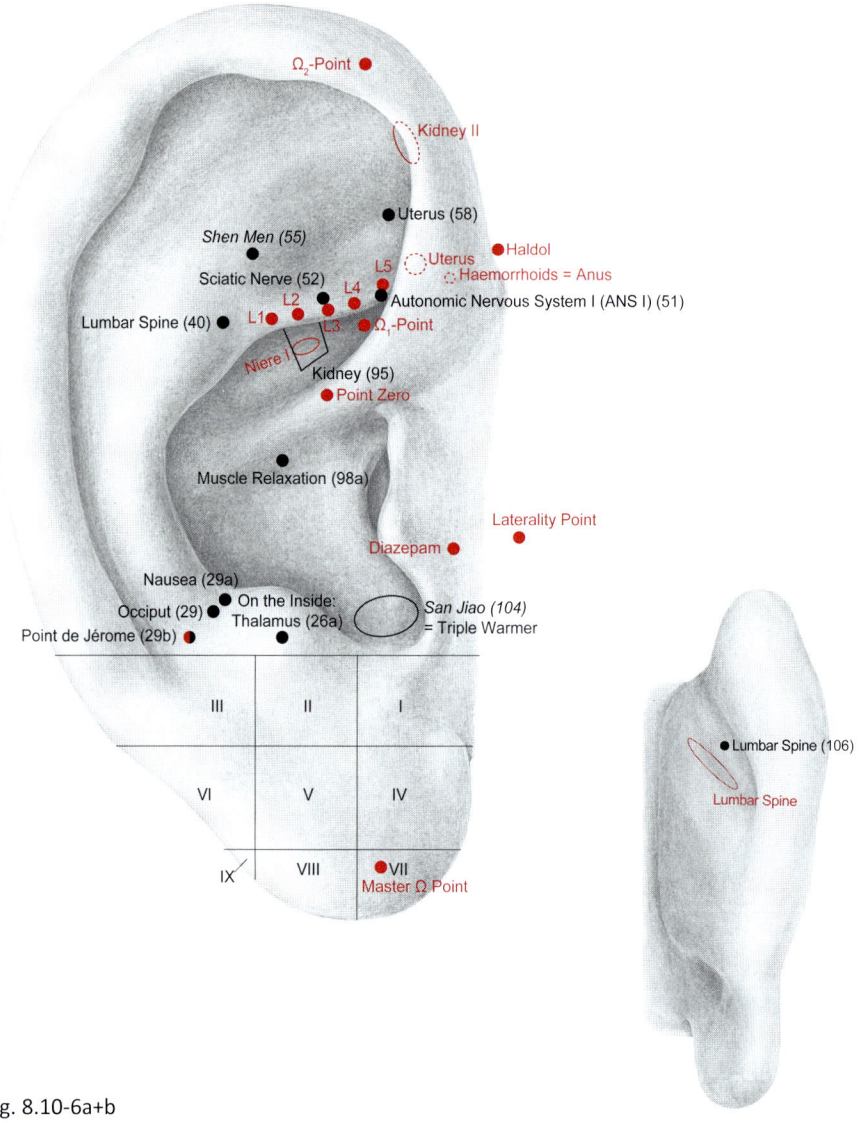

Fig. 8.10-6a+b

Description

- Nausea to the point of vomiting, especially during the first trimester
- Tendency to preterm birth, cervical insufficiency (incompetent cervix)
- Premature labour, abdominal pain radiating to the inguinal area
- Causes:
  - often Kidney deficiency

- often in combination with Spleen deficiency
- less commonly rising of Liver-*yang*
- oedema in the lower limbs, varicosities, haemorrhoids with weak connective tissue
- sciatica (› 8.1.3) caused by problems in finding a comfortable position, especially with history of sciatica

Point Prescription

French points

- Local points for accompanying problems: **Anus/Haemorrhoids** (› 6.4.3); **L1–5** (› 6.1.1), **Lumbar Spine** on the posterior ear (› 6.11.1), **Uterus** (› 6.5.2)
- Stabilising points during pregnancy: **Point Zero** (› 6.10.3), **Laterality Point** (› 6.8.6), **Kidney I** (› 6.5.1), **Kidney II** (› 6.5.4)
- Relaxing point, especially just before or during birth: **Diazepam** (› 6.7.3)
- Psychological points: **Omega Axis** (› 6.12.1), **Haldol** (› 6.8.6)

Chinese points

- Local points for accompanying problems: **Lumbar Spine (40)** (› 6.1.1), **Lumbar Spine (106)** on the posterior ear (› 6.11.1) **Sciatic Nerve (52)** (› 6.1.1), **Uterus (58)** (› 6.5.4)
- Analgesic points: **Thalamus (26a)** (› 6.7.4) **Occiput (29)** (› 6.7.4)
- Psychological points: **Point de Jérome (29b)** (› 6.8.2), **ANS I (51)** (› 6.6.5)
- Stabilising areas or points: **Kidney (95)** (› 6.5.1), **Triple Warmer (104)** (› 6.10.1) **Nausea (29a)** (› 6.3.3)
- Relaxing points: **Muscle Relaxation (98a)** (› 6.1.3), *Shen Men* **(55)** (› 6.7.2)

Treatment Intervals

- **Pregnancy without acute symptoms:** once monthly for stabilisation, support, and relaxation; during the final month once weekly in preparation for a harmonious and relaxed birth and, if required, for support in cases of foetal malposition
- **Acute symptoms:** 1–3 times weekly until there is a significant reduction in pain (e.g. with sciatica); once weekly for symptoms without pain such as nausea (especially during the first trimester), haemorrhoids, varicose veins, oedema of the lower limbs
- **Birth:** just before or during the due date semi-permanent needles, especially at relaxation points

The following body acupuncture points are also often used: BL-67 (premature labour, malposition of the foetus, difficulties during birth), BL-62 (foetal malposition), ST-36 (supporting the pregnancy), GB-41 (supporting the pregnancy), TH-4 (nausea/vomiting during pregnancy)

Treatment Course and Prognosis

- **During pregnancy:** for pregnancies without complications, reducing risk factors (such as premature labour, uterine bleeding)
- **During childbirth:** for a harmonious and relaxed birth, turning a malpositioned foetus
- **Acute symptoms:** generally symptoms improve or disappear completely within days after their initial occurrence

8.10.7 Endometriosis

Description

- Painful chronic disease caused by the presence of endometrial tissue outside of the uterus, generally on the peritoneum or in the lower pelvic cavity, especially around the ovaries; may occasionally affect the intestines and vaginal wall, only rarely the lungs or brain
- Ectopic endometrium (i.e. in an abnormal place) is also subject to the menstrual cycle
- May cause infertility
- Affects 10 % of women
- Causes unclear; there are various explanatory models regarding pathogenesis:
  - transplantation theory: transplantation of endometrial cells via fallopian tubes, blood, lymphatic vessels, or surgery
  - metaplasia theory: development of endometrial growths from localised embryonic cells in the pelvic cavity
  - genetic predisposition
  - environmental toxins (PCB, DDT, dioxin, oestrogen)
  - other causes (immunological, ANS-related) are debated

Point Prescription

French points
- Local points: **Ovaries** (› 6.5.2), **Colon** (› 6.4.1), **Uterus** (› 6.5.2), **Bladder** (› 6.5.1)
- Analgesic points: **PGE$_1$/Thymus** (› 6.7.6), **Thalamus** (› 6.7.4)
- Supporting points: **Point Zero** (› 6.10.3), **Kidney I** (› 6.5.1), **Laterality Point** (› 6.4.1)
- Psychological points: **Omega Axis** (› 6.12.1), **Diazepam** (› 6.7.3), **Frustration** (› 6.8.3), **Antidepressant Point** (› 6.8.5)

Chinese points
- Local points: **Pelvic Cavity (56)** (› 6.2.3), **Ovaries (23)** (› 6.5.1)
- Supporting point: **Triple Warmer (104)** (› 6.10.1)
- Relaxing point: **Muscle Relaxation (98a)** (› 6.1.3)

Treatment Intervals

- **Acute symptoms or acute progression:** 1–2 times weekly for 2–3 menstrual cycles until the menstrual pain has reduced significantly
- **Chronic symptoms:** every 3–4 weeks as preventative measure

Treatment Course and Prognosis

- **Acute symptoms:** symptoms often improve after only a few treatments; complete remission from symptoms may require treatments for up to 1 year
- **Chronic symptoms:** sustained relief from symptoms is possible with regular preventative treatments

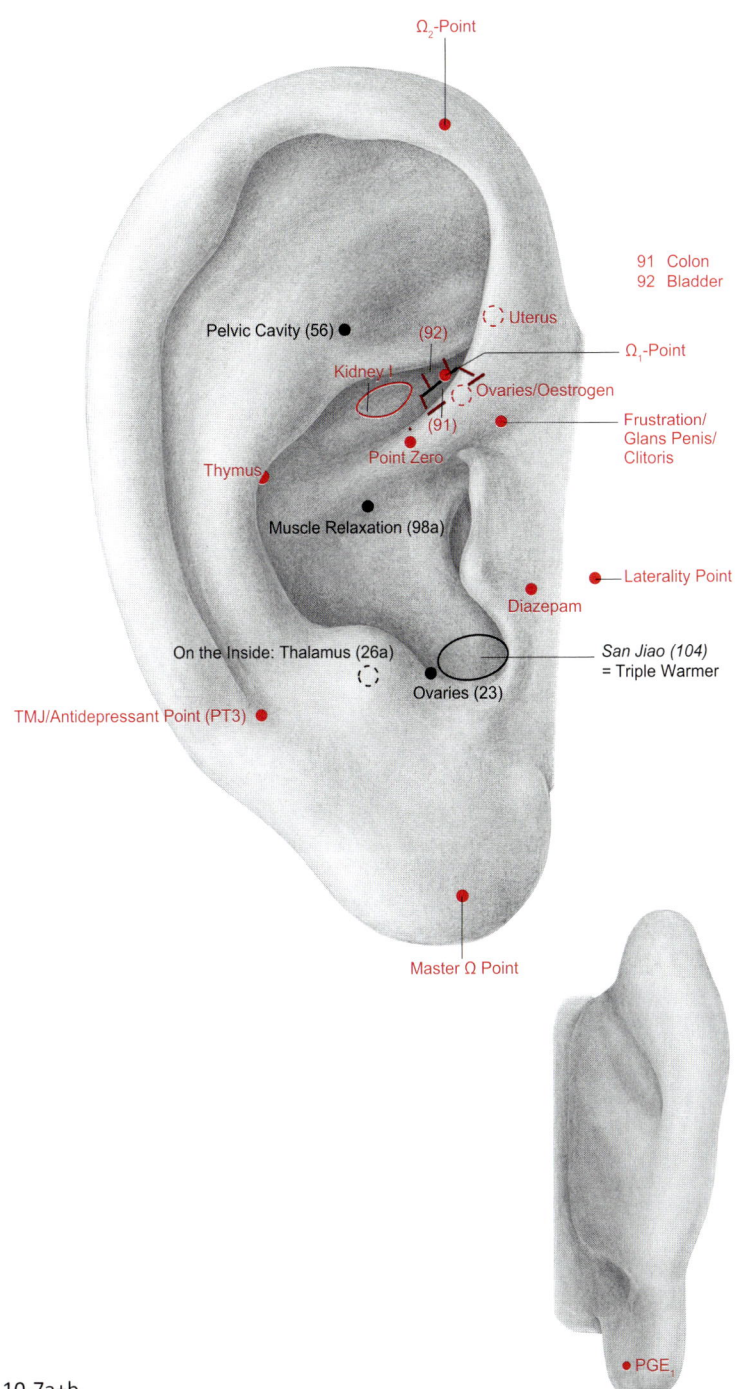

Ω₂-Point

91 Colon
92 Bladder

Pelvic Cavity (56)

(92)

Uterus

Ω₁-Point

Kidney I

Ovaries/Oestrogen

(91)

Frustration/
Glans Penis/
Clitoris

Point Zero

Thymus

Muscle Relaxation (98a)

Laterality Point

Diazepam

On the Inside: Thalamus (26a)

San Jiao (104)
= Triple Warmer

Ovaries (23)

TMJ/Antidepressant Point (PT3)

Master Ω Point

PGE₁

Fig. 8.10-7a+b

8.11 Neurological Disorders

8.11.1 Multiple Sclerosis (Encephalomyelitis Disseminata)

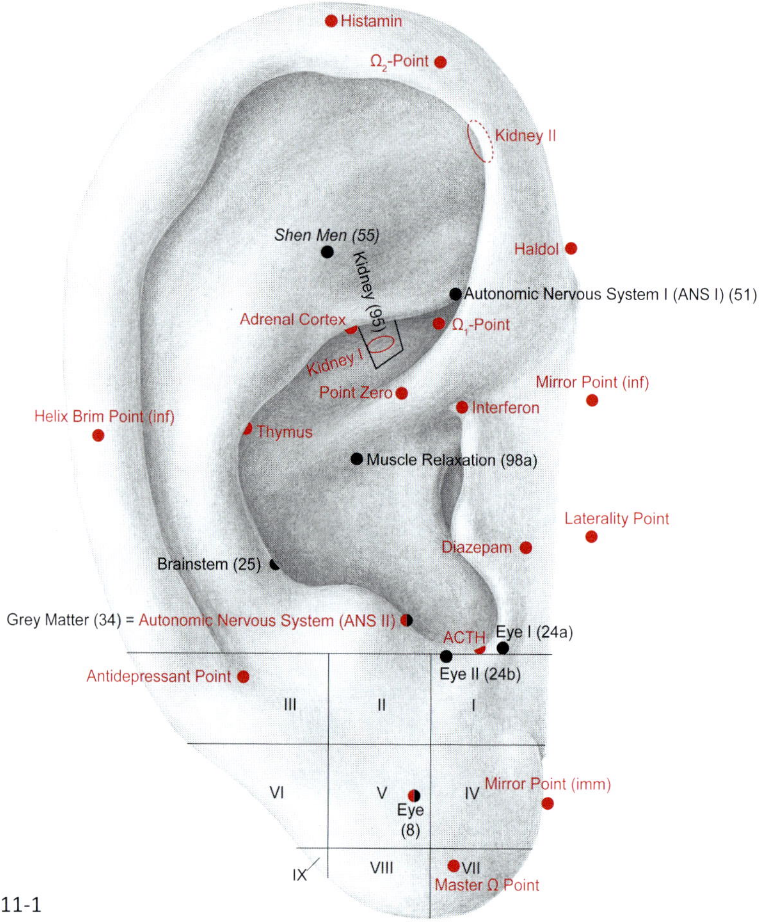

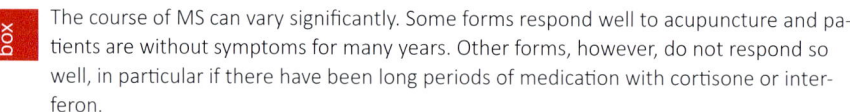

Histamin

Ω_2-Point

Kidney II

Shen Men (55)

Kidney (95)

Haldol

Autonomic Nervous System I (ANS I) (51)

Adrenal Cortex

Ω_1-Point

Kidney I

Mirror Point (inf)

Point Zero

Interferon

Helix Brim Point (inf)

Thymus

Muscle Relaxation (98a)

Laterality Point

Brainstem (25)

Diazepam

Grey Matter (34) = Autonomic Nervous System (ANS II)

ACTH Eye I (24a)

Antidepressant Point

Eye II (24b)

III

II

I

VI

V
Eye
(8)

IV Mirror Point (imm)

IX

VIII

VII
Master Ω Point

Fig. 8.11-1

> The course of MS can vary significantly. Some forms respond well to acupuncture and pa-
> tients are without symptoms for many years. Other forms, however, do not respond so
> well, in particular if there have been long periods of medication with cortisone or inter-
> feron.

Description

- Inflammatory disease of the central nervous system with focal areas of demyelination
- Onset primarily between ages 20–40, especially in women; 15 % of cases with higher
  familial incidence

- Positive diagnosis based on the presence of oligoclonal IgG bands (OCB) with electrophoresis (95 %) as well as demyelinating plaques on MRI scan
- Symptoms: sensory disturbance, ataxia, tremors, paralysis, retrobulbar neuritis with visual disturbances
- Causes:
  - autoimmune disease with genetic predisposition
  - viral; onset following immunisations is debated
  - environmental factors

Point Prescription

French points
- Immunostimulant points: **Immune Axis** (› 6.12.3), **Infection Axis** (› 6.12.4), **Interferon** (› 6.7.3), **ACTH** (› 6.6.6), **Adrenal Cortex** (› 6.6.1), **Thymus** (› 6.6.1)
- Stabilising points: **Point Zero** (› 6.10.3), **Laterality Point** (› 6.8.6), **Kidney I** (› 6.5.1), **Kidney II** (› 6.5.4)
- Relaxing point: **Diazepam** (› 6.7.3)
- Psychological points: **Omega Axis** (› 6.12.1), **Haldol** (› 6.8.6), **Antidepressant Point** (› 6.8.5)

Chinese points
- Local points: **Brainstem (25)** (› 6.10.4), **Grey Matter/ANS II (34)** (› 6.7.4), **Eye I (24a)** (› 6.3.4), **Eye II (24b)** (› 6.3.4), **Eye (8)** (› 6.3.4)
- Stabilising areas/points: **Kidney (95)** (› 6.5.1), **ANS I (51)** (› 6.6.5)
- Relaxing points: **Muscle Relaxation (98a)** (› 6.1.3), *Shen Men* **(55)** (› 6.7.2)

Treatment Intervals
- **Acute symptoms, relapse:** 2–3 times weekly until symptoms have improved significantly
- **Chronic symptoms:** 2–3 times monthly until symptoms have become stable at a decreased level; during symptom-free intervals monthly preventative treatments

Treatment Course and Prognosis
- **Acute symptoms:** symptoms often subside or disappear completely within 4 weeks
- **Chronic symptoms:** complete remission is possible but depends on the stage and severity of symptoms; symptoms may subside completely for many years but a relapse can never be excluded

8.11.2 Parkinson's Disease

Description

- Affects approximately 1 % of the population over age 60
- Bradykinesia, also akinesia, hypophonia, hypomimia, micrographia
- Rigor
- Tremor
- Causes:
  - degeneration of dopaminergic neurons in the substantia nigra
  - causes are often not clear: possibly medication side effects, poisoning (e.g. methylated spirits), infections (e.g. following encephalitis, Creutzfeld-Jakob disease), environmental factors are also debated (e.g. stress)

Point Prescription

French points

- Relaxing point: **Diazepam** (› 6.7.3)
- Psychological points: **Omega Axis** (› 6.12.1), **Antidepressant Axis** (› 6.12.6), **Frustration** (› 6.8.3)
- Stabilising point: **Laterality Point** (› 6.8.6)

Chinese points

- Local points: **Brainstem (25)** (› 6.10.4) **ANS II/Subcortex (34)** (› 6.7.4)
- Stabilising points: **Occiput (29)** (› 6.7.4), **ANS I (51)** (› 6.6.5)
- Relaxing point: **Muscle Relaxation (98a)** (› 6.1.3)

Treatment Intervals

- **Acute progression of symptoms:** 1–3 times weekly until symptoms have improved significantly and there is no further progression; existing medication can be reduced once there is a sustained improvement of symptoms
- **Chronic symptoms:** 1–3 times monthly, depending on how sustained treatment results are

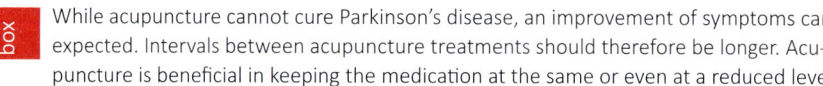

While acupuncture cannot cure Parkinson's disease, an improvement of symptoms can be expected. Intervals between acupuncture treatments should therefore be longer. Acupuncture is beneficial in keeping the medication at the same or even at a reduced level.

Treatment Course and Prognosis

- **Acute symptoms:** improvement often within 4 weeks
- **Chronic symptoms:** complete remission is not possible but a significant relaxation and improvement of symptoms can be achieved within 4–6 weeks; medication can sometimes be reduced while increases in dosage can often be slowed down. The subjective perception of symptoms is frequently better after the first treatment.

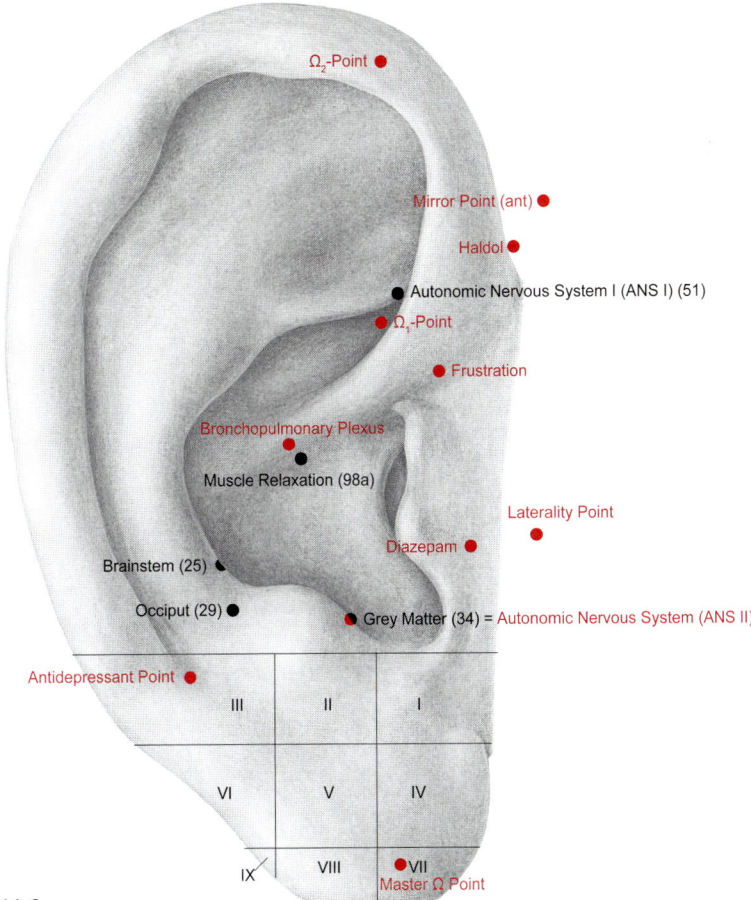

Ω₂-Point ●

Mirror Point (ant) ●

Haldol ●

● Autonomic Nervous System I (ANS I) (51)

● Ω₁-Point

● Frustration

Bronchopulmonary Plexus ●

● Muscle Relaxation (98a)

Laterality Point ●

Diazepam ●

Brainstem (25) ●

Occiput (29) ●

● Grey Matter (34) = Autonomic Nervous System (ANS II)

Antidepressant Point ●

III   II   I

VI   V   IV

IX   VIII   VII
Master Ω Point

Fig. 8.11-2

8.11.3 Cerebral Ischaemia (Stroke)

Description

- Hemiparesis
- One-sided sensory disturbances
- Aphasia
- Severity of symptoms can vary significantly
- Causes:
  - disturbed arterial perfusion of the brain caused by embolism, stenosis or cerebral microangiopathy (e.g. with hypertension); mainly affects the area supplied by the middle cerebral artery (80 % of cases with a death rate of 20 %)
  - intracerebral haemorrhage due to arteriovenous malformation, hypertension, or arteriosclerosis; often occurs in the area of the basal ganglia (20 % of cases with a death rate of 50 %)

Point Prescription

French points

- Local points (selection): **Upper arm** (› 6.2.1), **Thigh** (› 6.2.3), **Tongue** (› 6.3.4), **Motor and Sensory Pathway of the Spinal Cord** (› 6.9.3)
- Stabilising point: **Laterality Point** (› 6.8.6)
- Psychological points: **Omega Axis** (› 6.12.1), **Antidepressant Point** (› 6.8.5), **Haldol** (› 6.8.6)

Chinese points

- Local points: **Brainstem (25)** (› 6.10.4), **ANS II/Grey Matter (34)** (› 6.7.4)
- Relaxing point: **ANS I (51)** (› 6.6.5)

Treatment Intervals

- **Acute symptoms:** in the 1st week after the insult once daily, then approximately 2–3 times weekly until symptoms improve significantly, e.g. a lessening of the paralysis or improved speech
- **Chronic symptoms:** 2–3 times monthly until symptoms disappear or until there is a sustained improvement of symptoms

- Combining auricular acupuncture with body acupuncture is highly recommended. Treatment of the unaffected side should be given preference since it carries much more *Qi*.
- Possible acupuncture points include: PC-6, TH-5, LI-11, BL-62 , GV-20, LR-3.

Treatment Course and Prognosis

- **Acute symptoms:** generally significant improvement within 4 weeks
- **Chronic symptoms:** complete remission within 3–6 months depending on the severity and extent of the damage; in severe cases residual symptoms have to be accepted. The

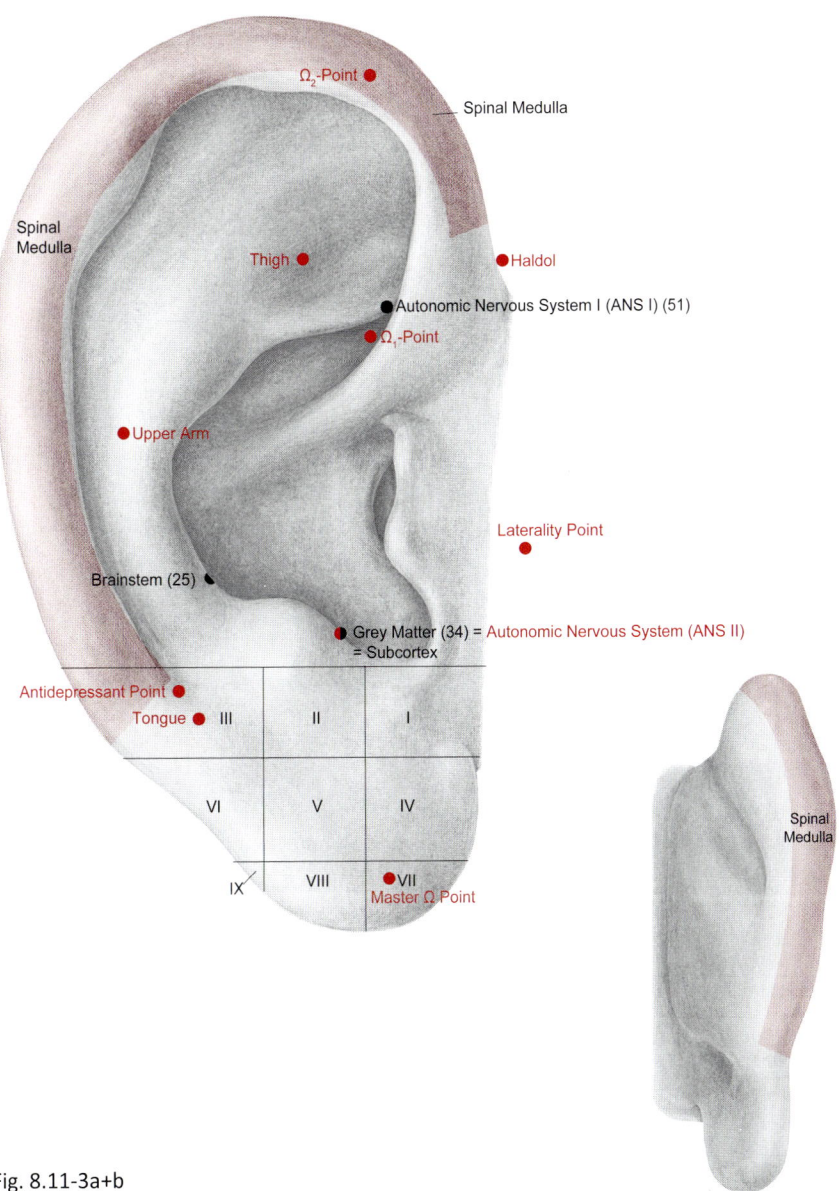

Fig. 8.11-3a+b

younger the patient, the better unaffected areas of the brain can take over functions of damaged areas. This process can be positively influenced by acupuncture. For these reasons acupuncture treatments should be concluded only when there is no further noticable progress.

8.11.4 Tourette Syndrome (Gilles de la Tourette Syndrome)

Description

- Neuropsychiatric disorder characterized by motor tics; classified as extrapyramidal hyperkinesia
- Sudden, generally involuntary, partially vehement, abrupt movements of a wide range of muscle groups
- Also verbal disturbances with unintentional utterances or noises
- Causes: not yet known

Point Prescription

French points

- Local points: **C1-7** (› 6.1.1), **Shoulder** (› 6.2.1) **Elbow** (› 6.2.1); **Hip** (› 6.2.3), **Knee** (› 6.2.3)
- Relaxing points: **Diazepam** (› 6.7.3), **PGE$_1$/Thymus** (› 6.7.6)
- Psychological points: **Omega Axis** (› 6.12.1), **Frustration** (› 6.8.3), **Antidepressant Point** (› 6.8.5)

Chinese points

- Local points: **Cervical Spine (37)** (› 6.1.1)
- Analgesic points: **Sun (35)**, **Occiput (29)**, **Thalamus (26a)** (› 6.7.4)
- Relaxing point: **Muscle Relaxation (98a)** (› 6.1.3)

Treatment Intervals

- **Acute symptoms or acute progression:** once daily until symptoms have reduced significantly, then once weekly until there is a general improvement or complete remission
- **Chronic symptoms:** once weekly until there is a significant improvement; then every 2–3 weeks until symptoms have subsided completely

> **box** Since neither analgesic nor glucocorticoid medication can alleviate pain, acupuncture is an important therapeutic option for pain management. Sufficient sleep supports acupuncture treatments. Beneficial adjuvant therapies include Feldenkrais, autogenic training, or osteopathy.

Treatment Course and Prognosis

- **Acute symptoms:** improvement generally within 4 weeks
- **Chronic symptoms:** complete remission generally only after long-term treatments, depending on the severity of the symptoms up to several years; significant relaxation often within 4–6 weeks

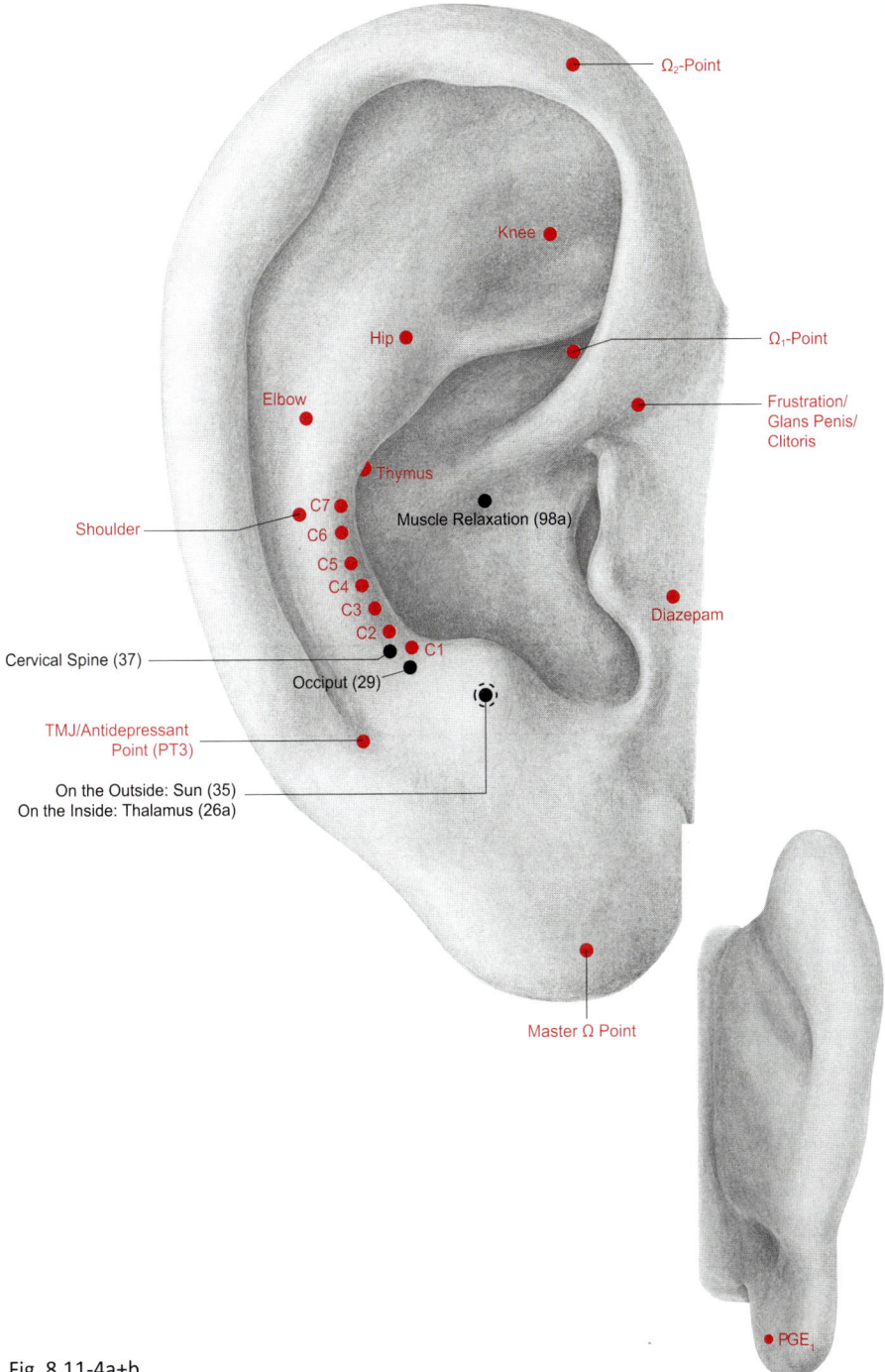

Ω₂-Point

Knee

Hip

Ω₁-Point

Elbow

Frustration/
Glans Penis/
Clitoris

Thymus

C7

C6

Muscle Relaxation (98a)

Shoulder

C5

C4

C3

C2

Diazepam

C1

Cervical Spine (37)

Occiput (29)

TMJ/Antidepressant
Point (PT3)

On the Outside: Sun (35)
On the Inside: Thalamus (26a)

Master Ω Point

PGE₁

Fig. 8.11-4a+b

8.12 Neurovegetative Disorders

8.12.1 Insomnia

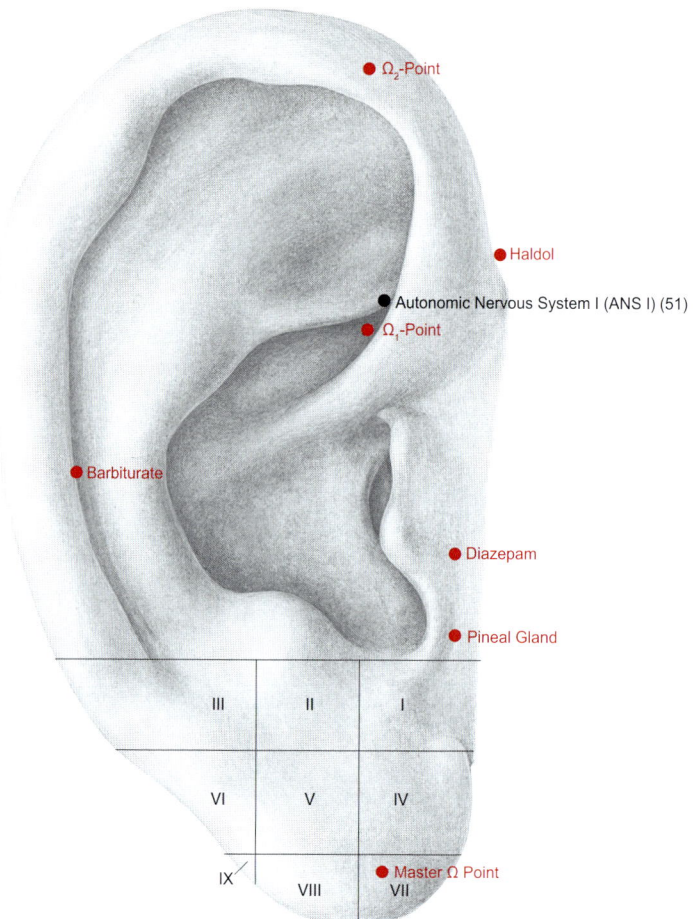

Fig. 8.12-1

Description

- Difficulty falling asleep: > 30 minutes to fall asleep
- Difficulty staying asleep: early waking after < 6 hours sleep for > 3 times weekly
- Causes: primary insomnia (caused by psychosocial stress etc.) or secondary insomnia (caused by psychiatric or organic diseases). **NB:** external causes such as shift work or noise have to be considered!
- Age-related sleep changes: shortened sleep rhythms, lighter sleep with more frequent waking, reduction of total sleep time

Point Prescription

French points
- Calming points: **Diazepam** (› 6.7.3), **Barbiturate** (› 6.7.1), **Haldol** (› 6.8.6), **Omega Axis** (› 6.12.1)
- Stabilising point: **Pineal Gland** (› 6.8.4)

Chinese points
- Stabilising point: **ANS I (51)** (› 6.6.5)

Treatment Intervals
- Initially 1–2 times weekly until symptoms have improved; the best treatment time is towards the evening (**NB**: patient may feel tired directly after the treatment)
- Then 2–3 times monthly until symptoms have disappeared

Treatment Course and Prognosis
The more long-standing the sleeping problem, the longer treatments will be required.
- **Acute insomnia:** approximately 4 weeks until symptoms disappear
- **Chronic insomnia:** treatments required for approximately 3–4 months until symptoms have disappeared

 Insomnia due to psychosocial causes can be alleviated, but not cured, by auricular acupuncture. It is essential that the patient changes the contributing circumstances and/or habits.

8.12.2 Vertigo

Description

- Causes:
  - otogenic, e.g. Menière's disease accompanied by hearing loss and tinnitus (> 8.12.6); with benign paroxysmal positional vertigo and vestibular neuropathy
  - vertebrogenic, e.g. degenerative changes of the cervical spine
  - disturbed blood circulation, e.g. cerebral arteriosclerosis, especially vertebrobasilar insufficiency, hypotension, increased intracranial pressure
  - neorological, e.g. acoustic neuroma
  - ophthalmological, e.g. refractive anomalies
  - psychological, e.g. anxiety disorders
- Forms of vertigo:
  - rotatory (objective) vertigo; psychogenic vertigo; sensation of being dragged upwards in an elevator; diffuse vertigo; positional vertigo (triggered by change in position); recurrent or permanent

Point Prescription

The same treatment protocol applies to all forms of vertigo; RAC-palpation (> 3.1.4) is the determining factor:

French points

- Local point: **Atlanto-occipital Joint** (> 6.1.1)
- Psychological point: **Anxiety** (> 6.8.5)
- Stabilising point: **Vertigo Line** (> 6.10.6)

Chinese points

- Local point: **Inner Ear (9)** (> 6.3.4)
- Stabilising point: ***Shen Men* (55)** (> 6.7.2)
- **Sensory Line** (> 6.10.6) with **Occiput (29)** (> 6.7.4), **Sun (35)** (> 6.7.4), **Forehead (33)** (> 6.3.3)

 Before treating with acupuncture it is essential that the patient is diagnosed by conventional medicine.

Treatment Intervals

- Initially once weekly until symptoms improve
- Then twice/month until symptoms have disappeared

Treatment Course and Prognosis

Depending on the cause:

- **Otogenic:**
  - provided there is no structural cause approximately 6–8 weeks until symptoms improve
  - generally 3–6 months until symptoms have disappeared

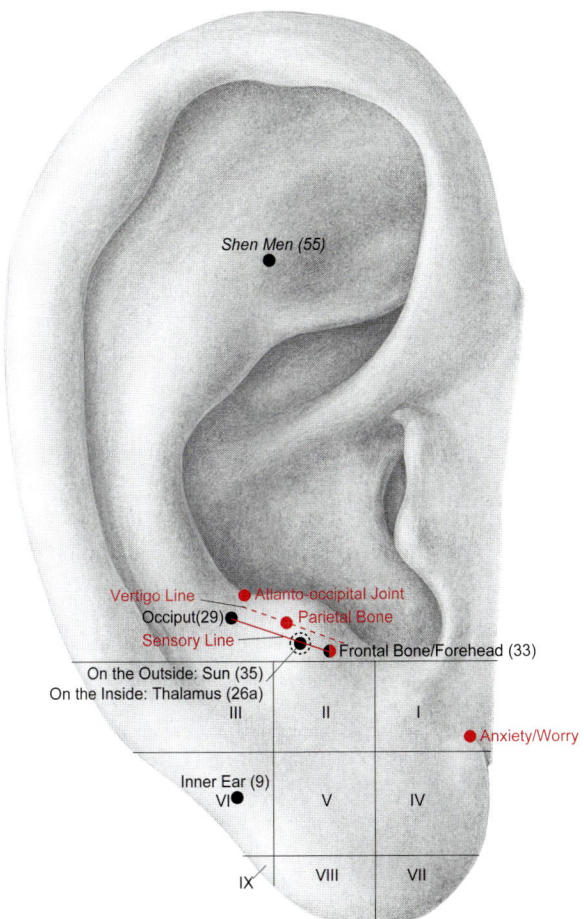

Fig. 8.12-2

- **Vertebral:**
  - irrespective of the extent of the degenerative changes approximately 2–4 weeks until symptoms improve
  - usually 2–3 months until symptoms disappear
- **Impaired circulation:**
  - approximately 2–3 months until symptoms improve (unless there are significant structural changes, e.g. pronounced arteriosclerosis)
  - generally 6–12 months until symptoms disappear (unless there are significant structural changes, e.g. pronounced arteriosclerosis)
- **Psychogenic:**
  - approximately 2–4 weeks until symptoms improve
  - approximately 3–6 months until symptoms disappear

8.12.3 Hiccups (Singultus)

Description

- Short-term involuntary diaphragmatic contractions; only rarely a permanent accompanying symptom of an underlying disorder (pathological singultus)
- Pathologic causes of hiccups:
  - localized irritation of the diaphragm caused by peritonitis, lung disease, abdominal surgery etc.
  - brain damage (basilar artery thrombosis, encephalitis, or alcohol intoxication)
  - medication side effects (e.g. anti-epileptic drugs)
  - allergic reaction (e.g. to certain foods)
  - psychogenic

Point Prescription

Hiccups, irrespective of their cause, can be treated with the following acupuncture points albeit with varying prognoses.

French points

- Local point: **Stomach** (› 6.11.3) on the posterior ear
- Stabilising point: **Point Zero** (› 6.10.3)
- Psychological points: **Diazepam** (› 6.7.3), **Haldol** (› 6.8.6), **Omega Axis** (› 6.12.1)

Chinese points

- Local points: **Stomach (87)**, **Cardia (86)** (› 6.4.1)

Treatment Intervals

- **Palliative**, e.g. hiccups caused by organic brain diseases, irritation of the diaphragm, or medication side effects:
  - 3 times weekly until symptoms improve
  - complete recovery is possible only if the underlying disorder can be resolved
- **Curative**, e.g. psychogenic or allergic hiccups:
  - initially 3 times weekly until symptoms improve
  - then 1–2 times weekly until symptoms have disappeared

Treatment Course and Prognosis

- Symptoms generally improve after approximately 4 weeks, irrespective of the cause
- Complete recovery: only with psychogenic or allergic hiccups, generally after 2–3 months

> Acupuncture can alleviate, but not cure hiccups with a mechanical or nerve-related pathogenesis.

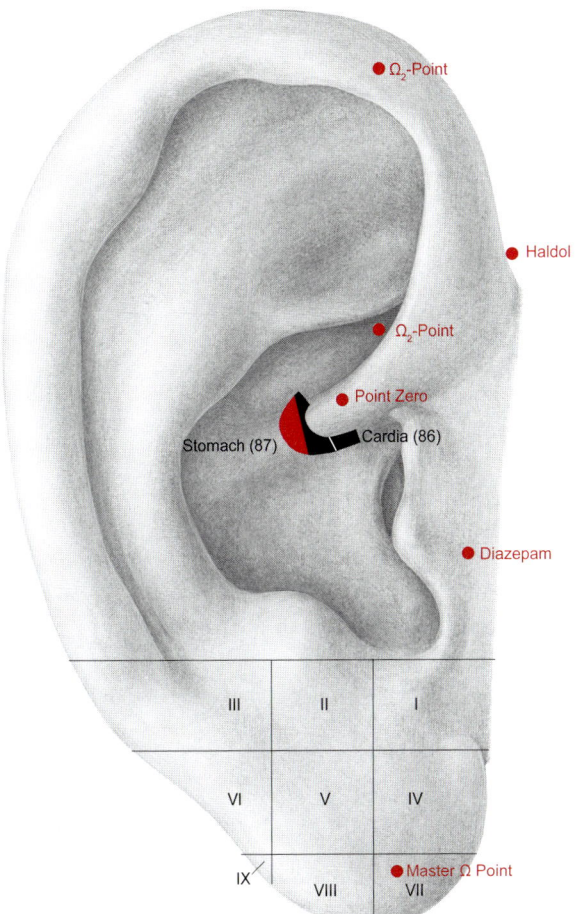

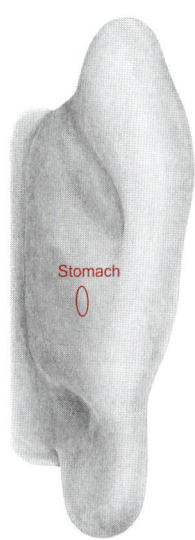

Fig. 8.12-3a+b

8.12.4 Motion Sickness (Travel Sickness, Kinetosis)

Description

- Irritation of the vestibular system, e.g. caused by travelling by car, bus, ship, plane, or railway
- Symptoms: dizziness, nausea to the point of vomiting, pallor, sweating, possibly drop in blood pressure, and headaches

Point Prescription

French points

- Local point: **Stomach** (› 6.11.3) on the posterior ear
- Stabilising point: **Point Zero** (› 6.10.3)
- Sedating point: **Diazepam** (› 6.7.3)

Chinese points

- Local points: **Stomach (87)**, **Cardia (86)** (› 6.4.1), **Inner Ear (9)** (› 6.3.4)

Treatment Intervals

- One acupuncture treatment, ideally on or 1 day before the day of travel; 2–3 semi-permanent needles may be added, e.g. on the points **Stomach** and **Anxiety**
- Repeat treatments prior to subsequent travels are recommended. If there are no symptoms on 3–4 journeys further acupuncture treatments are generally not required.

Treatment Course and Prognosis

- Symptoms generally disappear after one single treatment.
- In case of residual symptoms: 4 weekly treatments prior to the next journey

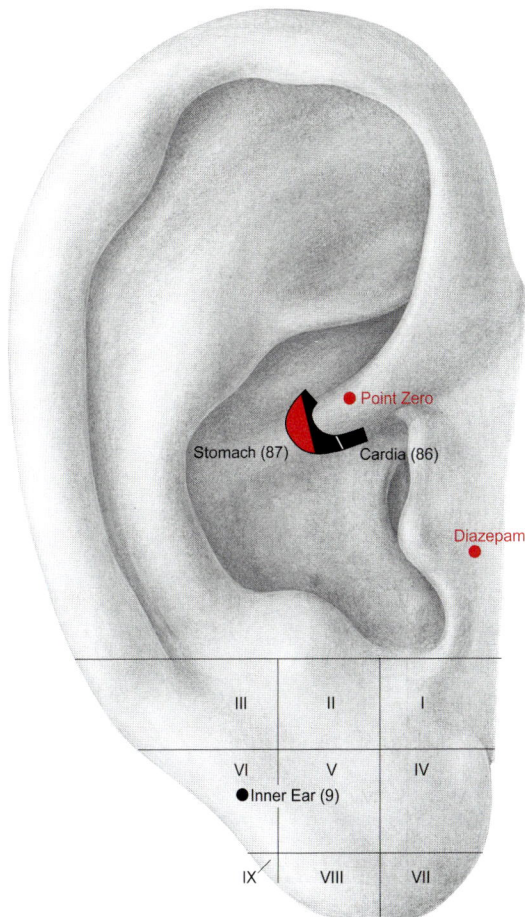

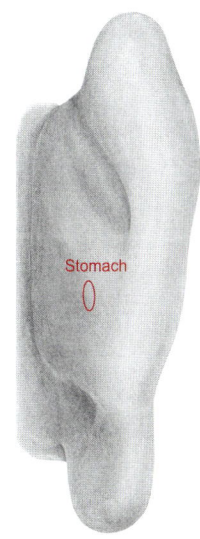

Fig. 8.12-4a+b

8.12.5 Jet Lag (Desynchronosis)

Description

- Circadian rhythm disturbance affecting normal functioning of the body
- Affects sleep-wake rhythm
- Causes:
  – crossing several time zones (air travel)
  – night shifts, shift work

Point Prescription

French points

- Local point: **Pineal Gland** (› 6.8.4)
- Stabilising points: **Laterality Point** (› 6.8.6), **Point Zero** (› 6.10.3)
- Relaxing points: **Diazepam** (› 6.7.3), **Omega Axis** (› 6.12.1)

Chinese points

- Stabilising points: **Occiput (29)** (› 6.7.4), **Sensorial Line** (› 6.10.6), *Shen Men* **(55)** (› 6.7.2), **ANS I (51)** (› 6.6.5), **ANS II (34)** (› 6.7.4)
- Relaxing point: **Muscle Relaxation (98a)** (› 6.1.3)

> **box**
> In a study conducted by the US Air Force five crew members were treated with auricular acupuncture as follows: electro-stimulation at *Shen Men* (55), ANS I (51), ANS II (34), Point Zero, and Pineal Gland. All five subjects reported calm and restful sleep after the treatment (Medical Acupuncture, 1999/2000, vol. 11, No. 2).

Treatment Intervals

- **Acute symptoms**, especially in conjunction with air travel: daily treatments until the circadian rhythm has been restored
- **Chronic symptoms**, especially with shift work: 2–3 times weekly for approximately 4 weeks to restore the patient's rhythm, or until the sleep disorder has resolved; then 1–2 times monthly to maintain treatment results

> **box**
> Shift work, especially with changing shift times, permanently affects the circadian rhythm. After an initial stabilisation regular monthly treatments are necessary for continuous support of the rhythm.

Treatment Course and Prognosis

- **Acute symptoms:** symptoms generally subside within a few days
- **Chronic symptoms:** significant relaxation and better regulation of the circadian rhythm within 4–6 weeks, possibly longer, depending on the severity of the disorder; if the causative factors persist long-term treatment is essential

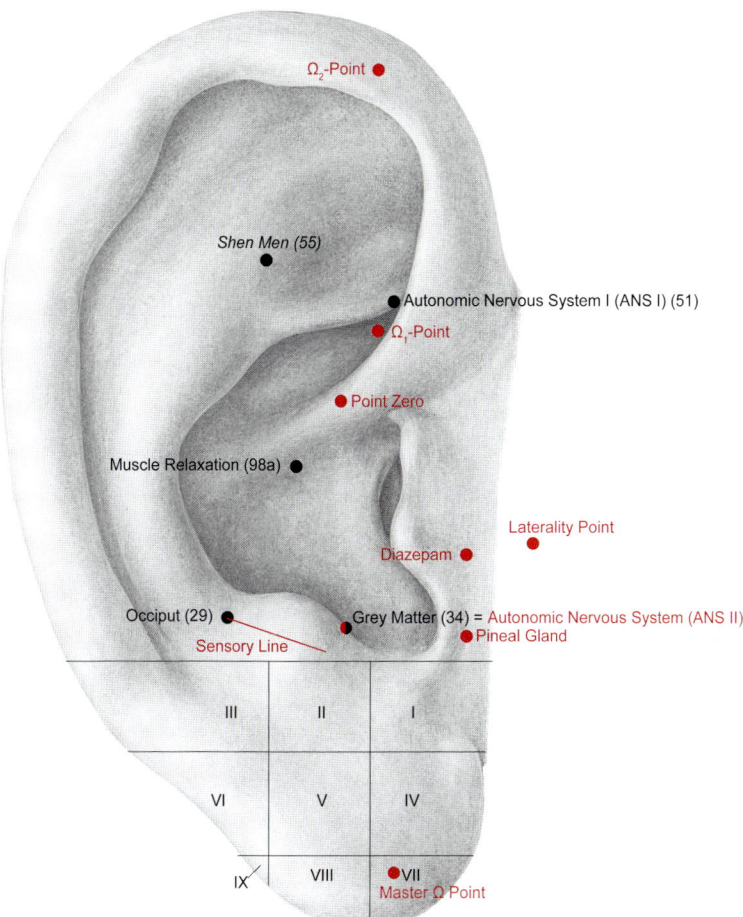

Fig. 8.12-5

8.12.6 Tinnitus

Description

- Perception of noise with widely varying characteristics in one's ear, e.g. buzzing, gushing, ringing, or whistling noises; may be continuous or intermittent; even or pulsatile forms
- Causes:
  - altered blood flow: mainly pulsatile forms
  - exposure to loud noises
  - ear disorders, e.g. otosclerosis, secretory otitis media, acute hearing loss (› 8.12.7)
  - neurological disorders, e.g. acoustic neuroma, multiple sclerosis
- May be triggered or exacerbated by stress

 Tinnitus may be exacerbated by psychological factors.

Point Prescription

If occurring together with sudden hearing loss, use the treatment protocol under › 8.12.7

French points

- Local points: **Sensorial Line** (› 6.10.6), **Atlanto-occipital Joint** (› 6.1.1)
- Psychological points: **Anti-Aggression** (› 6.8.5), **Haldol** (› 6.8.6)

Chinese points

- Local point: **Inner Ear** (› 6.3.4)
- Stabilising point: *Shen Men* **(55)** (› 6.7.2)

 Diagnosis (of exclusion) by a relevant consultant is essential before treating with auricular acupuncture.

Treatment Intervals

- **Acute tinnitus:** 3 times weekly, generally only the affected side is treated (but RAC-palpation is the determining factor [› 3.1.4])
- **Chronic cases** and with improved symptoms: once weekly, generally only the affected side is treated

Treatment Course and Prognosis

- Good prognosis for recent onset tinnitus; poor prognosis for symptoms for > 6 months
- Reduced volume or changed pitch generally within 4 weeks; otherwise little chance of improvement
- If there is an improvement, it takes about 6 months until symptoms disappear completely.

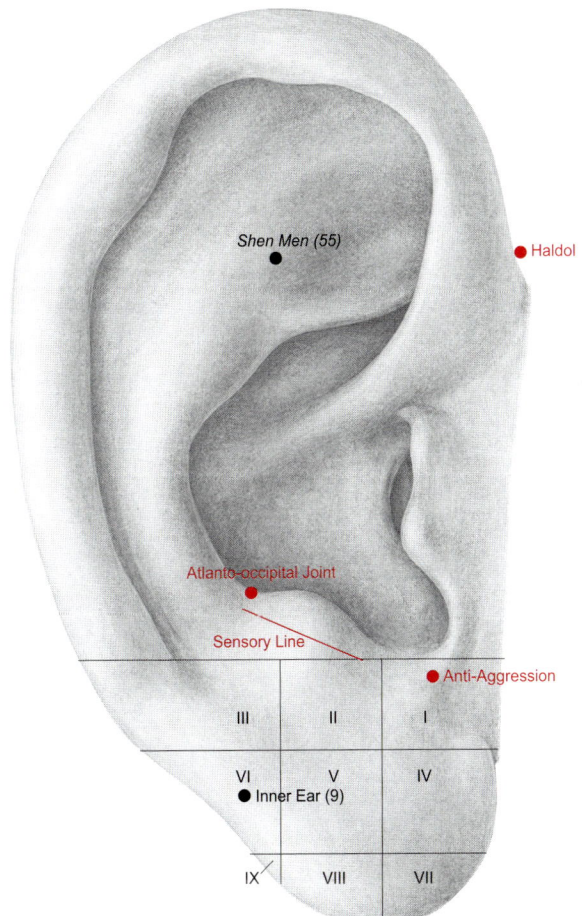

Fig. 8.12-6

8.12.7 Acute Hearing Loss

Description

- Mostly one-sided; typically characterized by an initial sensation of pressure followed by sudden hearing loss, possibly accompanied by tinnitus (› 8.12.6) and vertigo (› 8.12.2)
- Causes: to date no clear explanation, possibly caused by spasms of the arterial vessels in the inner ear, infections, and stress. Differential diagnosis: acoustic neuroma, inflammatory disorder of the middle and inner ear, zoster oticus, multiple sclerosis

Point Prescription

 Examination by a consultant is essential before treating with auricular acupuncture.

French points

- Local points: **Statoacoustic nerve** (› 6.10.5), **Sensorial Line** (› 6.10.6), **Vertigo Line** (› 6.10.6)
- Stabilising points: **Kidney I** (› 6.5.1), **Liver** (› 6.4.1)
- Psychological points: **Anti-Aggression** (› 6.8.5), **Haldol** (› 6.8.6), **Diazepam** (› 6.7.3), **Barbiturate** (› 6.7.1), **Point de Jérome (29b)** (› 6.8.2), **Antidepressant Point** (› 6.8.5)

Chinese points

- Local points: **Inner ear (9)** (› 6.3.4), **Occiput (29)**
- Stabilising point: ***Shen Men (55)*** (› 6.7.2)

- In addition to auricular acupuncture, body acupuncture or conventional treatments (e.g. infusions, pressure chamber) are essential, especially if there is no significant short-term improvement (within 2–3 treatments).
- Stress and other strain should be reduced to ensure a long-term treatment effect. A change of environment during the treatment course is often beneficial.

Treatment Intervals

- **Acute cases:** 3 times weekly
- **Chronic cases** and with improved symptoms: once weekly

Treatment Course and Prognosis

- Improved hearing within 4 weeks, otherwise poor prognosis
- Symptoms generally disappear completely after approximately 1–3 months
- Poorer prognosis if accompanied by tinnitus

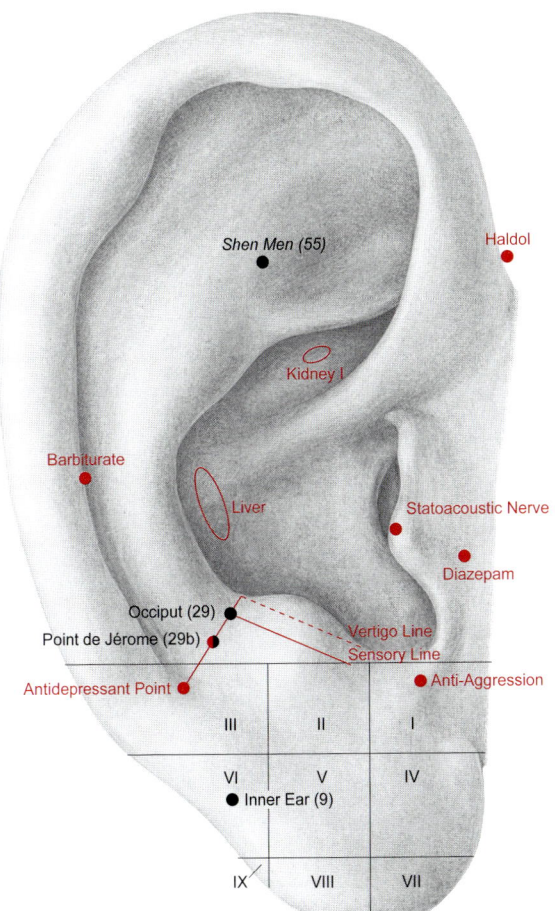

Fig. 8.12-7

8.13 Psychological Disorders

8.13.1 Depression

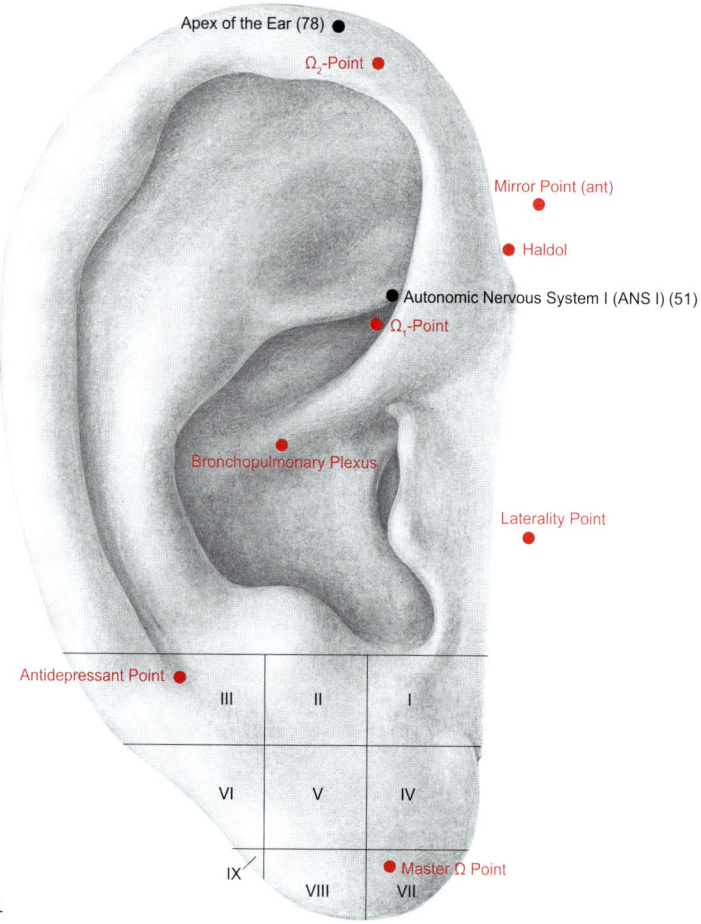

Apex of the Ear (78)

Ω_2-Point

Mirror Point (ant)

Haldol

Autonomic Nervous System I (ANS I) (51)

Ω_1-Point

Bronchopulmonary Plexus

Laterality Point

Antidepressant Point

III   II   I

VI   V   IV

IX   VIII   VII

Master Ω Point

Fig. 8.13-1

Description

- Various forms:
    - psychogenic depression
    - reactive depression
    - neurotic depression (dysthymia)
    - masked depression
    - psychotic depression
    - endogenous depression

- Core symptoms: depressive mood, indifference, bleak mood, easily fatigued, lack of motivation
- Secondary symptoms include: loss of appetite, loss of libido, difficulty concentrating; feeling worthless and stuck, feelings of guilt

Point Prescription

The same treatment protocol applies for the different forms of depression. RAC-palpation determines the point prescription (› 3.1.4).

French points

- Psychological points: **Antidepressant Axis** (› 6.12.6), **Omega Axis** (› 6.12.1), **Antidepressant Point** (› 6.8.5), **Haldol** (› 6.8.6), **Bronchopulmonary Plexus** (› 6.10.1)
- Stabilising point: **Laterality Point** (› 6.8.6)

Chinese points

- Stabilising points: **Apex of the Ear (78)** (› 6.10.3), **ANS I (51)** (› 6.6.5)

Treatment Intervals

- **Depressive Phase:** once daily or every other day; suicide risk requires close monitoring of the patient
- **Remission with few or no symptoms:** once weekly until there is a sustained relief from symptoms for > 4 weeks

- If there is a risk of suicide the patient should be hospitalised.
- While acupuncture can improve the client's motivation the level of depression may not diminish. It is therefore possible that the treatments will not result in a decrease of any suicidal tendencies.

Treatment Course and Prognosis

- **Reactive, psychogenic and neurotic depression:**
  - acute depression: 1–2 weeks until symptoms improve significantly and symptom-free intervals become longer
  - initial depressive episode (< 6 months): approximately 1–3 months until symptoms disappear
  - depression for > 6 months: treatments for up to 1 year until symptoms disappear
- **Endogenous and masked depression** (generally requires the combination with body acupuncture and Chinese herbal medicine):
  - 3–6 months for a sustained improvement
  - provided the patient responds well to treatments: > 1 year until there is a sustained recovery

8.13.2 Difficulty Concentrating

Description

- Causes include: feeling overwhelmed, fatigue, mental retardation, depression (› 8.13.1), poisoning (e.g. amphetamines), trauma
- Symptoms:
  – easily distracted
  – unable to complete a task or chore
  – recurring thoughts
  – slow perception

 The ability to concentrate varies significantly from individual to individual. It can be difficult, especially in children, to differentiate between pathological and physiological conditions.

Point Prescription

Difficulty concentrating can be an accompanying symptom of depression (› 8.13.1).

French points

- Stabilising points: **Point Zero** (› 6.10.3), **Laterality Point** (› 6.8.6)
- Psychological points: **Haldol** (› 6.8.6), **Diazepam** (› 6.7.3), **Omega Axis** (› 6.12.1)

Chinese points

- Stabilising point: **Tip of the Apex (78)** (› 6.10.3)

Treatment Intervals

- Initially once weekly until symptoms improve
- Then twice monthly for at least 2–3 months to consolidate treatment effects

Treatment Course and Prognosis

- 4 weeks until symptoms improve

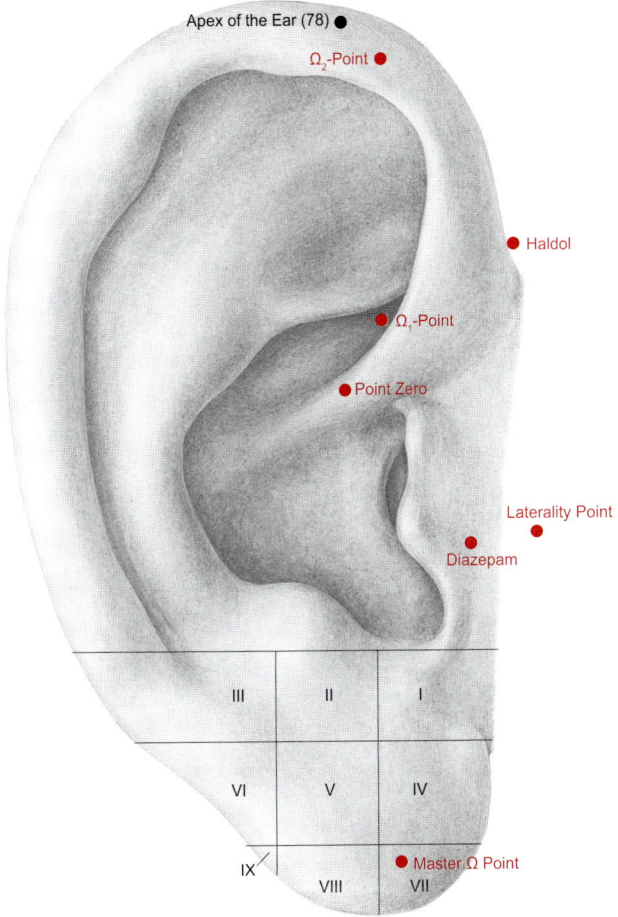

Apex of the Ear (78) ●

Ω₂-Point ●

● Haldol

● Ω₁-Point

● Point Zero

Laterality Point ●

● Diazepam

III II I

VI V IV

IX

VIII VII

● Master Ω Point

Fig. 8.13-2

8.13.3 Cardiac Neurosis

Description

- Recurrent attacks of 'heart pain' combined with restlessness, anxiety, fear of heart disease (e.g. myocardial infarction), and sometimes hyperventilation
- No verifiable anatomical or physiological correlation
- Causes include:
  - psychological trauma (e.g. death of spouse)
  - frustration
  - pent-up aggression

Point Prescription

French points

- Local points: **Heart II** (› 6.4.2), β-**Receptor** (› 6.7.1)
- Stabilising point: **Laterality Point** (› 6.8.6)
- Psychological points: **Omega Axis** (› 6.12.1), **Haldol** (› 6.8.6)

Chinese points

- Local point: **Heart I (100)** (› 6.4.1)
- Stabilising point: **Tip of the Apex (78)** (› 6.10.3), **ANS I (51)** (› 6.6.5)

> **box** Before starting treatments with auricular acupuncture any anatomical or physiological causes have to be excluded by a conventional medical examination.

Treatment Intervals

- Daily occurrence: once daily or every other day
- With improved symptoms once weekly until symptoms have disappeared

Treatment Course and Prognosis

- Generally significant improvement within 2 weeks
- Symptoms often subside completely after 2–3 months

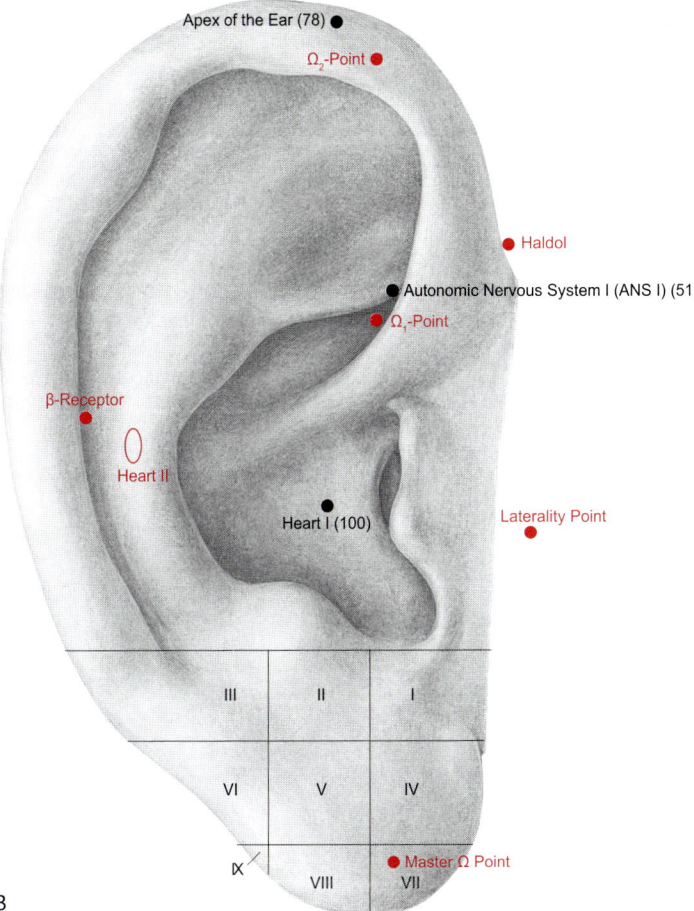

Apex of the Ear (78) ●

Ω₂-Point ●

● Haldol

● Autonomic Nervous System I (ANS I) (51)

● Ω₁-Point

β-Receptor ●

Heart II

Heart I (100) ●

Laterality Point ●

III   II   I

VI   V   IV

IX   VIII   VII

● Master Ω Point

Fig. 8.13-3

8.13.4 Anorexia Nervosa

Description

- Psychogenic eating disorder characterised by a refusal to eat: weight loss to the point of cachexia and starvation
- Onset generally during puberty, affects mainly women
- Psychodynamics: problematic relationship with the mother, rejection of femininity, sexual abuse
- May develop into or alternate with bulimia nervosa (› 8.13.5)

- If the condition is life-threatening the patient has to be hospitalised immediately.
- Milder forms can be treated with psychotherapy in an out-patient setting. Support with auricular acupuncture is in such cases of considerable benefit.

Point Prescription

French points

- Local points: **Gullet Point** (› 6.4.1), **Neural Stomach Point** (› 6.9.2)
- Psychological points: **Anti-Aggression** (› 6.8.5), **Haldol** (› 6.8.6), **Omega Axis** (› 6.12.1)
- Stabilising points: **Point Zero** (› 6.10.3), **Laterality Point** (› 6.8.6)
- Hormonal points: **Ovaries** (› 6.5.2), **Progesterone** (› 6.6.3), **Gonadotropin** (› 6.6.7), **Gynaecological Axis** (› 6.12.5)

Chinese points

- Local point: **Mouth (84)** (› 6.4.1)
- Stabilising point: **Hunger (18)** (› 6.10.5)

Treatment Intervals

- Initially once weekly until there is weight gain
- Then 2–3 times monthly

Treatment Course and Prognosis

Prognosis varies greatly from person to person:
- Total treatment duration is generally 1–2 years
- A change in eating habits and weight gain can be expected after 3–6 months

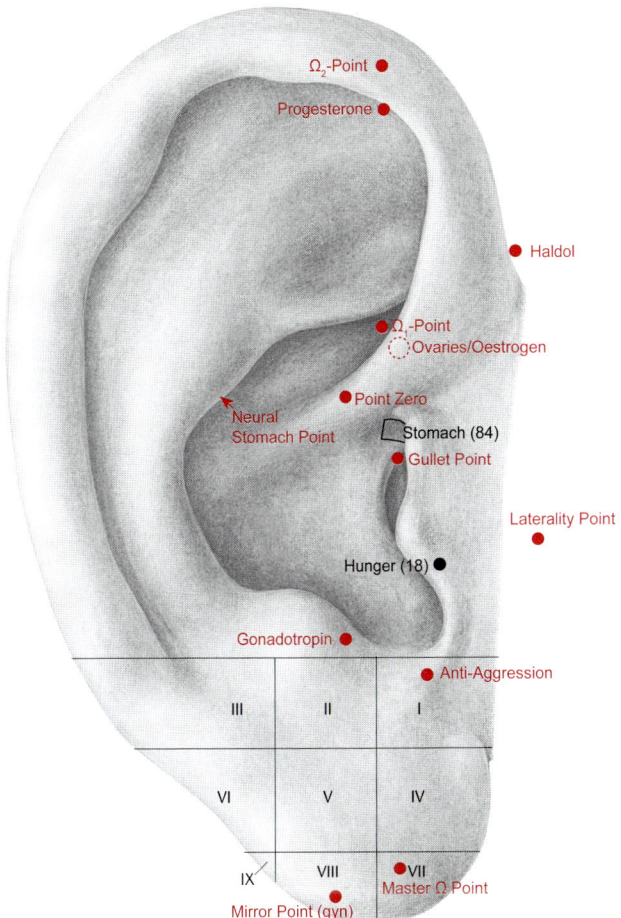

Fig. 8.13-4

8.13.5 Bulimia Nervosa

Description

- Psychogenic eating disorder: binge eating followed by measures to avoid weight gain (induced vomiting and/or abuse of laxatives and diuretics)
- Fear of weight gain while objectively being of normal weight
- Predominantly affects women

Point Prescription

French points

- Local points: **Gullet Point** (› 6.4.1), **Neural Stomach Point** (› 6.9.2)
- Psychological points: **Desire (29c)** (› 6.8.3), **Anti-Aggression** (› 6.8.5), **Haldol** (› 6.8.6), **Omega Axis** (› 6.12.1)
- Stabilising points: **Point Zero** (› 6.10.3), **Laterality Point** (› 6.8.6)

Chinese points

- Local point: **Mouth (84)** (› 6.4.1)
- Stabilising point: **Hunger (18)** (› 6.10.5)

 Psychotherapy is absolutely essential. Auricular acupuncture can provide additional support.

Treatment Intervals

- Initially once weekly until binge eating has stopped
- Then 2–3 times monthly until eating habits can be consciously controlled

Treatment Course and Prognosis

Prognosis varies greatly from person to person:

- A change in eating habits can be expected after 3–6 months
- Treatments generally necessary for 1–2 years; treatment results are not always satisfactory

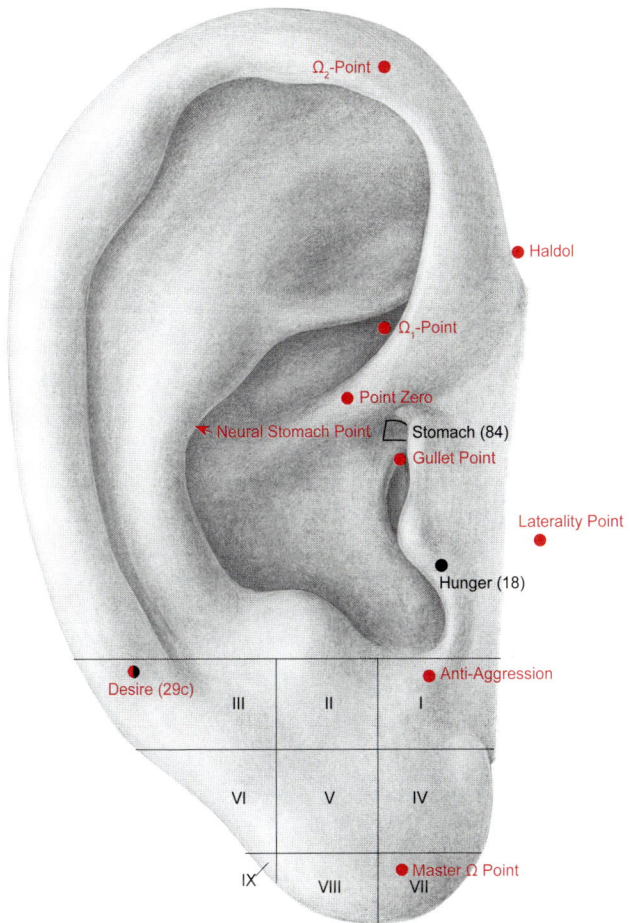

Ω₂-Point

Haldol

Ω₁-Point

Point Zero

Neural Stomach Point Stomach (84)

Gullet Point

Laterality Point

Hunger (18)

Desire (29c)

III II I

Anti-Aggression

VI V IV

IX VIII VII

Master Ω Point

Fig. 8.13-5

8.14 Anxiety Disorders

8.14.1 Exam Nerves

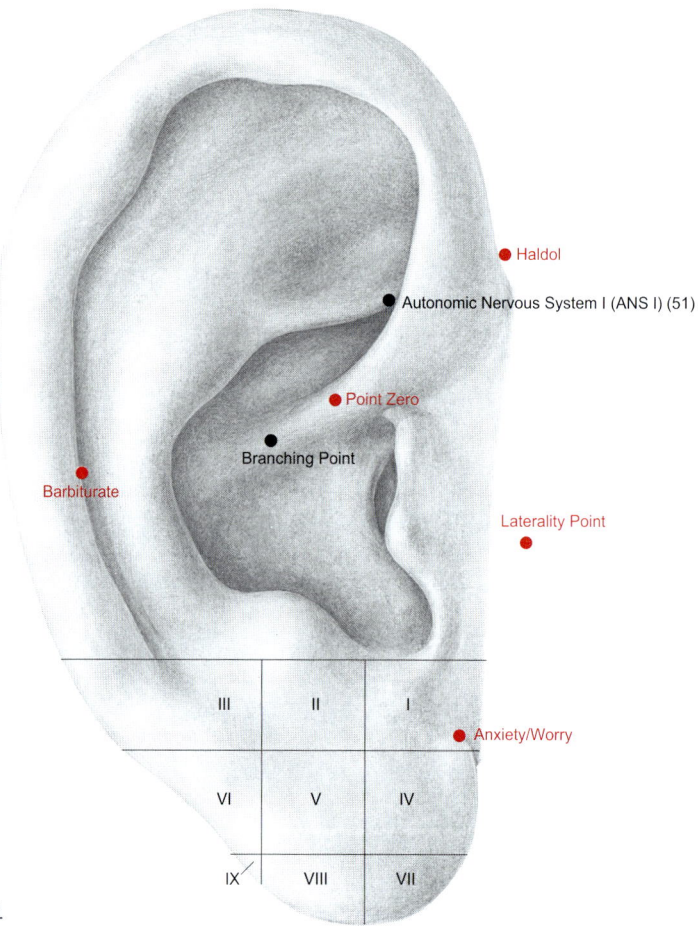

Haldol

Autonomic Nervous System I (ANS I) (51)

Point Zero

Branching Point

Barbiturate

Laterality Point

III   II   I

Anxiety/Worry

VI   V   IV

IX   VIII   VII

Fig. 8.14-1

Description

- Mental block during exam situations
- Irrespective of the degree of preparation (generally prepared well above average)

Point Prescription

French points

- Psychological points: **Anxiety** (dominant ear) **Worry** (non-dominant ear) (› 6.8.5)
- Calming points: **Barbiturate** (› 6.7.1), **Haldol** (› 6.8.6)
- Stabilising points: **Laterality Point** (› 6.8.6), **Point Zero** (› 6.10.3)

Chinese points

- Stabilising points: **Branching Point (83)** (› 6.10.1), **ANS I (51)** (› 6.6.5)

Treatment Intervals

- 2–3 days before the exam: once daily
- Several exams over a longer period of time: additionally once weekly

- Inserting 1–2 semi-permanent needles during the week of the exam can provide further assurance.
- If the patient suffers from other forms of anxiety (e.g. diffuse anxiety), this will delay or limit the therapeutic results.

Treatment Course and Prognosis

- Good; generally one treatment course is sufficient; a positive exam experience will in itself further reduce exam nerves.
- Repeat treatments may be necessary, especially if subsequent exams take place only months or years later.

8.14.2 Fear of Flying (Aerophobia)

Description

- Generally a concrete fear of a plane crash
- Only rarely combined with claustrophobia
- Sometimes triggered by a negative experience during the first flight (turbulences etc.)

Point Prescription

French points

- Psychological points: **Anxiety** (› 6.8.5), **Pineal Gland** (› 6.8.4)
- Sedating points: **Master-Ω-Point** (› 6.8.5), **Diazepam** (› 6.7.3)
- Stabilising point: **Laterality Point** (› 6.8.6)

Chinese points

- Stabilising points: Shen **Men (55)** (› 6.7.2), **Apex of the Ear (78)** (› 6.10.3)

Treatment Intervals

- Start of treatments 4 weeks before flying: once weekly for 3 weeks
- During the week before the flight: 2–3 times weekly

 1–2 semi-permanent needles should be inserted a few days before the flight as additional support.

Treatment Course and Prognosis

- Good, especially if the patient does not suffer from other forms of anxiety or phobias.
- If the patient also suffers from claustrophobia the prognosis is poorer and the time required for treatment is longer (up to approximately 6 months).

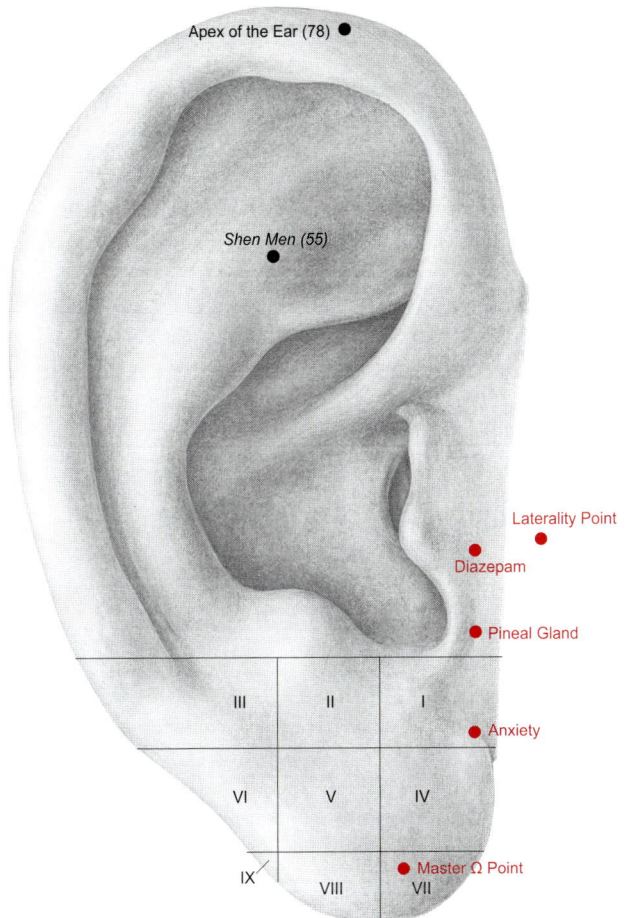

Fig. 8.14-2

8.14.3 Anxiety

Description

- Diffuse anxiety without a concrete reason or threat; usually in the form of attacks of varying duration, lasting minutes to hours, only rarely for days
- Accompanying symptoms:
  - physical symptoms such as sweating, thoracic pain, abdominal pain, nausea

Point Prescription

French points

- Psychological points: **Anxiety** (› 6.8.5)
- Sedating points: **Diazepam** (› 6.7.3), **Barbiturate** (› 6.7.1), **Haldol** (› 6.8.6), **Omega Axis** (› 6.12.1)
- Stabilising points: **Spleen** (› 6.11.3), **Heart II** (› 6.4.2), **Laterality Point** (› 6.8.6)

Chinese points

- Stabilising points: **Branching Point (83)** (› 6.10.1), **Apex of the Ear (78)** (› 6.10.3), **Spleen (98)** (› 6.4.1)

Treatment Intervals

- **Acute stage** (several anxiety attacks per week): 2–3 times weekly
- Once the **acute phase has subsided**: once weekly until there is sustained relief from symptoms

Treatment Course and Prognosis

- Good; approximately 1–2 months until symptom-free intervals become longer and the intensity of the anxiety attacks has reduced; medication can generally be discontinued at this stage
- If the patient responds well to acupuncture, approximately 3–6 months until symptoms have disappeared.

box
Complete abstinence from alcohol and drugs is generally required for good treatment results.

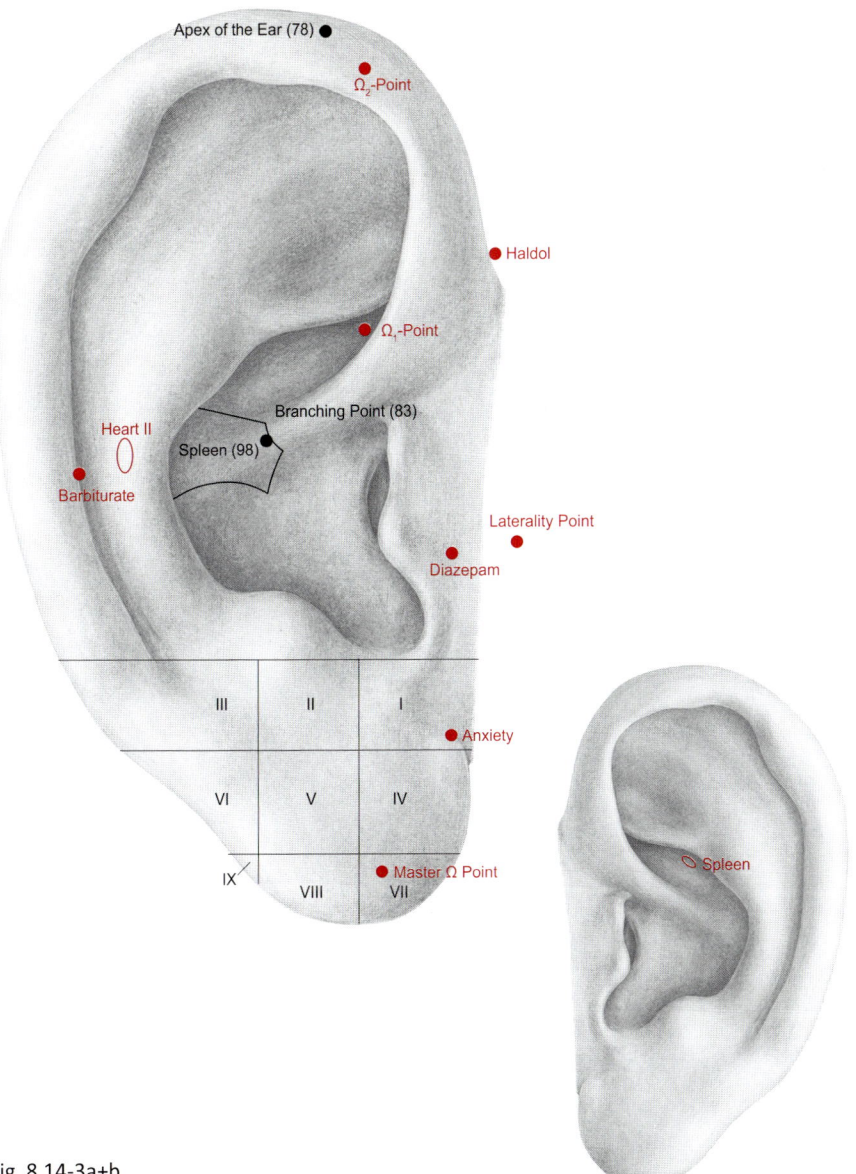

Apex of the Ear (78)

Ω₂-Point

Haldol

Ω₁-Point

Branching Point (83)

Heart II

Spleen (98)

Barbiturate

Laterality Point

Diazepam

III   II   I

Anxiety

VI   V   IV

IX   VIII   VII   Master Ω Point

Spleen

Fig. 8.14-3a+b

8.15 Paediatric Disorders

In children all points are, in principle, treated with laser only.

8.15.1 Otitis Media with Effusion (OME, Glue Ear)

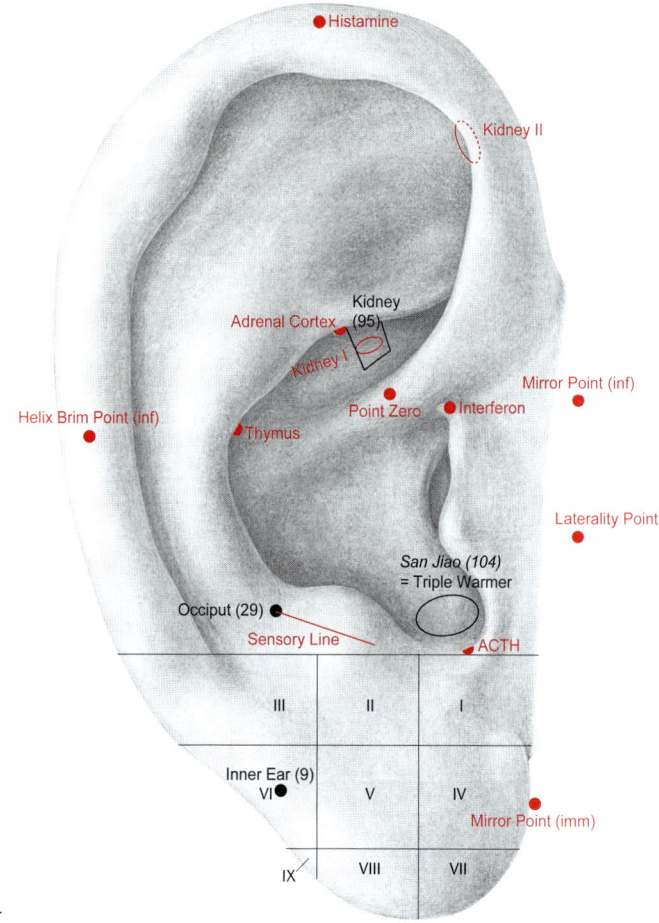

Fig. 8.15-1

Description

- Functional disorder of the eustachian tube with accumulation of fluids in the middle ear
- By otoscopy the fluid level is visible behind the ear drum
- Tympanometric evaluation often shows an altered impedance curve

- Hearing loss
- Pressure sensation in the ear
- May affect one or both ears
- Causes:
  - acute infections (rhinitis, sinusitis, tonsillitis etc.)
  - acute or chronic otitis media
  - in TCM: congenital weakness of the Kidneys

Point Prescription

French points
- Stabilising points: **Point Zero** (› 6.10.3), **Laterality Point** (› 6.8.6), **Sensorial Line** (› 6.10.6), **Kidney I** (› 6.5.1), **Kidney II** (› 6.5.4)
- Immunostimulant points: **Immune Axis** (› 6.12.3), **Infection Axis** (› 6.12.4), **Thymus** (› 6.6.1)

Chinese points
- Local point: **Inner Ear (9)** (› 6.3.4)
- Stabilising points: **Kidney (95)** (› 6.5.1), **Triple Warmer (104)** (› 6.10.1)
- Analgesic point: **Occiput (29)** (› 6.7.4)

Treatment Intervals

- **Acute symptoms:** 2–3 times weekly until there is a significant improvement in hearing or a reduction of fluid, or the infection has subsided
- **Chronic symptoms:** 2–3 times weekly for approximately 4 weeks until symptoms disappear; then 1–2 times monthly until there is a sustained relief from symptoms

Treatment Course and Prognosis

- **Acute symptoms:** generally symptoms disappear within 2–4 weeks
- **Chronic symptoms:** generally both hearing loss and fluid accumulation improve within 4–6 weeks depending on the severity of the case; if there is Kidney deficiency it will take up to 6 months until there is a sustained improvement, sometimes also longer

8.15.2 Enuresis (Bedwetting)

Description

- Bedwetting in children over age 5
- Differentiation between primary and secondary enuresis (after the child was dry for a period of time)
- Causes:
  - recurrent urinary tract infections
  - developmental delay of neural bladder control
  - disturbed day-night rhythm
  - psycho-social problems

Point Prescription

French points

- Local points: **Bladder** (› 6.5.1) on the anterior ear; **Bladder** (› 6.11.3) on the posterior ear
- Psychological points: **Diazepam** (› 6.7.3), **Omega Axis** (› 6.12.1), **Anti-Aggression** (› 6.8.5), **Anxiety/Worry** (› 6.8.5)
- Stabilising points: **Kidney I** (› 6.5.1), **Kidney II** (› 6.5.4) **Laterality Point** (› 6.8.6), **Pineal Gland** (› 6.8.4)
- Immunostimulant points: **Immune Axis** (› 6.12.3), **Infection Axis** (› 6.12.4), **Thymus** (› 6.6.1)

Chinese points

- Local points: **Bladder (92)** (› 6.5.1), **Kidney (95)** (› 6.5.1)
- Stabilising points: *Shen Men* **(55)** (› 6.7.2), **ANS I (51)** (› 6.6.5)

Treatment Intervals

- 1–2 times weekly until there are dry nights during treatment intervals; intervals can then be extended by weekly increments to fortnightly initially, then every 3 weeks and finally every 4 weeks, provided the child stays dry during the intervals. Staying dry for 4 weeks is considered a sustained therapeutic success and treatments can be concluded.

 Before starting treatments any urological anomalies as well as chronic urinary tract infections have to be excluded since they will not respond to auricular acupuncture.

Treatment Course and Prognosis

- Generally improvement within 4 weeks
- Sustained relief within a few months and up to one year, depending on the complexity of the case; psychosocial components can significantly delay the treatment progress as the child may reject any treatment success.
- The focus of both diagnosis and treatment is Kidney deficiency as the cause for enuresis. The deficiency may be congenital but it can also be acquired, e.g. disturbed day/night cycle, traumatic events etc. (› 8.4.7)

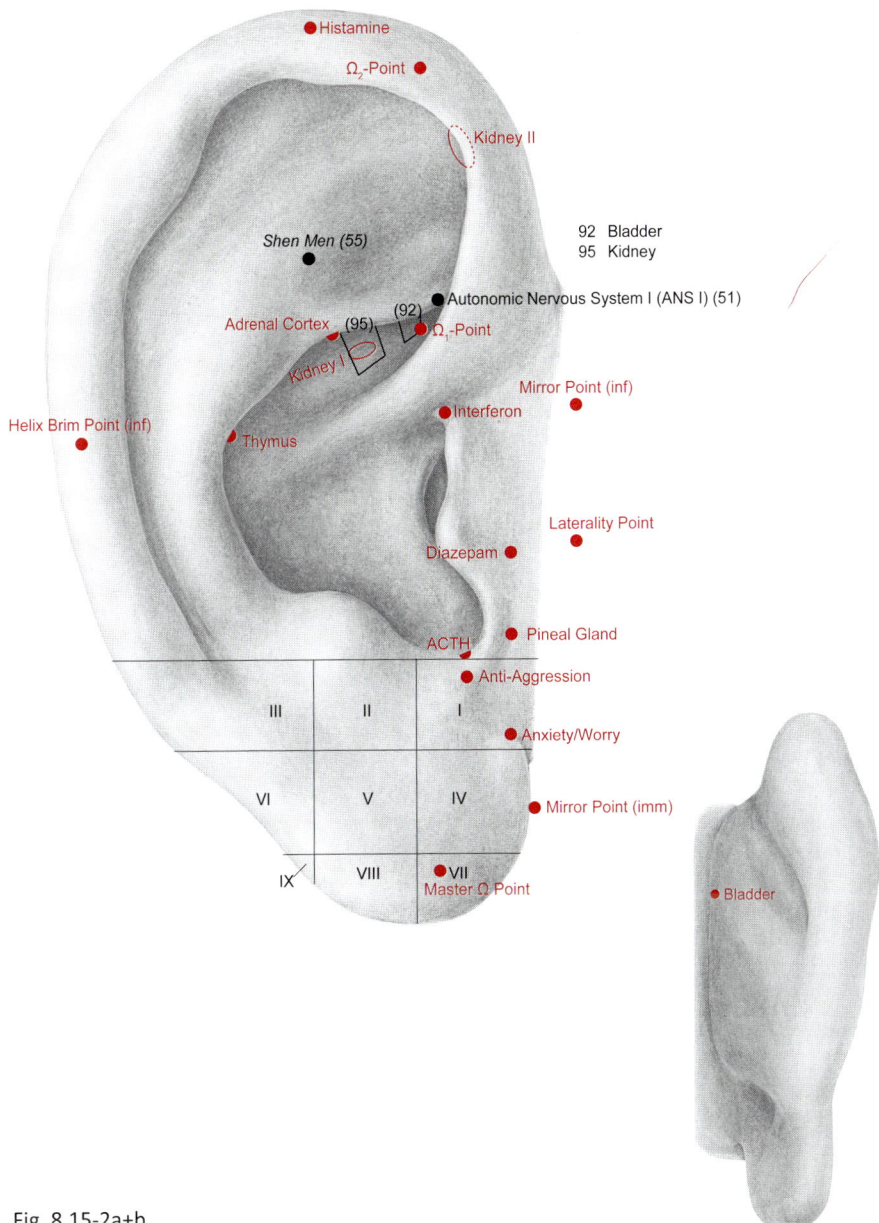

- Histamine
- Ω₂-Point
- Kidney II

Shen Men (55)

92 Bladder
95 Kidney

- Autonomic Nervous System I (ANS I) (51)

Adrenal Cortex (95) (92)
- Ω₁-Point
Kidney I
- Mirror Point (inf)
Helix Brim Point (inf)
- Interferon
- Thymus

- Laterality Point

Diazepam

ACTH
- Pineal Gland
- Anti-Aggression

III   II   I
- Anxiety/Worry

VI   V   IV
- Mirror Point (imm)

IX VIII VII
Master Ω Point

- Bladder

Fig. 8.15-2a+b

8.15.3 Attention Deficit Hyperactivity Disorder (ADHD)

Description

- Attention deficit disorder, often in combination with hyperactive, impulsive behaviour
- Onset before age 7, more prevalent in boys
- Affects approximately 5 % of school-age children
- Causes:
  - constitutional factors
  - psychosocial factors
  - children of above average intelligence who are insufficiently challenged or misunderstood

Point Prescription

French points

- Psychological points: **Omega Axis** (› 6.12.1), **Resentment** (› 6.8.1), **Anti-Aggression** (› 6.8.5), **Diazepam** (› 6.7.3), **Haldol** (› 6.8.6)
- Stabilising points: **Kidney I** (› 6.5.1), **Kidney II** (› 6.5.4), **Laterality Point** (› 6.8.6), **Point Zero** (› 6.10.3)

Chinese points

- Stabilising points: **Shen Men (55)** (› 6.7.2), **ANS I (51)** (› 6.6.5), **Kidney (95)** (› 6.5.1)

Treatment Intervals

- **Initial phase:** 1–2 times weekly until symptoms have calmed down and the ability to concentrate has improved
- **Subsequent treatments:** 2–3 times monthly until the child is more stable and balanced for extended periods of time; this, in turn, will often result in better marks in school

> **box** Above-average aptitude that is not recognised or encouraged, resulting in a low frustration threshold and acting out, is often diagnosed as ADD/ADHD. Affected children do not require treatment but encouragement and understanding, and symptoms will improve. Psychotropic drugs such as Ritalin should certainly not be prescribed!

Treatment Course and Prognosis

- **Initial phase:** symptoms generally improve within 4 weeks
- **Further treatment course:** it may take half a year or longer until the child is completely stable and balanced. Relapses may occur, e.g. due to stressful situations, but usually respond well to short-term treatments.

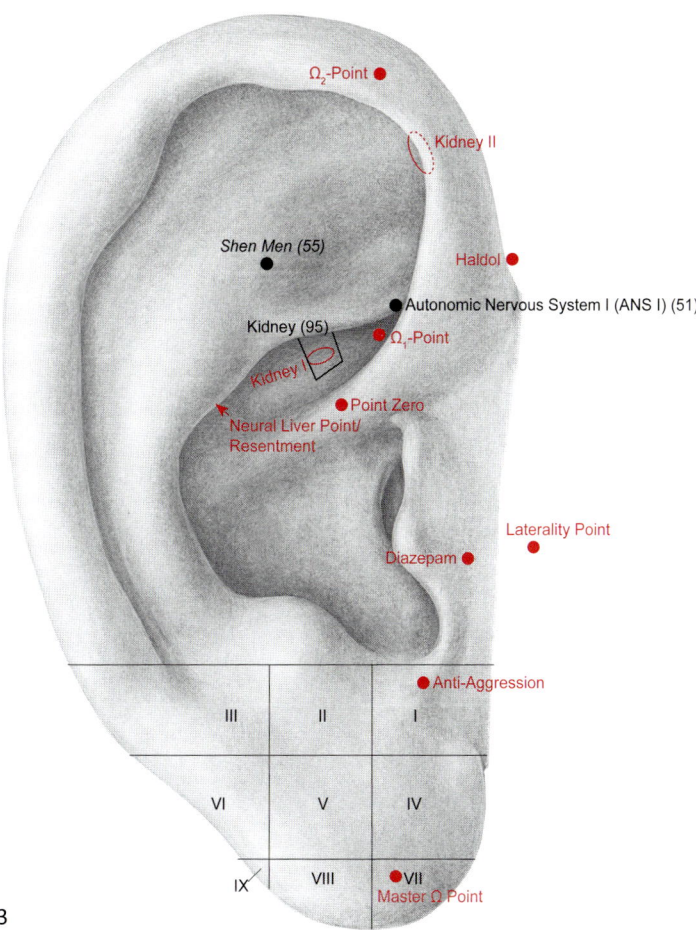

Ω₂-Point ●

Kidney II

Shen Men (55) ●

Haldol ●

●Autonomic Nervous System I (ANS I) (51)

Kidney (95)
●Ω₁-Point

Kidney I

●Point Zero

Neural Liver Point/
Resentment

Laterality Point
●

Diazepam ●

●Anti-Aggression

III	II	I
VI	V	IV
IX	VIII	VII

●VII
Master Ω Point

Fig. 8.15-3

9 Practice of Auricular Acupuncture by Different Schools

9.1 Differences

(› Fig. 9.1-1)

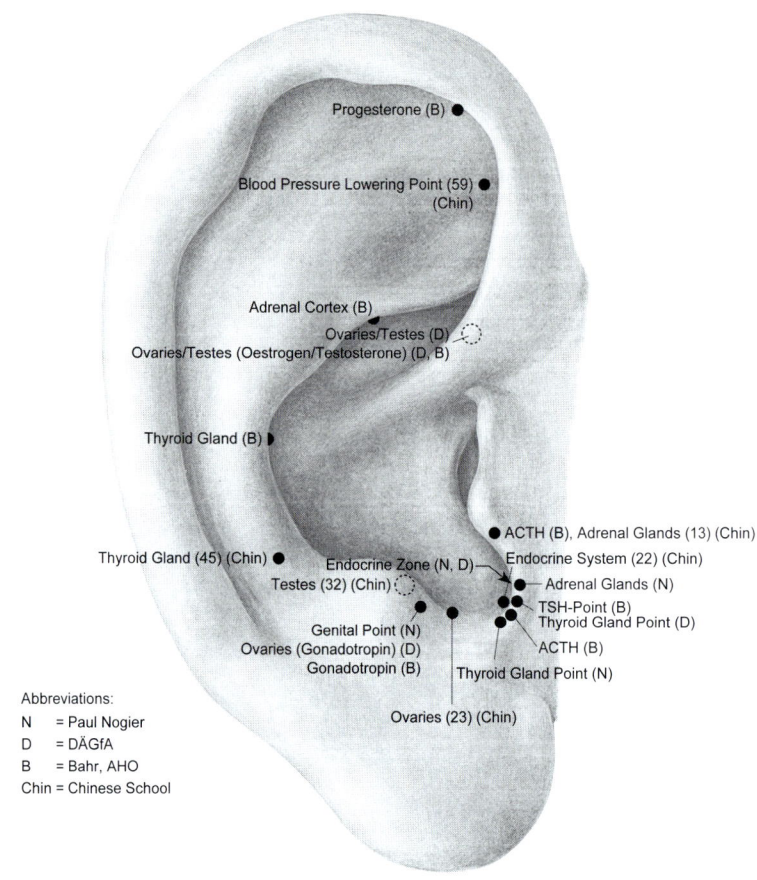

Fig. 9.1-1

Paul Nogier

- **Adrenal Cortex Point:** slightly superior to the intertragic notch
- **Thyroid Point:** slightly lateral to the intertragic notch
- **Endocrine Zone:** on the inside of the intertragic notch, extending approximately 1 cm both laterally and medially; divided into the points Thyroid Gland, Parathyroid Gland, and Pituitary Gland
- **Genital Point:** on the medial tip of the antitragus, corresponds to the location of the points Gonadotropin (after Bahr) and Ovaries/Gonadotropin (after DÄGfA [German Association for Medical Acupuncture])

Deutsche Ärztegesellschaft für Akupunktur (DÄGfA, German Association for Medical Acupuncture, Jochen Gleditsch › 6.13)

- **ACTH Point:** on the median line between the midpoint of the tragus and intertragic notch; also referred to as Adrenal Cortex Point (13), corresponds to the Hypertension Point (19)
- **Thyroid Gland:** corresponds to the point TSH; located at the intertragic notch, slightly towards cranial and medial (not included in figure)
- **Endocrine Zone:** on the inside of the intertragic notch, extending approximately 1 cm both laterally and medially; indicated for general endocrine functional disorders, in particular those affecting the thyroid gland
- **Ovaries (Gonadotropin):** on the medial tip of the antitragus
- **Testes/Ovaries:** on the inside of the helix rim, approximately 1 transverse process inferior to the intersection between helix and antihelix, often a cartilaginous protrusion

Acupuncture Health Organisation (AHO, Frank Bahr)

- **ACTH Point:** at the intertragic notch
- **Thyroid Gland:** on the concha wall, level with the junction between the upper third and the two lower thirds, and level with C7, approximately at the intersection of a horizontal line through Point Zero and the concha wall
- **Endocrinium:** not applicable
- **Ovaries/Testes (Oestrogen/Testosterone):** on the inside of the helix rim, approximately 1 transverse process inferior to the intersection between the helix and antihelix, often a cartilaginous protrusion
- **Gonadotropin:** on the medial tip of the antitragus (when imagining the antihelix as a snake with the antitragus forming its head, the point corresponds to the eye of the snake)
- **Progesterone:** in the scapha, anterior to the Vegetative Groove, lateral to the points Renin-Angiotensin and Kidney II

Chinese School

- **Adrenal Cortex (13):** slightly inferior to the midpoint of the tragus, on its edge
- **Hypertension (19):** on the median line between the midpoint of the tragus and the intertragic notch; the location corresponds to the point ACTH (after DÄGfA)
- **Thyroid Gland (45):** slightly lateral to the antihelix bulge, level with C2 and C3
- **Endocrine System (22):** an area in the concha inferior to the intertragic notch, medial to the point Ovaries (23)
- **Ovaries (23):** an area on the lateral intertragic notch, extending to the concha
- **Testes (23):** on the inside of the antitragus, on its medial aspect, adjacent and lateral to the area pertaining to the Ovaries (23)

9.2 Concurrences

(› Fig. 9.2-1)

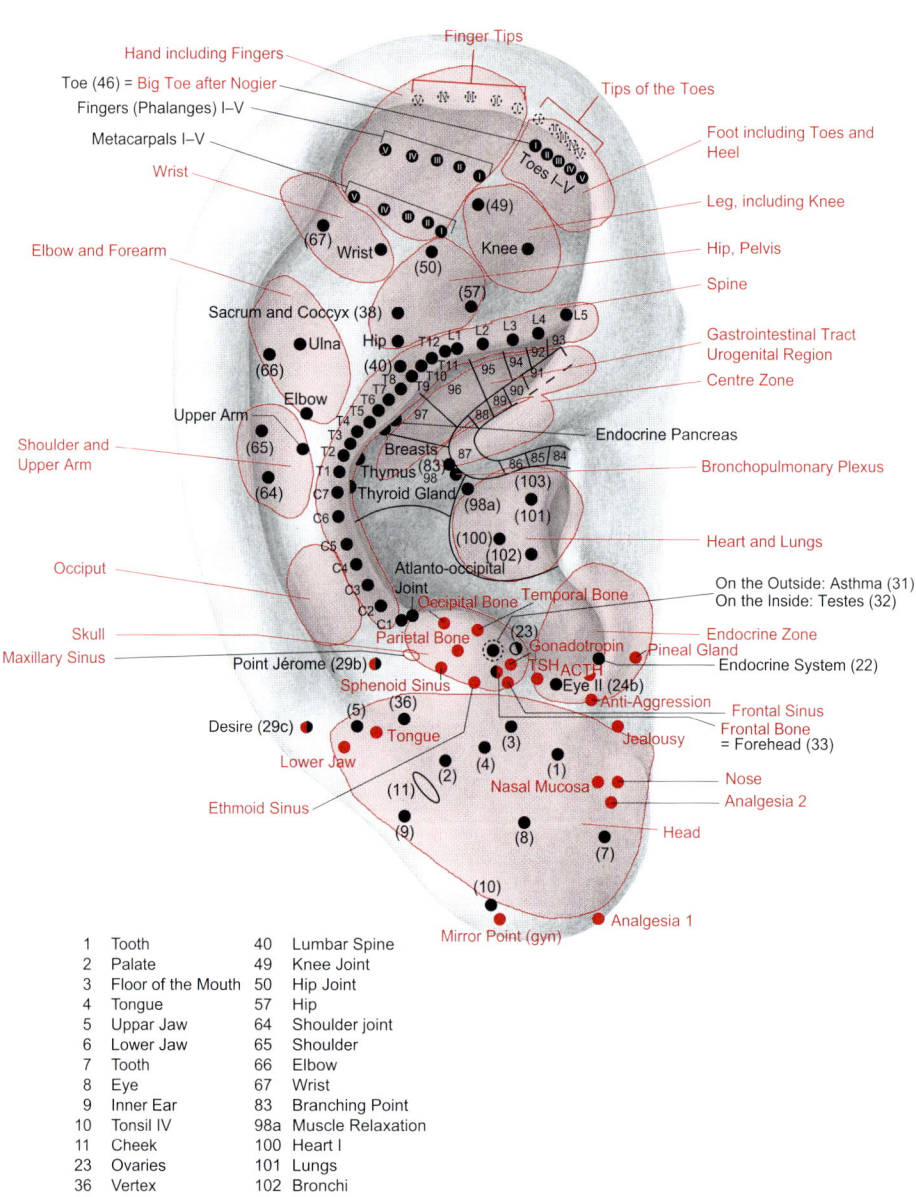

1	Tooth	40	Lumbar Spine
2	Palate	49	Knee Joint
3	Floor of the Mouth	50	Hip Joint
4	Tongue	57	Hip
5	Uppar Jaw	64	Shoulder joint
6	Lower Jaw	65	Shoulder
7	Tooth	66	Elbow
8	Eye	67	Wrist
9	Inner Ear	83	Branching Point
10	Tonsil IV	98a	Muscle Relaxation
11	Cheek	100	Heart I
23	Ovaries	101	Lungs
36	Vertex	102	Bronchi

Fig. 9.2-1

Spine

- Projection of the whole spine on the antihelix, with the cervical spine at the inferior end and the lumbar spine at the superior end
- Further differentiation of the spine according to muscles, vertebrae and discs

Upper Extremity

- **Occiput:** an area on the scapha between helix and antihelix, level with the projection of the cervical spine on the antihelix
- **Shoulders/Upper Arm:** an area on the scapha between helix and antihelix, level with the transition from the cervical to the thoracic spine on the antihelix
- **Elbow/Forearm:** an area on the scapha between helix and antihelix, level with the projection of the thoracic spine on the antihelix
- **Wrist:** an area on the scapha, level with Darwin's tubercle
- **Hand, including Fingers:** on the superior part of the scapha, medially adjacent to the triangular fossa

Lower extremity

- **Hip/Pelvis:** an area at the apex of the triangular fossa, between the crura of the antihelix; a cartilaginous protrusion is often found in this area
- **Leg, including Knee:** an area in the middle third of the triangular fossa, slightly more towards the upper crus
- **Foot, including Heel and Toes:** an area in the superior third of the triangular fossa, slightly more towards the upper crus

Head

- Bony structures of the **Skull**: mostly in the area of the antitragus
- All other structures pertaining to the **Head**: on the ear lobe

Internal Organs

- **Heart/Lungs:** in the inferior concha, lateral to the ear canal
- **Gastro-intestinal tract and urogenital region:** in the upper third of the inferior concha

Endocrine System

Several points with an effect on the endocrine system; while their location varies from school to school (see above) they are essentially concentrated in the area between tragus and antitragus

Central Zone

Stabilising zone and central aspect of the ear, associated with Laterality Point, Point Zero and Diaphragm Point; located on the helix root towards the ascending helix.

9.3 Individual Specialties of various Schools

(> Fig. 9.3-1)

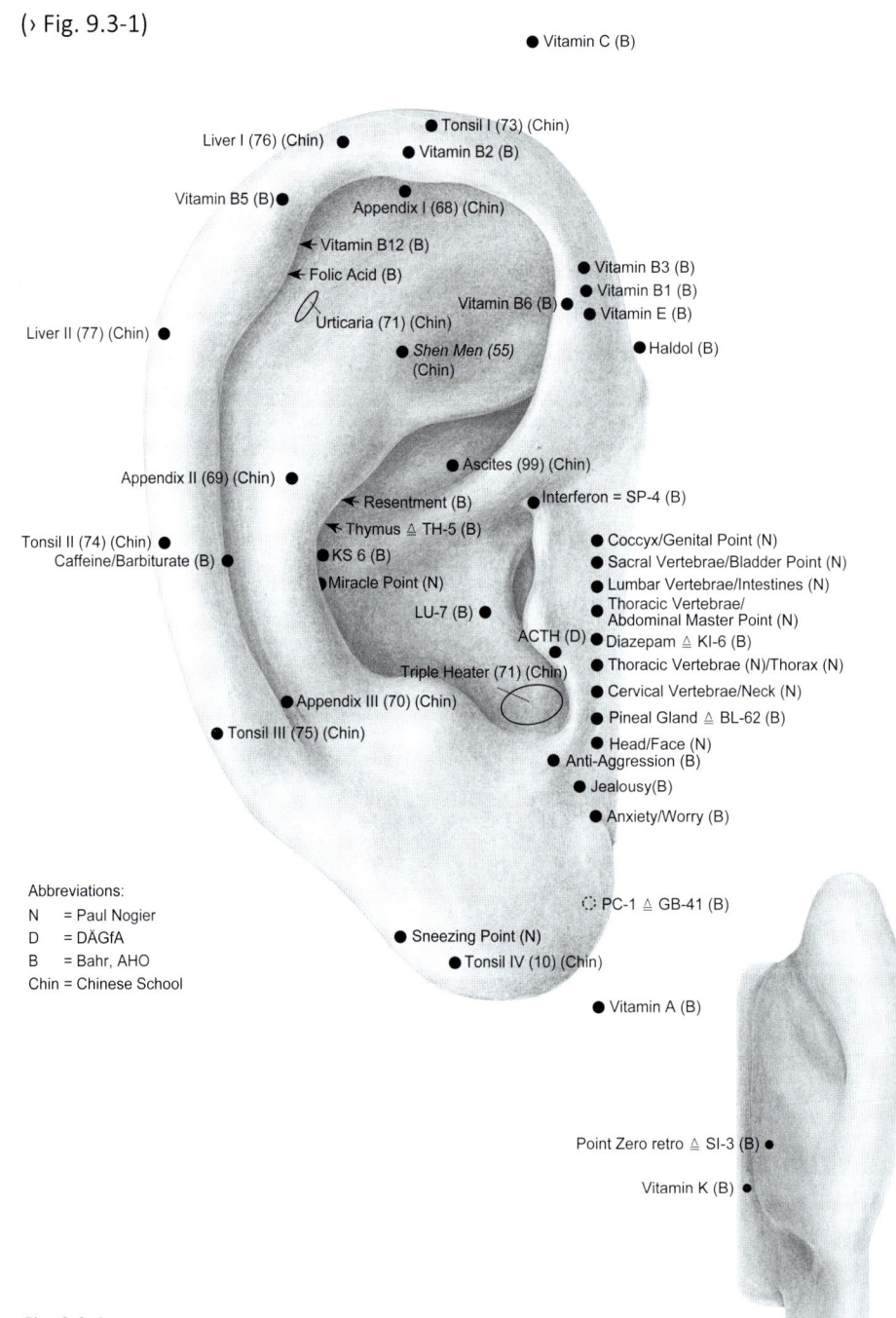

● Vitamin C (B)

● Tonsil I (73) (Chin)
Liver I (76) (Chin) ●
● Vitamin B2 (B)

Vitamin B5 (B) ●
Appendix I (68) (Chin)

← Vitamin B12 (B)
← Folic Acid (B)
● Vitamin B3 (B)
Vitamin B6 (B) ● ● Vitamin B1 (B)
● Vitamin E (B)
Urticaria (71) (Chin)
Liver II (77) (Chin) ●
● *Shen Men (55)* (Chin)
● Haldol (B)

● Ascites (99) (Chin)

Appendix II (69) (Chin) ●
● Interferon = SP-4 (B)
← Resentment (B)
← Thymus ≙ TH-5 (B)
Tonsil II (74) (Chin) ●
● Coccyx/Genital Point (N)
Caffeine/Barbiturate (B) ●
● KS 6 (B)
● Sacral Vertebrae/Bladder Point (N)
► Miracle Point (N)
● Lumbar Vertebrae/Intestines (N)
● Thoracic Vertebrae/
LU-7 (B) ●
   Abdominal Master Point (N)
ACTH (D) ● ● Diazepam ≙ KI-6 (B)
Triple Heater (71) (Chin) ● ● Thoracic Vertebrae (N)/Thorax (N)
● Cervical Vertebrae/Neck (N)
● Appendix III (70) (Chin)
● Pineal Gland ≙ BL-62 (B)
● Tonsil III (75) (Chin)
● Head/Face (N)
● Anti-Aggression (B)
● Jealousy(B)
● Anxiety/Worry (B)

Abbreviations:
N   = Paul Nogier
D   = DÄGfA
B   = Bahr, AHO
Chin = Chinese School

◌ PC-1 ≙ GB-41 (B)

● Sneezing Point (N)
● Tonsil IV (10) (Chin)

● Vitamin A (B)

Point Zero retro ≙ SI-3 (B) ●

Vitamin K (B) ●

Vitamin D (B) ●
PGE₁ ≙ GB-41 (B)

PGE$_1$ ≙ GB-41 (B)

Fig. 9.3-1

The list below contains the most important components or points of various schools but does not claim to be complete.

Paul Nogier

- **Points associated with the spine and organ areas**: on the medial border of the ear, in the groove medial to the tragus
- **Miracle point:** corresponds to the point Middle Cervical Ganglion (› 6.9.2) in the Sympathetic Groove
- **Sneezing Point:** on the lateral inferior border of the lobe, in the 9th zone, but medial to the area Trigeminal Nerve

Deutsche Ärztegesellschaft für Akupunktur (DÄGfA, German Association for Medical Acupuncture, Jochen Gleditsch)

- **ACTH Point:** on the median plane between the midpoint of the tragus and the inter-tragic notch; also referred to as Adrenal Cortex Point (16), equates the point Hypertension (19)
- **Very-Point Technique** (› 3.1.2): method for point location

Acupuncture Health Organisation (AHO, Frank Bahr › 6.13)

- **Psychological points:** Anxiety/Worry, Resentment, Jealousy, Anti-Aggression, and others
- **Medication-analogous Points:** Barbiturate/Caffeine, Diazepam, Haldol, and others
- Projection of so-called **Cardinal Points** (body meridian points) on the ear, which are arranged in pairs; the first point is needled on the right and the second point on the left:
  - **PC-6** (in the area of the Stellate Ganglion Point › 6.9.2) and **SP-4** (= Interferon Point 6.7.3)
  - **LU-7** (in the Lung area [101] › 6.4.1) and **KI-6** (= Diazepam Point › 6.7.3)
  - **GB-41** (= PGE_1 › 6.11.4) and **TH-5** (= Thymus Point › 6.6.1)
  - **SI-3** (= Point Zero on the posterior ear › 6.11.4) and **BL-62** (= Pineal Gland Point › 6.8.4)
- Projection of **vitamin deficiencies** on the ear:
  - **Vitamin A:** on the face, approximately 0,5 cm inferior to the lobe, on a line presenting a straight extension to the insertion of the ear lobe
  - **Vitamin C:** on the face, approximately 2 cm superior to the edge of the ear, on a straight line extending from the Ω_2-Point
  - **Vitamin D:** on the medial border of the posterior ear lobe, slightly inferior to the insertion of the ear lobe
  - **Vitamin K:** on the mastoid process behind the ear, approximately 2 cm superior to the insertion of the ear lobe
  - **Vitamin E:** on the medial border of the ear, on the ascending helix, slightly superior to the intersection between the helix and the antihelix
  - **Vitamin B_1:** on the helix rim, directly superior to the point Vitamin E
  - **Vitamin B_2:** slightly lateral to the Histamine point on the helix rim
  - **Vitamin B_3:** directly superior to the point Vitamin B_1 on the helix rim

– **Vitamin B$_5$:** slightly superior to Darwin's tubercle on the helix rim
– **Vitamin B$_6$:** slightly lateral to the points Vitamin B$_1$ and E on the helix rim
– **Vitamin B$_{12}$:** slightly inferior to the point Vitamin B$_5$ but in the Vegetative Groove in the scapha
– **Folic acid:** slightly inferior to the point vitamin B$_{12}$
- Projection of **trace elements**
- Attempts to detect the projection of Bach Flower Remedies on the ear

Chinese School

- Shen Men **(55):** slightly superior to the beginning of the superior crus (› 6.7.2)
- *San Jiao* **(Triple Warmer) (104):** in the most medial and inferior section of the concha (› 6.10.1)
- **Urticaria (71):** zone in the lateral concha, level with Darwin's tubercle (› 6.10.2)
- **Ascites (99):** in the concha, where the zones Duodenum (88), Small Intestine (89), Pancreas/Gallbladder (96), and Kidney (95) intersect

Further Points

The following points have not become established in auricular acupuncture as practiced in the West. Axel Rubach refers to these points as 'secondary points' or 'pseudo-locations', which may be used as points with an effect on only the lymphatic system (Rubach 2000).

- **Appendix I–III (68–70):** in the scapha (› 6.4.2)
- **Tonsils I–III (73–75):** on the helix rim (› 6.3.1)
- **Tonsils IV (10):** on the inferior aspect of the ear lobe (› 6.3.4)
- **Liver I–II (76–77):** on the helix rim (› 6.3.4)

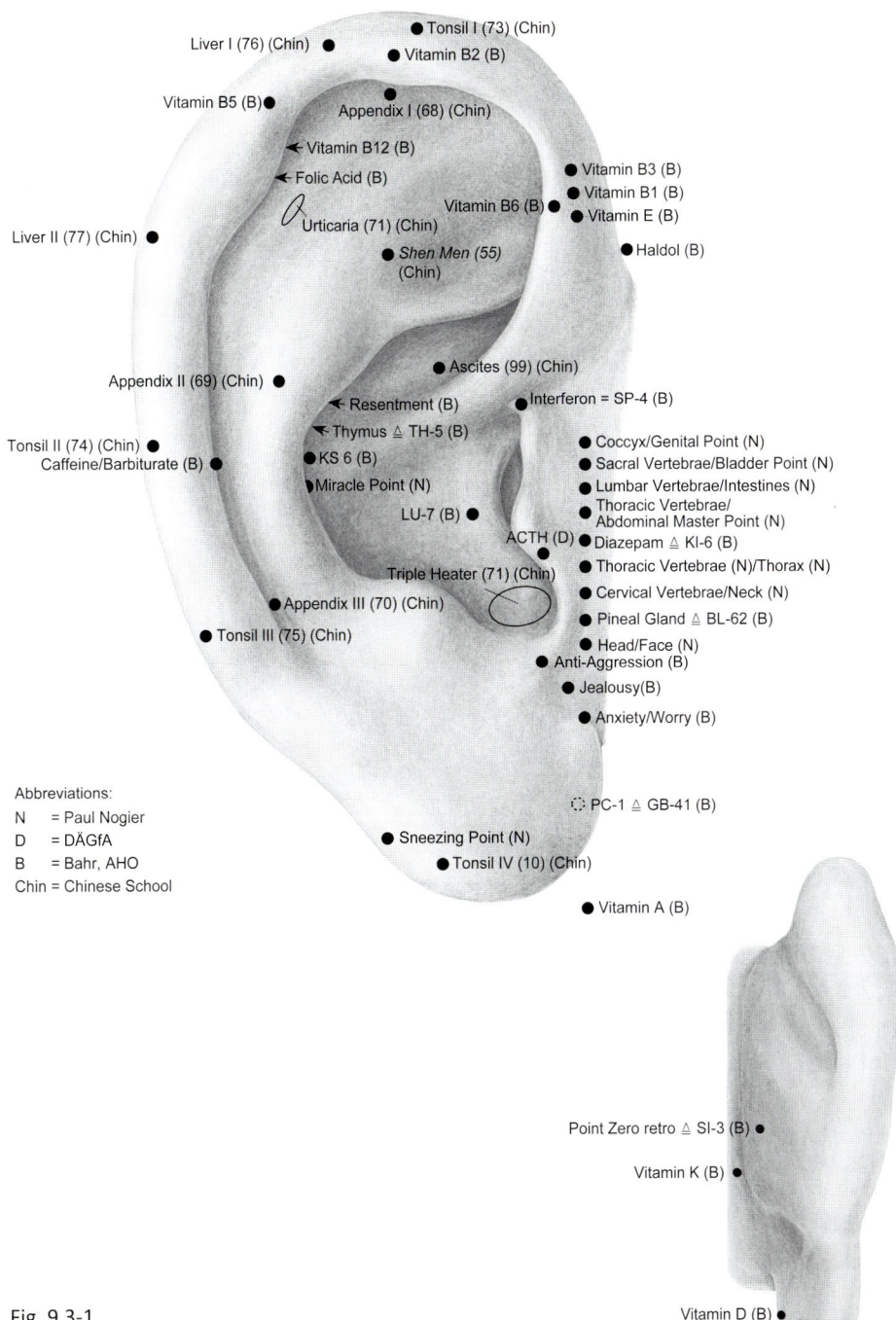

● Vitamin C (B)

● Tonsil I (73) (Chin)

Liver I (76) (Chin) ●

● Vitamin B2 (B)

Vitamin B5 (B)●

● Appendix I (68) (Chin)

←● Vitamin B12 (B)

←● Folic Acid (B)

Urticaria (71) (Chin)

Vitamin B6 (B) ●● Vitamin B3 (B)
●● Vitamin B1 (B)
●● Vitamin E (B)

Liver II (77) (Chin) ●

● Haldol (B)

● *Shen Men (55)* (Chin)

● Ascites (99) (Chin)

Appendix II (69) (Chin) ●

←● Resentment (B)

←● Thymus △ TH-5 (B)

● Interferon = SP-4 (B)

Tonsil II (74) (Chin) ●
Caffeine/Barbiturate (B) ●

● KS 6 (B)

Miracle Point (N)

LU-7 (B) ●

● Coccyx/Genital Point (N)
● Sacral Vertebrae/Bladder Point (N)
● Lumbar Vertebrae/Intestines (N)
● Thoracic Vertebrae/
  Abdominal Master Point (N)

ACTH (D) ● Diazepam △ KI-6 (B)

Triple Heater (71) (Chin)

● Thoracic Vertebrae (N)/Thorax (N)

● Cervical Vertebrae/Neck (N)

● Appendix III (70) (Chin)

● Pineal Gland △ BL-62 (B)

● Head/Face (N)

Tonsil III (75) (Chin) ●

● Anti-Aggression (B)

● Jealousy(B)

● Anxiety/Worry (B)

⊙ PC-1 △ GB-41 (B)

Abbreviations:
N   = Paul Nogier
D   = DÄGfA
B   = Bahr, AHO
Chin = Chinese School

● Sneezing Point (N)
● Tonsil IV (10) (Chin)

● Vitamin A (B)

Point Zero retro △ SI-3 (B) ●

Vitamin K (B) ●

Vitamin D (B) ●
PGE₁ △ GB-41 (B)

Fig. 9.3-1

10 Case Studies

The following case studies do not represent the average case load of everyday clinical practice, rather some outstanding and explicit cases have been chosen for the purpose of this book. Chronic disorders treated with acupuncture long-term for pain reduction cannot be described here since these treatments are not considered as concluded.

- Before the start of treatment patients were examined physically and diagnosed according to criteria based on Western conventional medicine. Any concurrent prescription medication taken by the patient is mentioned in the text (medical history).

- Acupuncture points used in body acupuncture are abbreviated (based on 'A Practical Dictionary of Chinese Medicine').

- Treatments were based on the principles of TCM. The explanations based on meridians and syndrome patterns are marked with a figure. These figures are referenced in the point prescription to establish a link between the chosen points and TCM criteria. Points not referenced by a figure correspond to treatment criteria of minor importance.

- When Chinese Herbal Medicine was used the individual herbs are listed with both the pinyin and Latin name. The prescribed herbs varied from treatment to treatment and not all herbs were prescribed at the one time. Generally, the herb combinations do not correspond to classical formulas.

10.1 Paediatric Migraine

R.S., 11-year-old female; treatment period: 4/10/2000 to 25/5/2001

Medical history

- Recurrent progressive headaches since age 4
- Generally lasting 1–2 days
- Occasionally in combination with sensitivity to light and noise, or abdominal pain
- Worse with foehn winds
- Additional finding: on rare occasions lower back pain due to scoliosis

TCM diagnosis

- Deficiency of the Middle
- Kidney deficiency
- Liver stagnation
- Wind evil

Treatment principle

Alleviate symptoms by
1. Tonifying deficient organs/meridians
2. Coursing the Liver
3. Relaxing tight spinal sections (cervical and lumbar spine)
4. Extinguishing Wind

Treatments (› Fig. 10.1-1)

This paediatric patient was treated with a Twin-Laser (Reimers & Janssen) with an output of 150/20 mW (infrared). All points were treated for approximately 2–5 seconds based on RAC-palpation.

Auricular acupuncture based on RAC-palpation

First treatment
- **Right side:** Omega Axis, C7 → **3**, L2 → **3**, Laterality Point → **1**, Liver → **2**, Kidney II → **1**
- **Left side:** Point Zero → **1**, Anti-Aggression → **1**, *Shen Men (55)* → **1**

Further points used in follow-up treatments
- **Right side:** Gallbladder → **2**, Frustration → **2**
- **Left side:** Diazepam → **3**, Infection Axis → **4**

Body acupuncture

First treatment
GV-20 → **1, 2**, GB-14 → **4**, LR-3 → **3**, KI-6 → **1, 2**

Further points used in follow-up treatments
TH-5 → **4**, TH-17 → **4**, ST-36 → **1**, LI-4 → **1, 4**

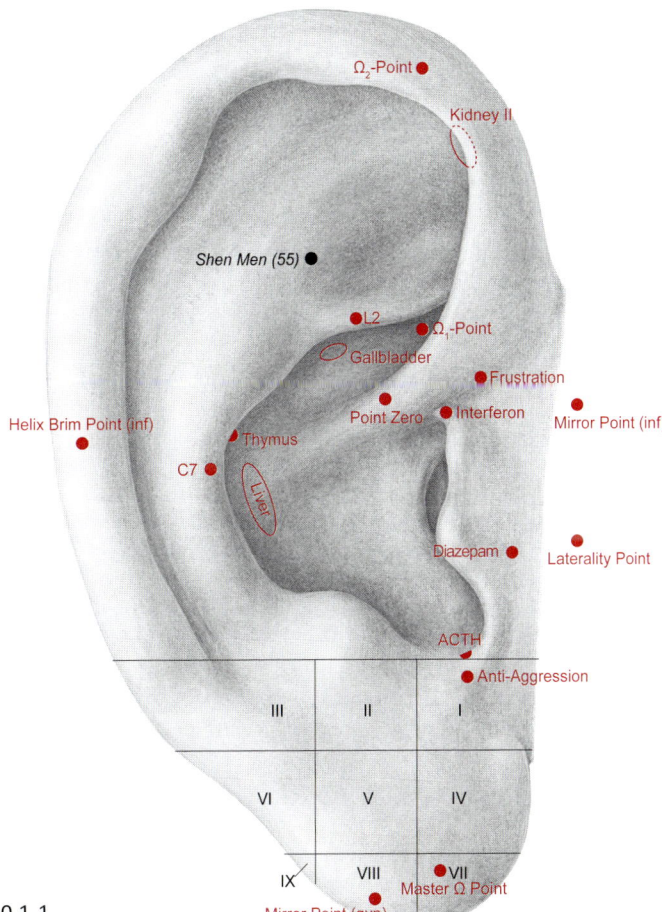

Ω_2-Point

Kidney II

Shen Men (55)

L2

Ω_1-Point

Gallbladder

Frustration

Helix Brim Point (inf)

Point Zero Interferon

Mirror Point (inf)

Thymus

C7

Liver

Diazepam

Laterality Point

ACTH

Anti-Aggression

III   II   I

VI   V   IV

IX   VIII   VII

Master Ω Point

Mirror Point (gyn)

Fig. 10.1-1

Treatment intervals

- 3 treatments once weekly
- 4 treatments once fortnightly
- 3 treatments at intervals of 3–4 weeks
- Treatments were concluded on 2/3/2001 when symptoms had subsided completely
- One further treatment due to mild headaches on 26/5/2001
- Sustained relief from symptoms (telephone conversation with the mother on 16/11/2001)

Summary

While headaches improved immediately after the first treatment they recurred at a reduced level; a flare-up occurred due to a pulmonary viral infection but this was quickly resolved. Eventually there was sustained relief from symptoms.

10.2 Atopic Dermatitis in a New Born Baby

B.J., 4-month-old, male; treatment period: 7/10/2002 to 22/12/2003

Medical history

- Cradle cap since birth
- Progressive eczema in the face and on the extensor sides of both arms and legs
- Additional findings: chronic rhinitis, recurrent ear aches, retractile testicle on the right side, undescended testicle on the left side

TCM diagnosis

- Deficiency of the Middle
- Kidney deficiency
- Channels blocked by Heat/Phlegm
- Wind evil

Treatment principle

Alleviate symptoms by
1. Tonifying deficient Organs/meridians
2. Clearing Heat stagnation
3. Eliminating Phlegm
4. Extinguishing Wind
5. Tonifying local points

Treatments (› Fig. 10.2-1)

This infant was treated with a Twin-Laser (Reimers & Janssen) with an output of 150/20 mW (infrared). All points were treated for approximately 2–5 seconds based on RAC-palpation.

Auricular acupuncture based on RAC-palpation

First treatment
- **Right side:** Immune Axis → **4**, Frontal and Maxillary Sinus → **5**, Bronchopulmonary Plexus → **1**, Point Zero → **1, (3)**
- **Left side:** Infection Axis → **4**, Frontal and Maxillary Sinus → **5**, Point Zero → **3, (1)**

Further points used in follow-up treatments
- **Right side:** Kidney I (95) → **1**, Kidney II → **1**
- **Left side:** Kidney I (95) → **1**, Kidney II → **1**

Body acupuncture

First treatment
BL-2 → **4**, LI-20 → **1, 4**, LI-4 → **1, 4**, LU-5 → **1, 2, 3**, ST-36 → **1**

Further points used in follow-up treatments
KI-6 → **1**, LR-3 → **1, 2**, GB-41, LI-11 → **2, 3, 4**

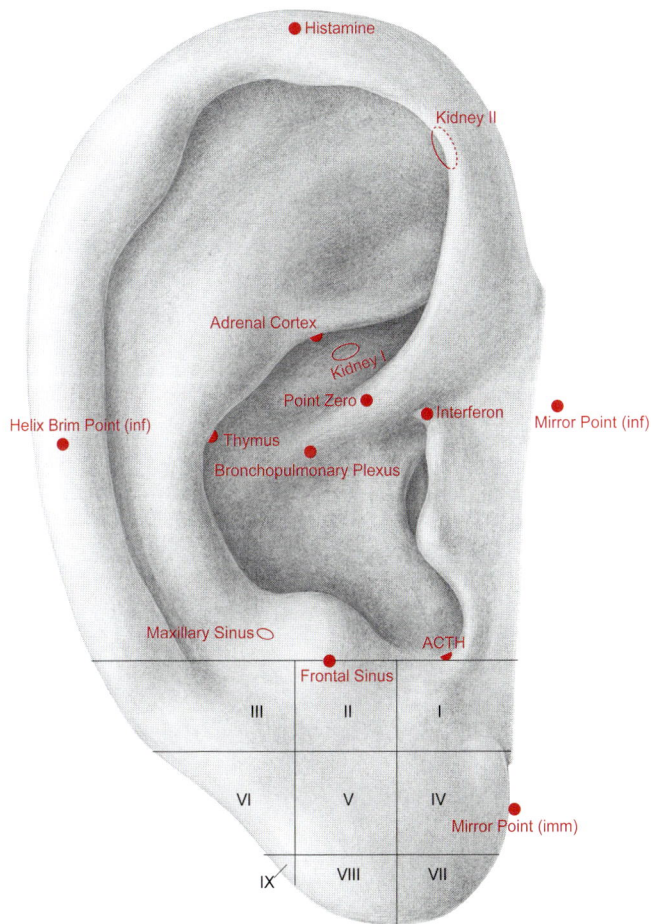

Fig. 10.2-1

Treatment intervals

- Every other week from start of treatments
- Treatment frequency was increased to once weekly during acute exacerbations (e.g. infection)
- Treatment intervals were increased to 3 weeks as symptoms improved
- Treatments were concluded on 22/12/2003 when symptoms had completely subsided

Summary

The eczema improved significantly after the 1st treatment but tended to recur, especially in conjunction with pulmonary infections. Inguinal testicle surgery during the final treatment phase worsened the dermatological symptoms only very little. This suggests a sustainable treatment result.

10.3 Macular Degeneration

M.P., 59-year-old male; treatment period: since 27/03/2001 (ongoing)

Medical history

- Macular degeneration (central geographic atrophy) in both eyes, episodes with rapid progression
- Dry form
- Onset of symptoms at the beginning of 1999, unable to work since 8/2000
- Vision at the time of the 1st treatment: right eye 50 %; left eye 20 % (with glasses)
- Further ophthalmic diagnoses: stereoamblyopia, myopia, presbyopia
- Secondary diagnoses: cervical myalgia, lower back pain

TCM diagnosis

- Liver deficiency
- Kidney deficiency
- Heat damage

Treatment principle

Arrest progression of the disorder and improve subjective vision by:
1. Tonifying deficient Organs/meridians
2. Tonifying local points
3. Cooling Heat

Treatments (› Fig. 10.3-1)

The patient was treated with both auricular and body acupuncture. The needles were retained for 20 minutes.

Auricular acupuncture based on RAC-palpation

First treatment

- **Right side:** Eye I (24a) → **2**, Eye II (24b) → **2**, Liver → **1**, Stellate Ganglion → **2**, C7 → **2**
- **Left side:** Eye I (24a) → **2**, Eye II (24b) → **2**, Eye (8) → **2**, *Shen Men* (55) → **1**, Frustration

Further points used in follow-up treatments

- **Right side:** Eye (8) → **2**, L2 → **2**, Point Zero
- **Left side:** Anti-Aggression, Diazepam

Body acupuncture

First treatment

Yu Yao → **2**, **3**, BL-1 → **2**, **3**, GB-14 → **2**, LR-3 → **1**, **3**, TH-3, ST-1 → **2**, **3**

Further points used in follow-up treatments

TH-6 → **1**, BL-20 → **2**, **3**, ST-36 → **1**, GB-37 → **1**, **2**

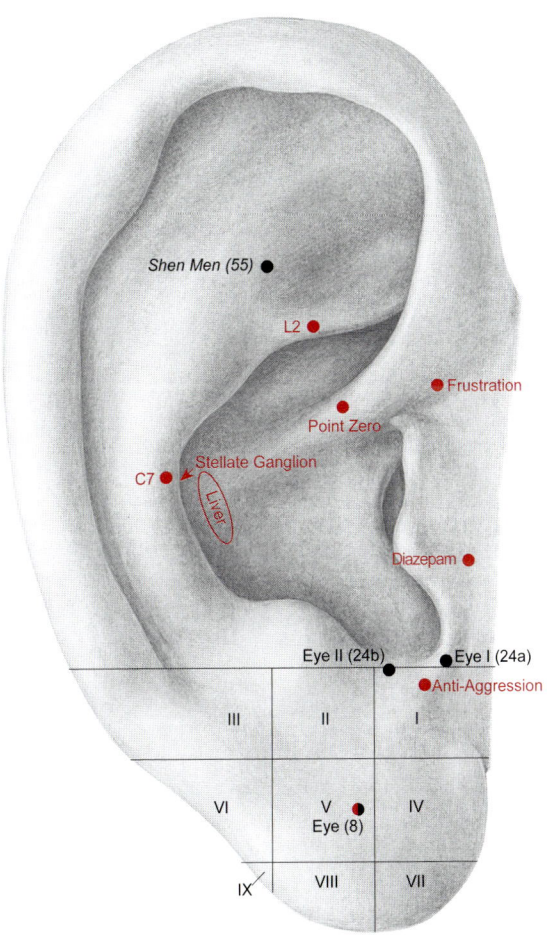

Fig. 10.3-1

Treatment intervals

- Once weekly for approximately 6 months
- Then every 2–3 weeks
- Upon no further subjective improvement of symptoms: once monthly to sustain treatment results

Summary

After the 1st treatment the patient reported a significant subjective improvement in night vision for one day; he further reported clearer vision during the day for 1–2 days. As treatments progressed, the patient's vision improved subjectively. This was particularly noticeable when reading. Objective eye tests by an ophthalmologist showed an improvement of 5 % in both eyes. In summary, it was possible to arrest the rapid progression of the disorder with acupuncture, while the subjective vision improved slightly but markedly.

10.4 Brain Tumours

The following section describes several forms of brain tumours with varying degrees of malignancy and their response to acupuncture treatments. As is typical for the treatment of tumours in general, there were surprising curative results in some cases while in others only palliative treatments were possible; some tumour patients died despite acupuncture treatments. However, in these cases it had been possible to extend the patients' life span and, more importantly, to significantly improve their quality of life. It seems that acupuncture can maximally mobilise the body's powers of self-healing; but once these are irreversibly exhausted patients will die within a few days or weeks. At least acupuncture can markedly reduce the period of suffering during the final phase of a tumour patient's life.

10.4.1 Astrocytoma

G.W., 34-year-old female; treatment period: since 18/11/1999

Medical history

- Spring 1996: epileptic seizures, subsequent diagnosis of a grade III astrocytoma
- Initial treatment: surgery, followed by 33 radiation treatments
- December 1998: recurrent episode; further surgery in January 1999, postoperative right-sided hemiparesis
- April 1999: further recurrence; hyperthermia therapy/chemotherapy; progressive tumour growth
- Further chemotherapy; tumour reduced by 20 % (residual size 6 cm)
- At this point: start of acupuncture treatments
- Secondary diagnoses at start of acupuncture treatments: partial paralysis of the right arm (side effect of cancer treatment, see above); altered sensitivity in the right arm (unable to differentiate between hot/cold), paraesthesia in the right leg.

TCM diagnosis

- Deficiency of the Middle, Kidney deficiency
- Phlegm obstruction of the Kidneys
- Impaired *Qi* circulation in the network vessels

Treatment principles

Relieve symptoms by

1. Tonifying deficient Organs/meridians
2. Resolving and eliminating Phlegm
3. Opening the network vessels
4. Coursing *Qi*
5. Tonifying local points

Treatments (› Fig. 10.4-1)

Disposable needles were used for both auricular and body acupuncture. These were retained for 20 minutes.

Auricular acupuncture based on RAC-palpation

First treatment

- **Right side:** Atlanto-occipital Joint → **5**, Shoulder → **5**, L2 → **5**, *Shen Men* (55) → **1**, Anxiety

- **Left side:** Occipital Bone → **4**, Brainstem (25) → **4**, Grey Matter(34) → **4**, Immune Axis, Diazepam

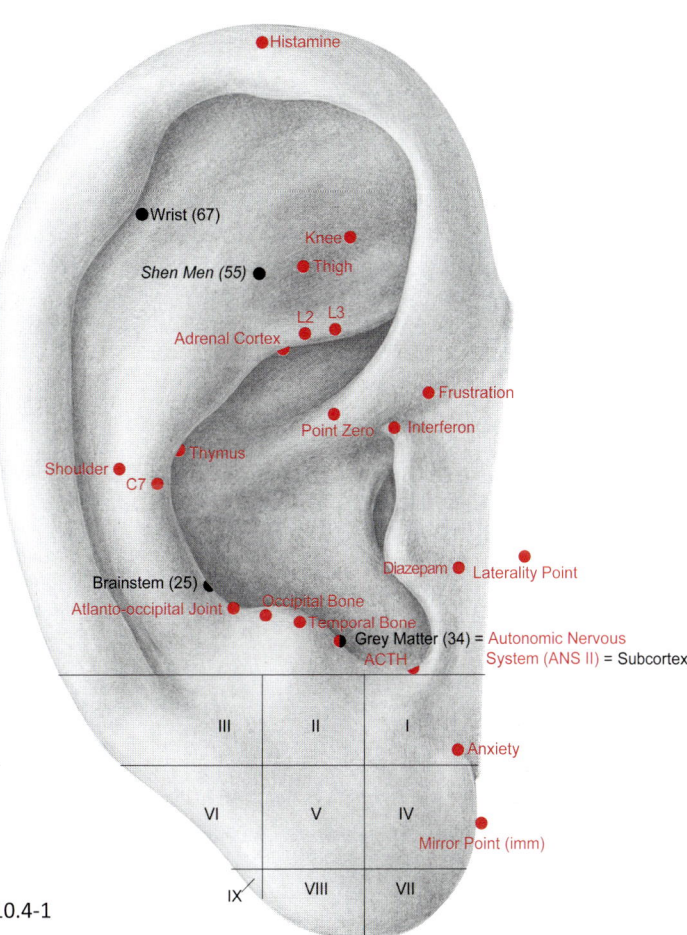

Fig. 10.4-1

Further points used in follow-up treatments
- **Right side:** Point Zero → **1, (2)**, L3 → **5**, Thigh → **4, 5**, Temporal Bone → **4**, Brainstem (25) → **4**
- **Left side:** Laterality Point → **1**, C7 → **5**, Point Zero → **2, (1)**, Knee → **4, 5**, Interferon, Thymus, Wrist (67) → **4, 5**, Frustration

Body acupuncture

First treatment
GV-20 → **1**, PC-6 → **1, 2, 4**, LR-3 → **1**, LI-11 → **2**, SP-4 → **1, 2**

Further points used in follow-up treatments
GB-20, GB-41, ST-36 → **1**, TH-5 → **3, 4**, BL-40 → **1, 5**, SP-3 → **2, 4**, KI-3 → **1, 5**, KI-6 → **1**

Treatment intervals

- Initially once weekly for 6 weeks
- Then every other week for approximately 6 months
- Then every 3–4 weeks until NMR spectroscopy findings were negative (February 2002)
- Ongoing sporadic treatments to further reduce residual sensory disturbances

Summary

After the first treatment the patient reported a subjective improvement, the acute shoulder pain had resolved. During the further treatment course the paraesthesia in the right leg as well as the partial paralysis in the right arm subsided almost completely. It took somewhat longer to regain the ability to differentiate between cold/warm in the right arm but this has now been nearly completely resolved. During a check-up with NMR spectroscopy complete remission was diagnosed for the first time; this was confirmed by a further check-up in October 2002. Since then the patient is considered to be free from tumours. To date (the beginning of 2011) the patient receives acupuncture every six weeks in order to treat minimal residual sensory symptoms.

10.4.2 Glioblastoma multiforme Grade IV

G.E., 29-year-old female; treatment period: 08/02/2002 to 04/08/2005. This rapidly progressive disorder has a very poor prognosis.

Primary medical history

- Vertigo attacks since 1999
- Since October 2001 progressively worse headaches; on 23 December 2001 diagnosis of occipito-parietal glioblastoma by NMR spectroscopy
- Initial treatment: surgery on 27/12/2001, followed by 34 radiation treatments
- Annual MRI check-ups until 2005; no indication of a relapse, only a dilation of the posterior horn of the lateral ventricle and parenchymal damage close to the surgical site
- Acupuncture treatments since 8/2/2002 during postoperative radiation treatments
- Pregnancy with C-section on 23/05/2005, no complications

TCM diagnosis

- Deficiency of the Middle and the Kidneys
- Phlegm obstruction of the Kidneys
- Impaired *Qi* circulation in the network vessels

Treatment principles

Relieve symptoms by
1. Tonifying deficient Organs/meridians
2. Resolving and eliminating Phlegm
3. Opening the network vessels
4. Coursing the *Qi*
5. Tonifying local points

Treatments (› Fig. 10.4-2)

Disposable needles were used for both auricular and body acupuncture. These were retained for 20 minutes.

Auricular acupuncture based on RAC-palpation

- **Right side:** Brainstem (25) → **5**, Immune Axis → **1**, Grey Matter (34) → **5**
- **Left side:** Brainstem (25) → **5**, *Shen Men* (55) → 4, Interferon → **1**, Thymus → **1**

Further points used in follow-up treatments

- **Right side:** Kidney I + II → **1**, Frustration, Point Zero → **1, (2)**, C7 → **5**, Anxiety
- **Left side:** Laterality Point → **1**, interferon→ **1**, Diazepam

Body acupuncture

First treatment
Yin Tang, *Tai Yang*, GV-20 → **4**, PC-6 → **1,4**, ST-36 → **1**, LR-3 → **1**

Further points used in follow-up treatments

LU-5 → **1**, GB-41 → **3** fertility disorder, KI-6 → **1**, KI-7 → **1**, HT-7 → 1,3, TH-4 → **3** (morning sickness)

Treatment intervals

- Initially once weekly for 6 weeks
- Then fortnightly treatments for approximately 1 month, followed by a 6-month treatment break during rehab (4/2002)
- Due to inconclusive MRI findings further treatments since 10/2002:
  - initially once weekly for 6 weeks
  - then every other week for approximately 3 months (11/2002 to 3/2003)
  - then 1–2 treatments per month for about 5 months (until 8/2003), followed by a treatment break until April 2004
- Further monthly treatments for fertility until September 2009 when the patient became pregnant; delivery by Caesarean section on 23 May 2005; prenatal MRI negative

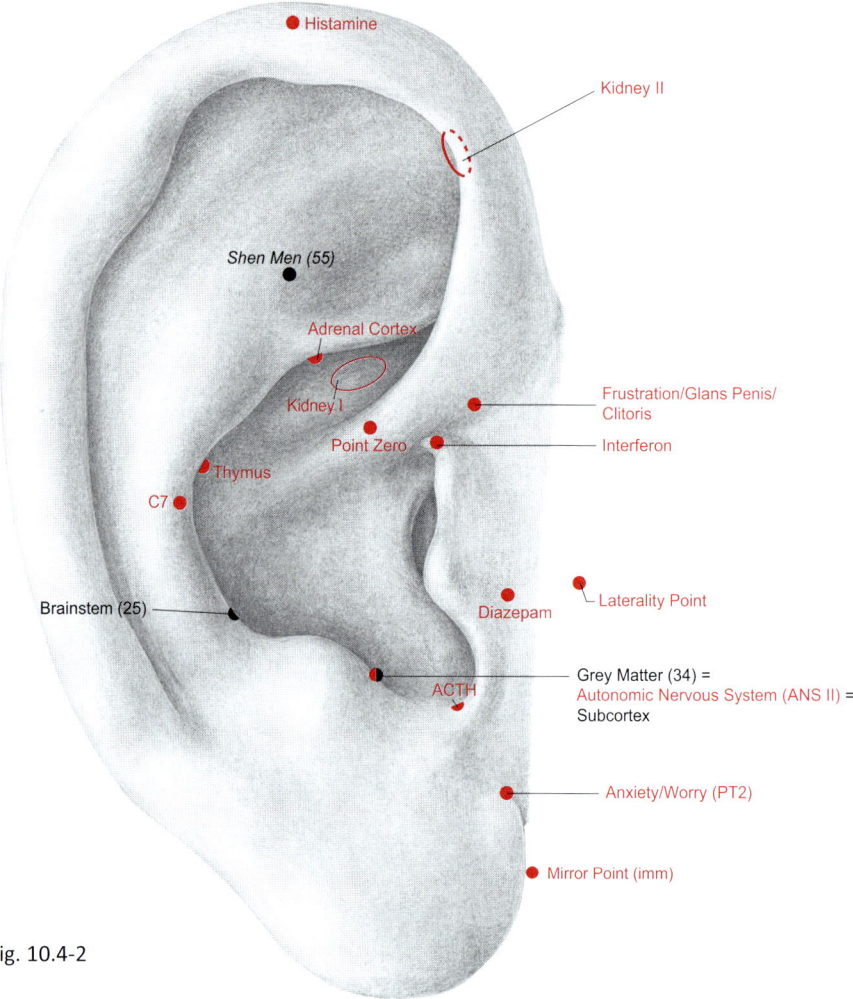

Fig. 10.4-2

Summary

The patient first came for acupuncture after surgery, during the early stages of radiation therapy. The side effects of the radiation therapy, in particular exhaustion, responded well to the treatments. Only the hyperaesthesia of the scalp and hair loss could not be prevented completely.

From April 2002 onwards the patient received chemotherapy for 12 months; she did not receive further treatments until October 2002. With inconclusive MRI findings in September 2002 acupuncture treatments were resumed in October 2002 and continued until August 2003. At that time she was preoccupied with letting go of her overprotective mother.

In January 2004 (after concluding chemotherapy) the patient reported that she would like to have a child. She consistently pursued conception since April 2004, becoming pregnant in August 2004; acupuncture treatments continued throughout her pregnancy until she gave birth by C-section on 23 May 2005. The last prepartal treatment took place on 19 May 2005.

On 4 August 2005 she returned for treatments for exhaustion. There were no other symptoms at that time. This suggests a continuous complete remission.

10.4.3 Pinealoma, Pineoblastoma WHO Grade III

M.Ch., 32-year-old male; treatments: 19/10/2004 until October 2009 (deceased). The course of the disease and the prognosis were uncertain due to liquorgenic metastasis of the pineal gland.

Primary medical history

- Following the death of his father in 2001 pressure pain in the left ear resulted in the diagnosis of a pineal gland tumour WHO III
- Surgery: ventriculocisternostomy for the treatment of hydrocephalus and removal of tumour on 6 March 2003, followed by radiation therapy (45.6 Gy) in August/September 2002
- Symptom-free until July 2004; during routine MRI check-up discovery of cerebellar metastases; gamma-knife radiosurgery on 15 September 2004
- Acupuncture treatments since 19 October 2004
- MRI scan on 16 February 2005: recurrent cerebellar tumour as well as multiple metastases in the spinal canal
- 30 radiation treatments of the head and spinal canal until 20 April 2005
- MRI scan in August 2005: findings unchanged; oncologist recommends chemotherapy and bone marrow transplant but the patient refuses treatment
- Since then acupuncture treatments
- Secondary diagnoses at start of treatment: altered sensation in the left leg, in particular at the knee and on the sole of the foot; sciatic pain on the left-hand side, unstable gait/dizziness; pressure pain in the anus following prostatitis; later increased salivation, tinnitus in the left ear

TCM diagnosis

- Deficiency of the Kidneys and the Middle
- Phlegm obstruction of the Kidneys
- Impaired *Qi* circulation in the network vessels

Treatment principle

Relieve symptoms by:
1. Tonifying deficient Organs/meridians
2. Resolving and eliminating Phlegm
3. Coursing the *Qi*
4. Tonifying local points

Treatments (› Fig. 10.4-3)

Disposable needles were used for both auricular and body acupuncture. These were retained for 20 minutes.

Auricular acupuncture based on RAC-palpation

First treatment
- **Right side:** Brainstem (25) → **4**, Immune Axis → **1**, Grey Matter(34) → **4**, *Shen Men* (55) → **3**
- **Left side:** Brainstem (25) → **4**, Point Zero → **1**, Laterality Point → **1**

Further points used in follow-up treatments
- **Right side:** Kidney I + II → **1**, Frustration, C7 → **4**, Medulla → **4**
- **Left side:** Interferon, Diazepam, Medulla → **4**, Spinal Points → **4**, Knee → **4**

Body acupuncture

First treatment
GV-20 → **1, 3**, BL-40 → **1**, BL-62 → **1, 3**, SP-9 → **2**, LR-3 → **1**

Further points used in follow-up treatments
LU-5 → **1**, GB-41 → **3**, KI-6 → **1**, KI-7 → **1, 3** TH-17, TH-3 → **3**, ST-36 → **1**

Treatment intervals

- Once weekly

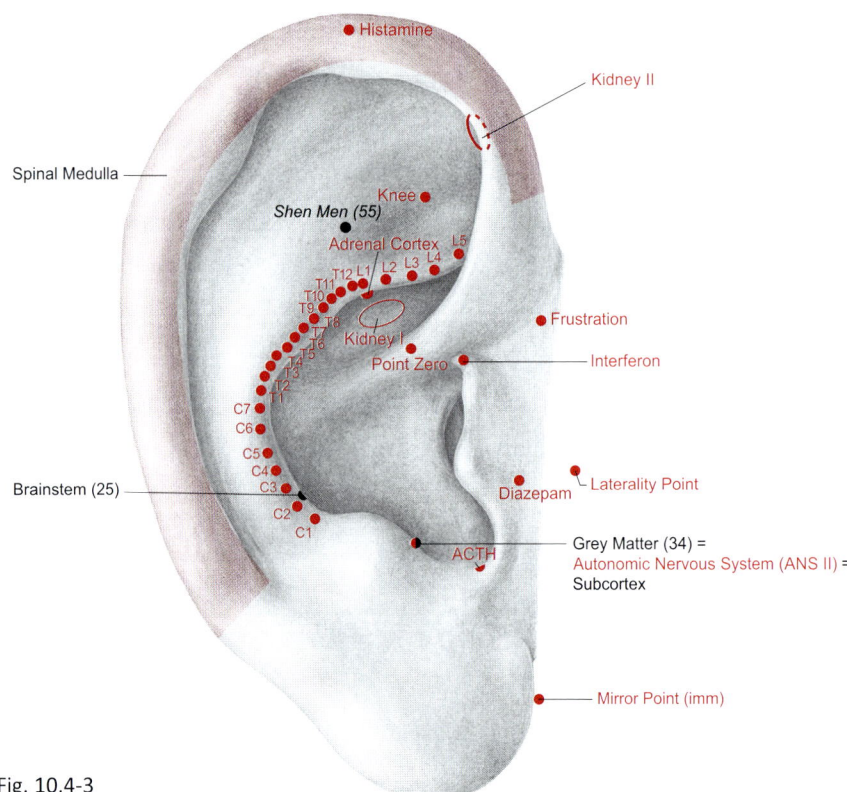

Fig. 10.4-3

Summary

The patient first came for acupuncture in October 2004 – 1½ years after a pineoblastoma diagnosis and subsequent surgery, radiation therapy as well as radiosurgery of a recurrent tumour in the cerebellum. The primary symptoms were altered sensations in the left leg, sciatic pain on the left side, anal pressure pain as well as disturbed balance when walking. These symptoms continuously improved with acupuncture until symptoms had almost completely subsided. The annual MRI check-up in February 2005 showed a recurrence of the cerebellar tumour as well as multiple spinal metastases. These were treated by radiation with a maximum dosis of 60 Gy. However, there was no significant reduction of the metastases, leaving this patient with no further treatment options.

The acupuncture treatments resulted in a further reduction of neurological symptoms, allowing the patient to lead an almost symptom-free life and to be physically active until the middle of 2009. This far exceeded the predicted life expectancy coupled with a good quality of life. From the middle of 2009: vertigo, gait, and the generalized debility worsened significantly. This was caused by a recurrent tumour growth which could not be controlled. The patient died in October 2009.

10.4.4 Meningioma, WHO Grade I

S.M., 48-year-old male; treatment since 16/05/2008. With surgery, slowly infiltrating mengingiomas have a good prognosis but a malignant degeneration is possible.

Primary medical history

- Following persistent cervical cephalgia and hearing loss on the left the treating osteopath recommended an MRI test
- Diagnosis of a petroclival mengingioma infiltrating the trigeminal nerve; surgical tumour enucleation on 28/01/2008
- Postoperative facial paralysis and numbness in the trigeminal area on the left, double vision
- Acupuncture treatments since 16/05/2008 for nerve irritation and prevention of a relapse
- Secondary findings: corneal ulcer in the left eye caused by the postoperative facial paralysis, amniotic membrane transplant on 04/02/2008

TCM diagnosis

- Deficiency of the Kidneys and the Middle
- Phlegm obstruction of the Kidneys
- Impaired *Qi* circulation in the network vessels

Treatment principle

Relieve symptoms by
1. Tonifying deficient Organs/meridians
2. Resolving and eliminating Phlegm
3. Coursing the *Qi*
4. Tonifying local points

Treatments (› Fig. 10.4-4)

Disposable needles were used for both auricular and body acupuncture. These were retained for 20 minutes.

Auricular acupuncture based on RAC-palpation

First treatment

- **Right side:** Immune Axis → **1**, Stellate Ganglion → **3**
- **Left side:** Brainstem (25) → **4**, Grey Matter (34) → **4**, *Shen Men* (55) → 1, Interferon → 1, Trigeminal Nerve → **4**, Diazepam

Further points used in follow-up treatments

- **Right side:** Point Zero → **1, (2)**, L3 → **4**, Thigh → **4**, Temporal Bone → **4**, Brainstem (25) → **4**

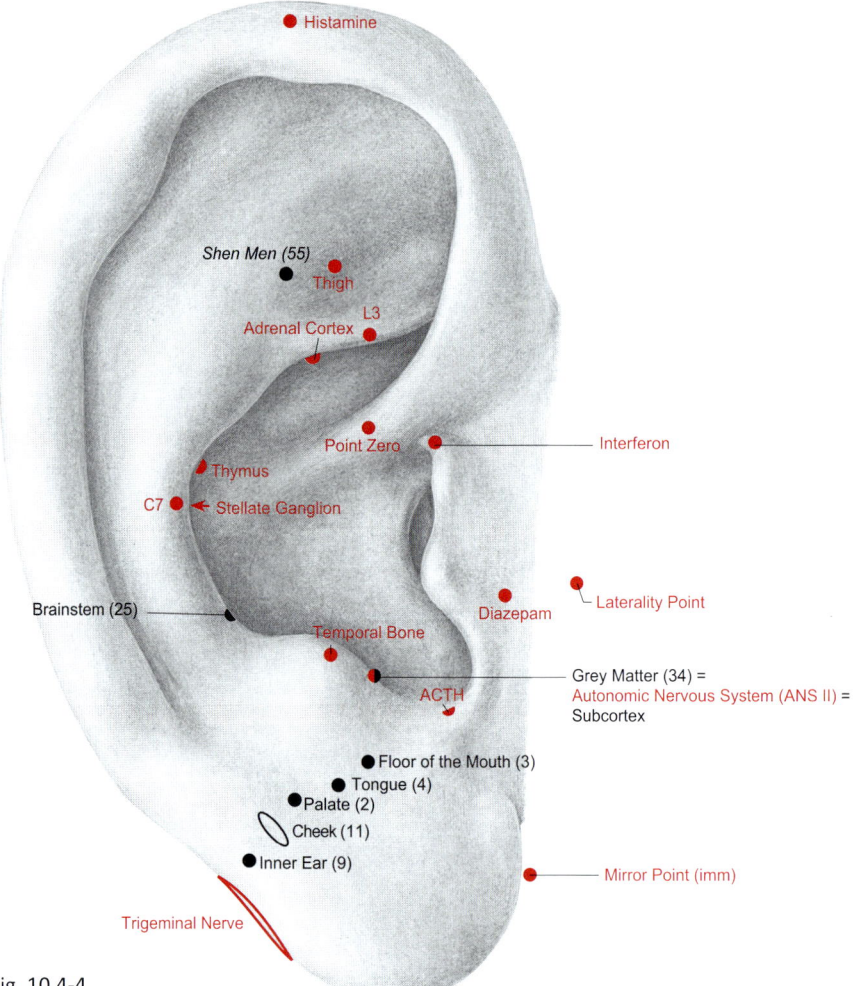

Fig. 10.4-4

- **Left side:** Floor of the Mouth (3) → **4**, Tongue (4) → **4**, Palate (2) → **4**, Cheek (11) → **4**, Inner Ear (9) → **4**, Laterality Point → **1**, C7 → **4**, Point Zero → **2**, Interferon → **1**, Thymus → **1**

Body acupuncture

First treatment
GV-20 → **1, 3**, PC-6 → **1, 2**, 3 E 17 → **3**, GB-14, ST-1 → **4**, LI-4 → **3**

Further points used in follow-up treatments
SI-19 → **3**, LR-3 → **1**, TH-5 → **3**, KI-6 → **1**, *Tai Yang* → **4**, BL-2 → **4**, LI-20 → **4**

Treatment intervals

- Once weekly

Summary

The patient first came for acupuncture on 16/05/2008 for the treatment of postoperative symptoms (facial paralysis, trigeminal irritation, double vision; amniotic membrane transplant) following the resection of a meningioma on 28/01/2008. Acupuncture was also intended as a prophylactic measure for the prevention of a relapse.

The facial paralysis improved after the first treatment. The patient reported improved sensation in his teeth and also in his tongue and lower jaw, as well as a tingling sensation in the left orbital area which previously had been numb. During the further treatment course symptoms reduced continually. The double vision which had forced the patient to cover his left eye to see clearly began to subside after the 4th treatment. His vision improved significantly and at the present time his vision in not impaired in any way. The creases on the forehead have returned to normal, as have the corners of the mouth (able to whistle). There are some residual sensory disturbances in the left half of the face.

10.4.5 Meningioma, WHO Grade I

W.I., 47-year-old female; treatments: 19/01/2001 to 27/09/2002. With surgery, slowly infiltrating meningiomas have a good prognosis but a malignant degeneration is possible. This patient further suffers from a selective IgG-immunopathy.

Primary medical history

- Chronic pancreatic insufficiency since 1992, Panzytrat 3 times daily (1-2-1) for nausea
- 1994 surgical treatment of a meningioma in the cerebral falx; since then carbamazepine for epilepsy
- Recurrent migraine headaches, treated with metamizole and diazepam
- Mild hemiparesis of the left-hand side
- In 1996 the investigation of chronically recurrent sinusitis resulted in a diagnosis of selective IgG-deficiency with subsequent monthly IgG substitution
- Syncope with injections, infusions, taking of blood samples, and acupuncture
- Secondary findings at the start of treatments: recurrent lower back pain following the fracture of a lumbar vertebra (in 1968)

TCM diagnosis

- Deficiency of the Middle and the Kidneys
- Phlegm obstruction of the Kidneys
- Impaired *Qi* circulation in the network vessels
- Rising Liver *Yang*

Treatment principle

Relieve symptoms by
1. Tonifying deficient Organs/meridians
2. Resolving and eliminating Phlegm
3. Opening the network vessels
4. Coursing the *Qi*
5. Tonifying local points
6. Calming Liver *Yang*

Treatments (› Fig. 10.4-5)

Disposable needles were used for both auricular and body acupuncture. These were retained for 20 minutes.

Auricular acupuncture based on RAC-palpation

First treatment
- **Right side:** Immune Axis → **1**, Liver → **6**, Point Zero → **1,2**, L2 → **5**
- **Left side:** Grey Matter (34) → **4**, Interferon → **1**, Thymus → **1**, Kidney I → **1**, L2 → **5**

Further points used in follow-up treatments
- **Right side:** Frontal Sinus → **5**, Maxillary Sinus → **5**, Thigh → **4, 5**, Temporal Bone → **4**, Brainstem (25) → **4**, Anxiety, Diazepam
- **Left side:** Frontal Sinus → **5**, Maxillary Sinus → **5**, Nose → **5**, Infection Axis → **1**, Anxiety Axis

Body acupuncture

First treatment
GV-20 → **1**, ST-36 → **1**, LR-3 → **6**, LI-4 → **2**

Further points used in follow-up treatments
BL-20 → **5**, LI-20 → **5**, GB-14, TH-6 → **3, 4**, BL-40 → **1, 5**, KI-7 → **1**, HT-7 → **1, 2, 4**, KI-3 → **1, 5**

Treatment intervals

- Initially fortnightly treatments for 1 month
- Then 1–2 treatments per month for approximately 4 months (June 2001)
- Once weekly from 08/06/2001 to 27/09/2001
- Then 1–2 monthly treatments until 27/09/2002

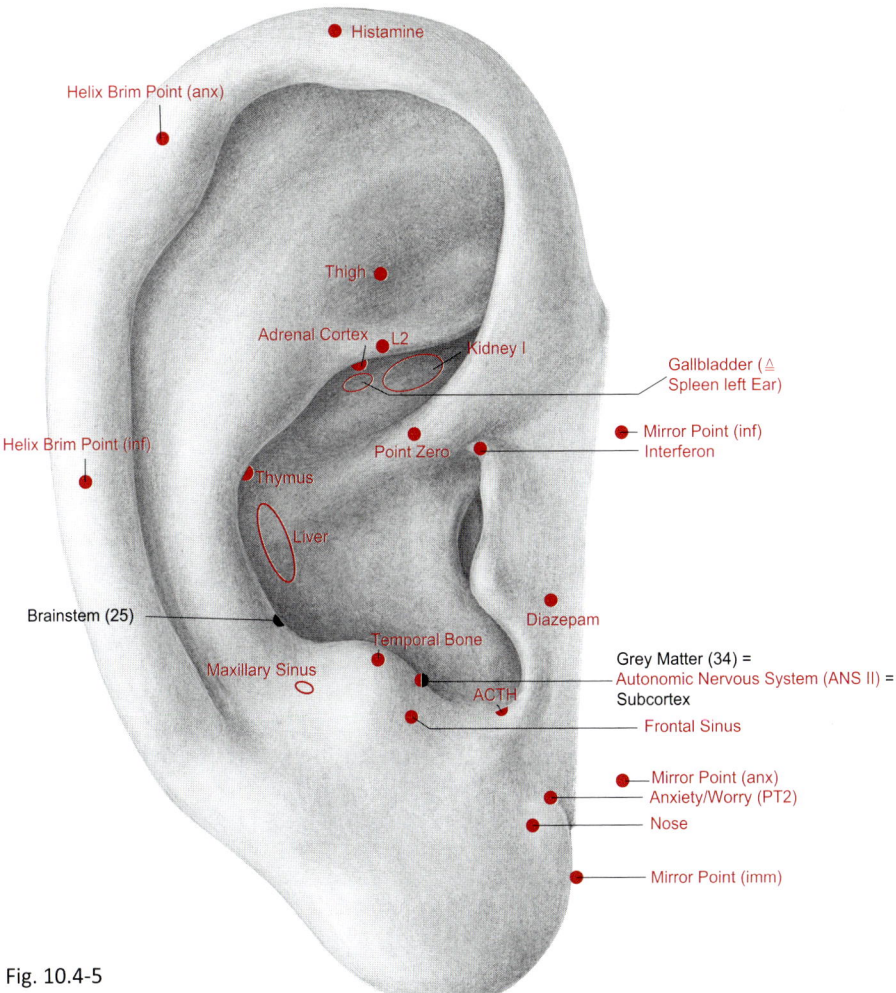

Fig. 10.4-5

Summary

Both sinusitis and nasal breathing already improved after the first treatment, despite the complex history and this multimorbid patient. Instead of a blocked nose there were now symptoms of rhinitis. However, there was only a short-lived relief from the recurrent migraine-like headaches caused by metamizole abuse.

To increase the effect of the acupuncture treatments the patient was treated once weekly since 08/06/2001. After 3 months elevated ACTH and cortisol levels were discovered during a routine check-up (test results from 21/09/2001, Medizinische Klinik Innenstadt, Munich).

	30/07/2001	17/09/2001
Cortisol (4.0–19.0 microg/dl)	20.8	29.0
ACTH-(15.0–50.0 picog/ml)	46.0	60.0

Since acromegaly could be excluded the elevated levels were probably a result of the acupuncture treatments.

 These two case studies (› 10.4.5 and 10.16) demonstrate that treating the Immune Axis can result in elevated blood cortisol levels. In the first example the actual cortisol levels were raised, while in the second example 17-α-hydroxyprogesterone was elevated since cortisol itself could not be synthesised due to the lack of 21-hydroxylase.

10.5 Epilepsy

L.M., 22-year-old male; treatment period: 13/09/2002 to 12/07/2003

Medical history

- June 2000: stretched piercing of the right ear lobe with a ring taking up nearly the whole lobe, stretching extending to the antitragus
- July 2000: acute cervical myalgia with headaches and eye pressure for one week, followed by an epileptic grand mal seizure (aura with coloured lights, drooling, convulsions, retrograde amnesia); initially no treatments
- Christmas 2000; second seizure with subsequent medication; despite medication seizures about every 2½ months; the cause of the seizures is unclear but according to EEG originating in both cerebral hemispheres; various unsuccessful attempts with different drugs to manage the seizures
- Since September 2002 acupuncture treatments
- Secondary findings: none

TCM diagnosis

- Kidney deficiency
- Liver stagnation
- Phlegm obstruction of the Kidneys
- *Qi* stagnation

Treatment principle

Relieve symptoms by
1. Resolving the interference field in the ear (caused by stretched piercing)
2. Tonifying deficient Organs/meridians
3. Coursing the Liver
4. Resolving Phlegm obstruction
5. Coursing *Qi*

Treatments (› Fig. 10.5-1)

Disposable needles were used for both auricular and body acupuncture. These were retained for 20 minutes.

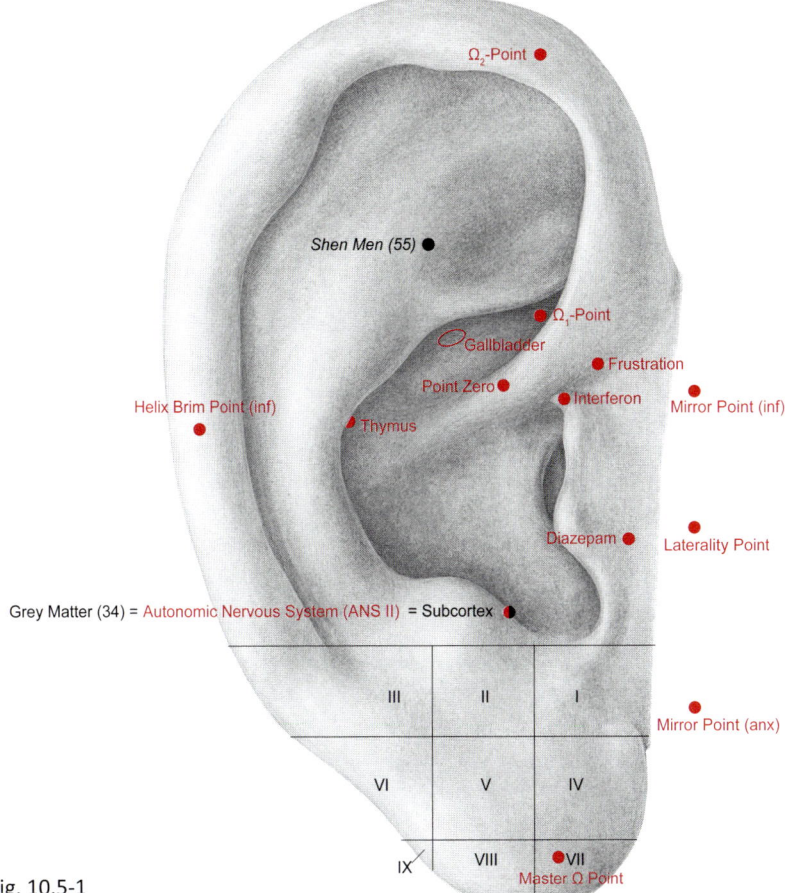

Fig. 10.5-1

Auricular acupuncture based on RAC-palpation

First treatment
- **Right side:** Brainstem (25) → **1**, Grey Matter (34) → **1**, *Shen Men* (55) → **3**, Omega Axis → **3**, Laterality Point → **4**
- **Left side:** Brainstem (25) → **1**, Grey Matter (34) → **1**, *Shen Men* (55) → **3**, Diazepam → **3**, Point Zero → **4**

Further points used in follow-up treatments
- **Right side:** Gallbladder → **3**, Frustration → **3**
- **Left side:** Diazepam → **3**, Infection Axis

Body acupuncture

First treatment
GV-20 → **2, 3**, PC-6 → **3, 4, 5**, LR-3 → **3**

Further points used in follow-up treatments
TH-10 → **4, 5**, PC-5 → **4, 5**, ST-40 → **4**, KI-6 → **2**

Chinese herbal medicine

Buthus (*quanxie*, descending, pacifies the Liver), Rhizoma gastrodiae (*tianma*, descending, pacifies the Liver), Ramulus et unci uncariae (*gouteng*, descending, pacifies the Liver), Tuber curcumae longae (*yujin*, regulates and invigorates *Xue*), Bambusae concretio siliceae (*tianzhuhuang*, cooling, transforms hot Phlegm), Fructus gleditsiae (*zaojiao*, transforms cold Phlegm), Fossilium ossis mastodi (*longgu*, descending, calms the spirit)

Treatment intervals

- Initially once weekly for 6 weeks
- Then irregular intervals (2–4 weeks) due to lack of patient compliance
- The patient did not return after his treatment on 12/07/2003.

Summary

After starting acupuncture treatments the patient was without symptoms for 8 weeks while continuing with medication. After forgetting to take his medication, coupled with exposure to a stressful situation, he again had a seizure. Subsequently he was free of symptoms for 4 months but missed 2 appointments. He returned for treatments after suffering another seizure in January 2003. The patient reported auras with coloured lights on two occasions but these did not develop into seizures. In April 2003, four months after the last seizure, the patient was in an extremely stressful situation triggering a seizure. While acupuncture treatments prevented further seizures the patient had several aura events. Despite being cautioned by his physician, the patient sometimes consumed up to 5 glasses of beer a day.

Note: there is a close connection in time between the piercing and the first seizure. The stretched piercing clearly affected areas of the ear representing various regions of the brain (occipital, frontal and temporal bones as well as Grey Matter [34]). Acupuncture treatments were able to significantly reduce the frequency of the seizures, and it was only after starting acupuncture that the auras experienced by the patient did not develop into seizures. The lack of patient compliance had an effect on the treatment success.

10.6 Chronic Polyarthritis

Z.G., 54-years-old female; treatment period: 27/03/1997 to 18/03/1999

Medical history

- January 1997: fracture of the left navicular bone; since February 1997 pain and swelling of the right ankle and forefoot; short-term improvement with anti-inflammatory medication and cortisone therapy
- In the following weeks and months the pain spread progressively to the spine, shoulders, knee joints as well as the joints of fingers and toes on both sides
- Blood tests: initially only elevated leukocyte count, later also elevated CRP
- Previous surgeries/diseases: hysterectomy, appendectomy, tonsillectomy, nephrolithiasis
- Secondary findings: collagenous colitis in1999

TCM diagnosis

- Deficiency of the Middle
- Liver stagnation
- *Bi*-syndrome with Phlegm and Cold obstruction, Heat damage
- Local *Qi* stagnation

Treatment principle

Relieve the complaint by
1. Tonifying deficient Organs/meridians
2. Coursing the Liver
3. Resolving Phlegm
4. Eliminating Cold and Heat damage
5. Coursing and relaxing the *Qi* locally

Treatments (› Fig. 10.6-1)

Disposable needles were used for both auricular and body acupuncture. These were retained for 20 minutes. On some occasions the interference fields (such as scars) were treated with semi-permanent needles, which were retained for about 1 week unless they spontaneously fell out beforehand.

Auricular acupuncture based on RAC-palpation

First treatment
- **Right side:** Immune Axis → **3, 4**, Atlanto-occipital Joint → **5**, C7 → **5**, Maxillary Sinus → **3**
- **Left side:** Infection Axis → **3, 4**, Frontal Sinus → **3**, Point Zero → **1, 3**, *Shen Men* (55) → **2**

Further points used in follow-up treatments
- **Right side:** Point Zero → **1, 3**, Kidney → **1**, Gallbladder → **2**, Pineal Gland, Ankle → **5**, Wrist → **5**, Hip → **5**, Knee → **5**, Shoulder → **5**, PGE$_1$, Tonsils → **5**, Uterus → **5**
- **Left side:** Anti-Aggression → **2**, Antidepressant Point, C3 → **5**, C7 → **5**, L2 → **5**, Laterality Point → **1**, Omega Axis → **2**, Haldol → **2**, Frustration, Thymus → **1**

Body acupuncture

First treatment
None.

Further points used in follow-up treatments
TH-5 → **4, 5**, SP-10, SP-3 → **3, 4**, ST-36 → **1, 3, 5**, LI-4 → **5**, LI-11 → **3, 4**, LR-3 → **2**, LU-5 → **1, 4**, GB-20 → **4**, HT-7 → **4, 5**, PC-6 → **3, 4, 5**

Chinese Herbal Medicine

Ramulus cassiae (*juemingzi*, cools the Liver), Radix angelicae dahuricae (*baizhi*, releases the surface, warming), Rhizoma atractylodis (*cangzhu*, aromatic herb, transforms dampness), Radix heraclei (*duhuo*, expels Wind, aromatically transforms Dampness, alleviates pain),

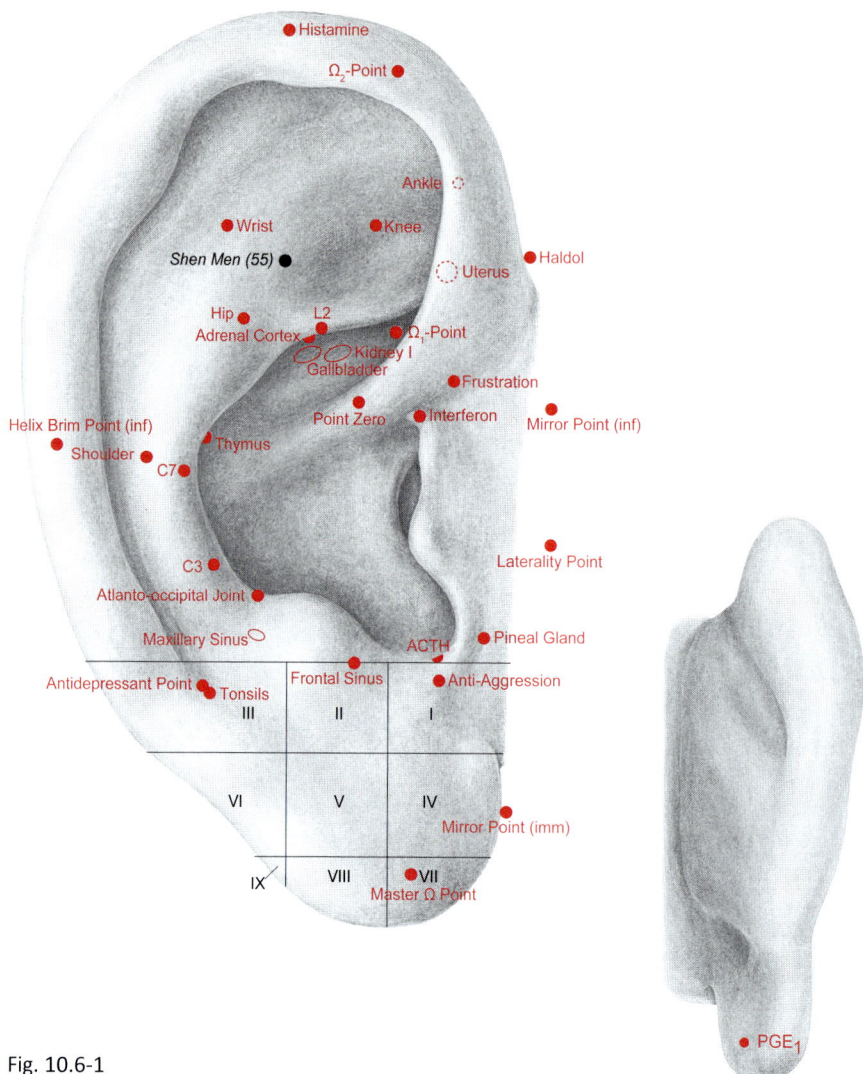

Fig. 10.6-1

Semen plantaginis (*cheqianzi*, promotes urination, transforms Dampness), Semen glycyrrhizae (*gancao*, tonifies *Qi*), Rhizoma curcumae longae (*jianghuang*, regulates and invigorates *Xue*), Radix salviae milthiorrhizae (*danshen*, regulates and invigorates *Xue*) etc.

Treatment intervals

- Initially about once weekly for half a year
- Followed by 1–2 treatments per fortnight, depending on the symptoms, for half a year
- Followed by 1–2 treatments per month until there was a sustained relief from symptoms

Summary

After the first treatment the patient felt significantly better overall and had no pain in her neck; however, the lower back pain as well as the joint pain had hardly improved. During the first half year of receiving treatments, symptoms fluctuated widely: there were symptomatic changes which could be correlated with the acupuncture treatments but the overall picture barely improved. However, during the next 6 months the symptoms improved significantly. Since August 1998 there was only occasional joint pain. At the same time the patient as well as the people around her noticed an increasingly aggressive behaviour in the patient. Treatments were concluded on 18/03/1999 when there was a sustained relief from symptoms.

Note: Chronic polyarthritis is an autoimmune disorder characterised by the body attacking its own tissue. As treatment results from acupuncture become more sustained, one can often observe that patients begin to direct previously suppressed feelings of aggression against their environment. In patients who won't allow this to happen this may delay treatment results.

10.7 Frozen Shoulder (Periarthritis humeroscapularis)

H.H., 64-year-old, male; treatment period: 07/04/1998 to 12/09/2000

Medical History

- Severe pain in the right shoulder following a fall on 22/07/1996 while playing tennis; rotator cuff tear on the right-hand side. An X-ray showed osteoarthritis secondary to the traumatic injury; 50 massage treatments and physiotherapy did not relieve the symptoms in any significant way.
- Following an osteopathic/chiropractic treatment on 18/02/1997 for the first time immediate symptomatic relief but significant residual symptoms
- Renewed check-up (X-ray) in March 1997 showed a bony avulsion of the supraspinatus tendon, treated surgically on 20/03/1997
- Postoperative physiotherapy did not achieve a complete relief from symptoms
- Residual pain at the start of acupuncture treatments: pain at the biceps tendon insertion with external rotation; pain with elevation of the right arm for more than 45°
- Secondary findings: type-2 diabetes mellitus, progressive spinal muscular dystrophy, umbilical hernia, nicotine abuse

TCM diagnosis

- Compensated deficiency of the Middle
- Compensated deficiency of the Kidneys
- Phlegm obstruction

Treatment principle

Relieve symptoms by
1. Tonifying deficient Organs/meridians
2. Resolving Phlegm obstruction
3. Local relaxation of the musculature

Treatments (› Fig. 10.7-1)

Disposable needles were used for both auricular and body acupuncture. These were retained for 20 minutes.

Auricular acupuncture based on RAC-palpation

First treatment
- **Right side:** Shoulder → **3**, C2 → **3**
- **Left side:** Point Zero → **1, 2**, Diazepam → **3**

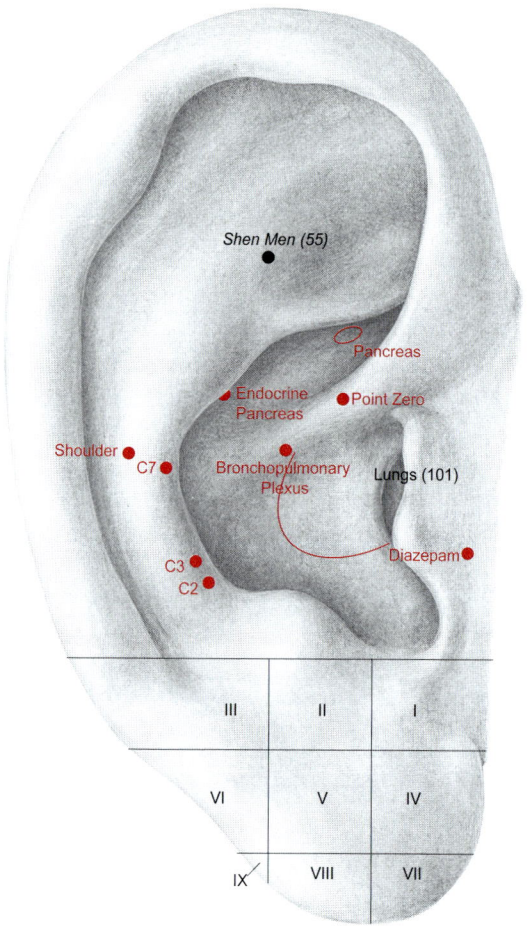

Shen Men (55)

Pancreas

Endocrine
Pancreas

Point Zero

Shoulder

C7

Bronchopulmonary
Plexus

Lungs (101)

C3

C2

Diazepam

III   II   I

VI   V   IV

IX   VIII   VII

Fig. 10.7-1

Further points used in follow-up treatments

- **Right side:** C3 → **3**, C7 → **3**, Point Zero → **1,** Endocrine Pancreas → **1,** *Shen Men* (55), Lung (101)
- **Left side:** Pancreas, Bronchopulmonary Plexus → **1, 2**

Body acupuncture

First treatment
SI-9 → **2, 3**, LI-11 → **2, 3**, TH-5

Further points used in follow-up treatments
LR-3, ST-36 → **1, 2**, LI-14 → **3**, GB-20 → **3**

Treatment intervals

- 2 treatments at 1-week intervals resulted in a sustained relief from symptoms
- Further treatments only to treat secondary findings and to stabilise the treatment effects

Summary

Despite the complications before the start of acupuncture treatments (see above) it was possible to resolve the main complaint within 2 treatments; after the second treatment the patient was again able to carry furniture, play tennis and participate in a sailing regatta. This would have seemed impossible before the treatments. When the patient last came to the clinic, on 12/09/2000, the right shoulder was completely symptom-free.

10.8 Lower Back Pain (Lumbago)

D.R., 51-year-old male; treatment period: 29/01/2003 to 10/07/2003

Medical history

- Chronic recurrent lower back pain from an early age
- Since 25/01/2003: following an extended pain-free period progressive lower back pain with pain increasingly radiating to the left testicle
- MRI of the lumbar spine: early stages of spondylosis affecting the facet joints of L4/5 and L5/S1, no disc protrusions, no spinal stenosis
- Seoncdary findings: fear of heights, nicotine abuse

TCM diagnosis

- Deficiency of the Middle
- Liver stagnation
- Wind damage
- Phlegm obstruction

Treatment principle

Relieve symptoms by

1. Tonifying deficient Organs/meridians
2. Coursing the Liver
3. Relaxing tense sections of the spine (cervical and lumbar spine)
4. Resolving Wind and Phlegm

Treatments (› Fig. 10.8-1)

Disposable needles were used for both auricular and body acupuncture. These were retained for 20 minutes.

Auricular acupuncture based on RAC-palpation

First treatment

- **Right side:** Point Zero → **1, 3**, L4 → **3**, L5 → **3**, *Shen Men* (55) → **2**
- **Left side:** L2 → **3**, S1 → **3**, Diazepam → **3**, Antidepressant Axis → **2**

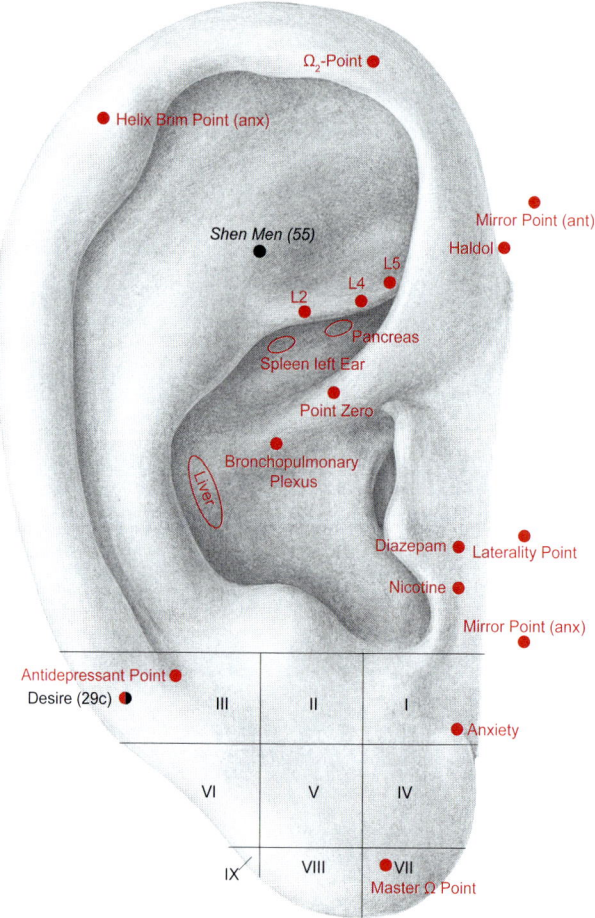

Fig. 10.8-1

Further points used in follow-up treatments
- **Right side:** Anxiety → **2**, Omega Axis → **2**, Laterality Point → **1**, Liver → **2**
- **Left side:** Desire, Nicotine, Anxiety Axis → **2**, Testes

Body acupuncture

First treatment

GV-20 → **2, 4**, BL-40 → **1, 2**, SP-9 → **4**, BL-62 → **2**, LR-3 → **2**

Further points used in follow-up treatments

HT-7 → **2**, GB-41 → **4**, SI-3 → **3, 4**, ST-9 → **3**, KI-6 → **1**

With acute progressive pain 0.1 ml-Xylonest 1 % was injected in addition to acupuncture at the auricular points Ω_1-Point and Lumbar Spine.

Treatment intervals

- Initially 1–2 times weekly until symptoms had improved significantly
- Followed by fortnightly treatments until symptoms had subsided completely

Summary

Due to the chronic nature of the lower back pain, the acute flare-up could not be stopped immediately. Initially, the condition worsened and the pain radiated to the left testicle so that an MRI scan of the lumbar spine was carried out. After the acupuncture treatment there was a short-lived improvement for a few days; however, longer symptom-free spells occurred only after 6 weeks of treatments. A stable, sustained relief from symptoms was achieved after 6 months. Since then the patient has had no relapses regarding his lower back pain. He continued with treatments for anxiety attacks which have also reduced significantly.

10.9 Infertility

M.D., 33-year-old female; treatment period: 12/07/1997 to 22/09/2001

Medical history

- Anorexia nervosa, worse from 1993–1996, eating disorder already present during puberty
- No period since 1993 despite hormone therapy
- Following psychosomatic treatment as inpatient until 10/96 normal body weight; periods returned for a short time with hormone therapy but stopped again when medication was discontinued in 1/97
- Married since 12/96, desire to have children
- Secondary findings: allergic rhinitis, Raynaud's syndrome, hypotension

TCM diagnosis

- Deficiency of the Middle
- Stagnation of the Liver
- Deficiency of Body Fluids

Treatment principle

To re-establish natural periods and create a stable condition for pregnancy by
1. Tonifying deficient Organs/meridians
2. Coursing the Liver
3. Harmonising Body Fluids

Treatments (› Fig. 10.9-1)

Disposable needles were used for both auricular and body acupuncture. These were retained for 20 minutes.

Auricular acupuncture based on RAC-palpation

First treatment
- **Right side:** Gynaecological Axis → **1**, Point Zero → **1**
- **Left side:** Kidney I → **1**

Further points used in follow-up treatments
- **Right side:** Gallbladder → **2**, Frustration → **2**
- **Left side:** Ovaries → **1**, Frustration → **2**, Point Zero → **1**, Gonadotropin Point → **3**, Laterality Point → **1, 2, 3**

Body acupuncture

First treatment
SP-10 → **3**, BL-40 → **1**

Further points used in follow-up treatments:
LU-5 → **1**, KI-7 → **1**, ST-36 → **1**, LR-3 → **2**

Chinese herbal medicine

Radix paeoniae lactiflorae (*baishao*, nourishes and tonifies *Xue*), Radix angelicae sinensis (*danggui*, nourishes and tonifies *Xue*), Semen persicae (*taoren*, regulates and invigorates *Xue*), Radix aconiti (*fuzi*, warms the interior), Cortex cinnamomi cassiae (*rougui*, warms the interior), Rhizoma cyperi (*xiangfu*, regulates the flow of *Qi*), Rhizoma ligustici (*chuanxiong*, regulates and invigorates *Xue*), Rhizoma scirpi seu sparganii (*sanleng*, regulates and invigorates *Xue*), Radix codonopsitis (*dangshen*, tonifies *Qi*), Herba epimedii (*yinyanghuo*, tonifies and fortifies *Yang*), Cortex eucommiae (*duzhong*, tonifies and fortifies *Yang*), Semen Zizyphi spinosae (*suanzaoren*, descending, quiets the spirit), Rhizoma zingiberis viridis (*shengjiang*, releases the surface, warming) etc.

Treatment intervals

- Initially 5 weekly treatments
- Followed by treatments at intervals of 2–3 weeks until the patient had a period on 23/12/1997
- Continuation with fortnightly treatments; 2nd period at the end of January, 3rd period in mid-March, followed by pregnancy; after week 15 the patient discontinued treatments
- Further treatments since 15/02/2001; following a miscarriage in week 8 the patient is again pregnant (week 7)
- Fortnightly treatments until week 39

Summary

After treatments with auricular acupuncture and TCM for half a year, the patient's condition had become sufficiently stable for a period to occur. This was at a time when her body weight had increased to 52 kg about which the patient was not very happy. The menstrual cycle was stable over a period of 3 months, the patient then became pregnant. She was treated with TCM up to week 15. Due to the positively experienced first pregnancy followed by a regular, 6-week cycle the patient did not come for acupuncture during her 2nd pregnancy. She miscarried after week 8. She returned for TCM and auricular acupuncture treatments during her 3rd pregnancy. This was without complications and she gave birth to a healthy baby.

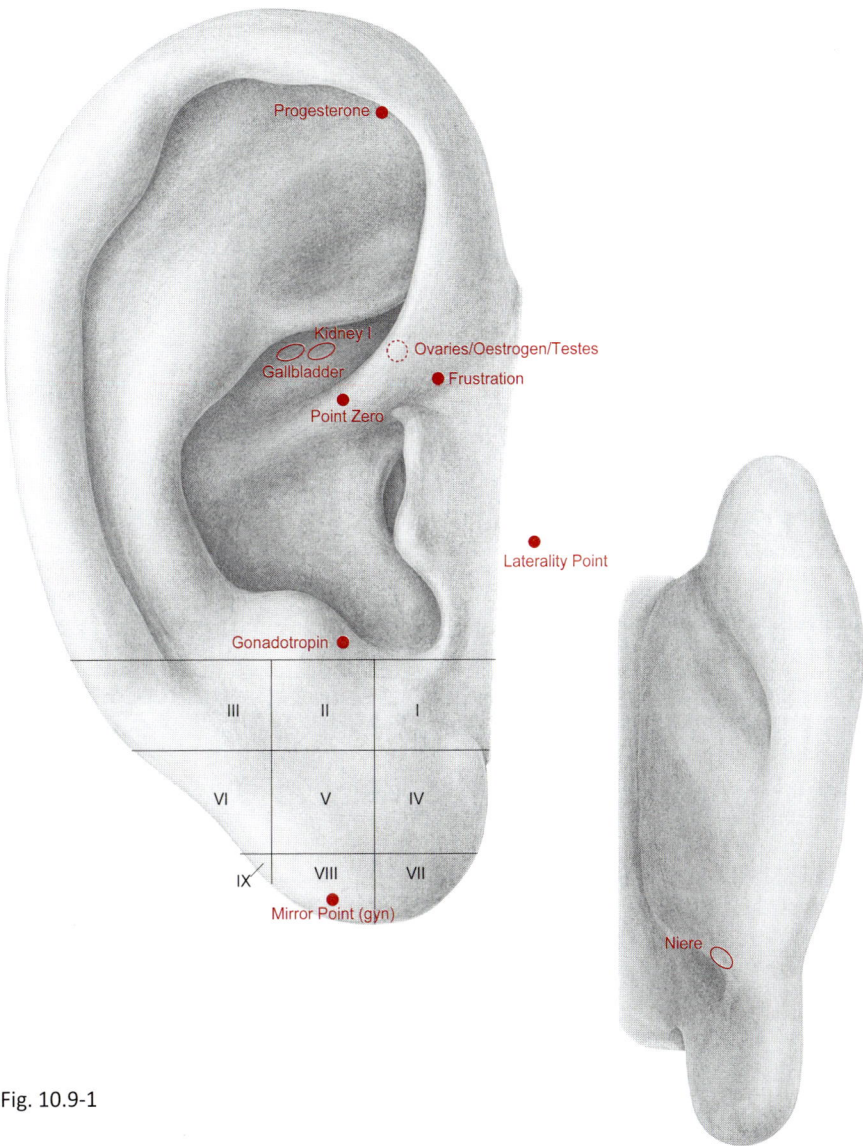

Fig. 10.9-1

10.10 Parkinson's Disease

I.W., 52-year-old female; treatment period: since 25/08/1996, for Parkinson's disease since 03/12/1999, no treatments from 27/06/2000 to 30/01/2002

Medical history

- Exhaustion due to stress, getting progressively worse over a period of several months, accompanied by increasing inner restlessness and tremor in all extremities, later becoming more pronounced on the right-hand side of the body
- Intensity of the exhaustion changing from day to day, initially to the point of being bedridden
- Occasionally the above symptoms are accompanied by sensory disturbances, especially in the right hand
- Significant impairment of the right hand, barely able to write, and occasionally not at all
- Walking significantly impaired due to tremor in the right leg, unstable gait
- Secondary findings: bilateral cervical myalgia, sciatica on the left

TCM diagnosis

- Deficiency of the Middle
- Kidney deficiency
- Heart deficiency
- Stagnation of the Liver
- Wind damage

Treatment principle

Relieve symptoms by
1. Tonifying deficient Organs/meridians
2. Coursing the Liver
3. Extinguishing Wind
4. Relaxing tense sections of the spine (cervical spine, lumbar spine)

Treatments (› Fig. 10.10-1)

Disposable needles were used for both auricular and body acupuncture. These were retained for 20 minutes.

Auricular acupuncture based on RAC-palpation

First treatment
- **Right side:** Laterality Point → 1, Antidepressant Axis, Anxiety, *Shen Men* (55) → 2
- **Left side:** Omega Axis → **2**, Anxiety Axis, *Shen Men* (55) → **2**

Further points used in follow-up treatments
- **Right side:** Omega Axis → **2**, Brainstem (25) → **1**, Grey Matter(34) → **1**, Frustration → **2**, Sciatic Nerve → **4**

- **Left side:** Diazepam → **4**, C5 → **4**, C7 → **4**, Atlanto-occipital Joint → **4**, Point Zero → **1**, Laterality Point → **1**, Brainstem (25) → **1**, Knee → **4**

Body acupuncture

First treatment
GV-20 → **2, 3**, GB-41 → **2**, HT-7 → **1**, BL-40 → **1, 4**, SP-9 → **4**

Further points used in follow-up treatments
LR-3 → **2, 3**, TH-5, GB-20 → **3**, ST-36 → **1**, LI-11 → **3**, KI-3 → **1**, LU-5 → **1**, SP-3, KI-6 → **1**, PC-6 → **1, 3**

Treatment intervals

- Once weekly for 3 weeks, followed by a 2-month break; in the meantime therapy with sifrol (0.35 mg 3 times daily)
- 21 treatments at irregular intervals of 1–2 weeks
- Treatment break until 30/01/2002
- Followed by treatments every 1–2 weeks

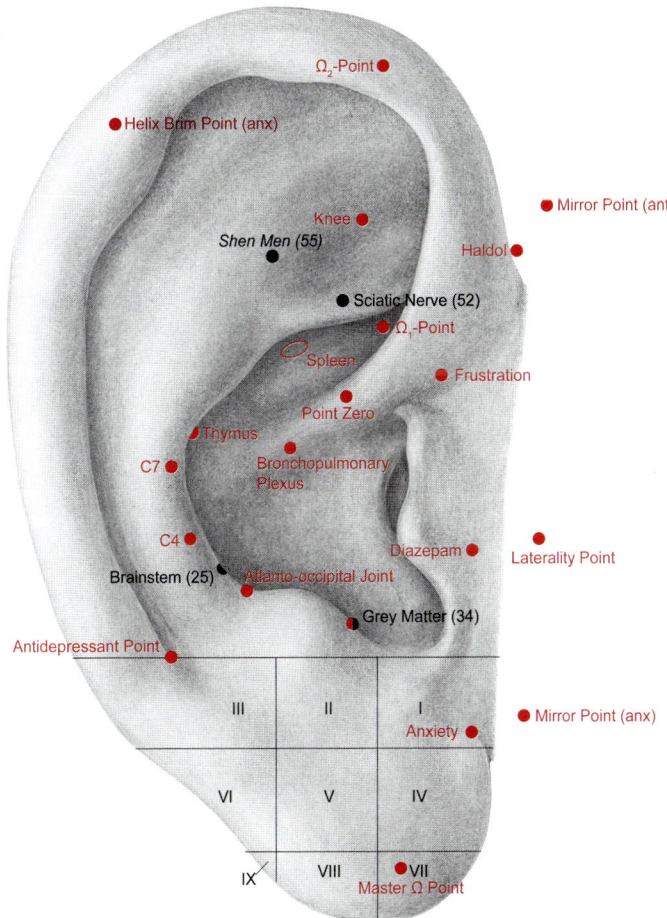

Fig. 10.10-1

Summary

At the start of treatments there was a minor improvement of symptoms but due to the continuous stress at her workplace the patient soon felt exhausted again. Despite this, the symptoms continued to lessen, albeit with relapses that can be attributed to a lack of patient compliance. Eventually the tremor in the right arm (to the point of being unable to write) and the right leg (unstable gait) improved so that the patient terminated treatments on 27/06/2000. At that point she was better but not symptom-free.

The clinical picture worsened markedly during the treatment break and required inpatient admission to a neurological ward. She was prescribed sifrol (0.35 mg 3 times daily) which stabilised her condition but did not resolve the tremor in her arm and leg (which was now also accompanied by sensory disturbances) as well as her impaired ability to write.

On 30/01/2002 the patient returned for acupuncture treatments – this time with much better compliance than before. Regular treatments (intervals of 1–2 weeks) and continued medication resulted in symptoms completely subsiding by February 2004. Her ability to walk and write was completely restored. It was now also possible to reduce her medication by a third without a worsening of symptoms. The patient is still receiving treatments. The treatment goal is to achieve a sustained relief from symptoms, if possible without medication.

10.11 Optic Neuritis

P.-R.A., 34-year-old female; treatment period: 04/03/2003 to 15/07/2003

Medical history

- Mild retro-orbital headache for 3 days, followed by an acute decrease in vision in the right eye since 17/02/2003
- When covering the right eye, only a dark grey fog can be seen with the left eye
- Visually evoked potentials: reduced P100 (both latency and amplitude) in the left eye
- Extracranial Doppler sonography: no findings
- Head MRI: minimal comma-shaped signal enhancement at the internal capsule on the right-hand side (demyelination?), otherwise no findings
- Secondary findings: cervical PAP smear III, arthritis in the left knee

TCM diagnosis

- Deficiency of the Middle
- Stagnation of the Liver
- Heat/Phlegm
- Localised weakness

Treatment principle

Relieve symptoms by
1. Tonifying deficient Organs/meridians
2. Coursing the Liver

3. Cooling Heat, resolving Phlegm
4. Tonifying areas of localised weakness, opening sensory orifices

Treatments (› Fig. 10.11-1)

Disposable needles were used for both auricular and body acupuncture. These were retained for 20 minutes.

Auricular acupuncture based on RAC-palpation

First treatment

- **Right side:** Immune Axis → **3**, Uterus → **3**, *Shen Men* (55) → **2**
- **Left side:** Point Zero → **1**, Interferon → **3**, Thymus → **3**, Eye I (24a) → **3, 4**, Eye II (24b) → **3, 4**, *Shen Men* (55) → **2**

Further points used in follow-up treatments

- **Right side:** Kidney I → **1**, Kidney II → **1**, Liver → **2**, Omega Axis → **2**
- **Left side:** Diazepam → **2**, Laterality Point → **1**, Eye (8) → **4**, Anti-Aggression → **2**, Knee → **2**, Knee Joint (49) → **2**

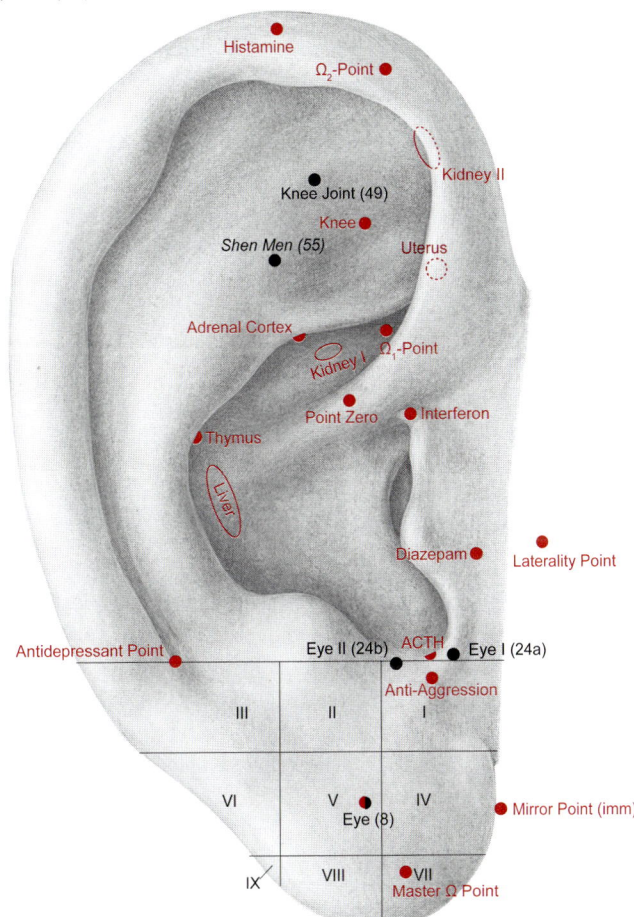

Fig. 10.11-1

Body acupuncture

First treatment

Yuyao (Extra point: Fish Waist) → **3, 4**, GB-1 → **3, 4**, BL-1 → **3, 4**, TH-3 → **4**, LR-3 → **2**, GB-41 → **2**

Further points used in follow-up treatments

GV-20 → **2, 4**, BL-40 → **3, 4**, ST-36 → **1, 4**, SP-9 → **3, 4**, KI-6 → **1, 3**, LR-8 → **4**

Treatment intervals

- 2 treatments within one week
- 2 treatments at weekly intervals
- 5 treatments at intervals of 2–4 weeks

Summary

In the two weeks following the onset of the disorder (but before starting acupuncture) the patient's visual impairment did not change. The patient refused to take glucocorticoids which I also considered not necessary. From the first treatment onward there was a significant subjective visual improvement. During the further treatment course the patient's vision continued to improve until symptoms had disappeared and vision was restored completely so that intervals between treatments could be extended. The patient received further treatments during her pregnancy until February 2004 when she reported a sustained relief from symptoms regarding her vision. No further treatment of the left eye was necessary since July 2003.

10.12 Psoriasis

S.G., 76-year-old male; treatment period: 13/09/1997 to 19/07/1999

Medical history

- Since approximately June 1993 scaling, itching rash, especially on the face and neck but also on the extremities and on the torso
- Constantly present since the onset but in varying degrees of intensity; as topical treatment with hydrocortisone brings only short-lived relief this was discontinued
- Occasional additional symptoms include light sensitivity and reddening of the eyes
- Secondary findings: surgeries: hiatus hernia, pelvic ring fracture, fracture of the right humerus, total hip replacement on the left; since 12/1992 oral anticoagulant therapy (warfarin) due to atrial fibrillation, hypertension, prostate adenoma
- Concurrent medication: Arelix (piretanide)→ low dosis, Novodigal (acetyldigoxin) → 0.2, enalapril → 5, warfarin →; as needed: Prospan (dry extract of ivy leaves) →, Tebonin forte (ginkgo biloba extract) → higher dosis

TCM diagnosis

- Deficiency of the Middle
- Liver stagnation

- Phlegm
- Wind damage
- Heat damage

Treatment principle

Relieve symptoms by

1. Tonifying deficient Organs/meridians
2. Coursing the Liver
3. Resolving Phlegm and extinguishing Wind
4. Cooling Heat
5. Relaxing tense sections of the spine (lumbar)

Treatments (› Fig. 10.12-1)

Disposable needles were used for both auricular and body acupuncture. These were retained for 20 minutes.

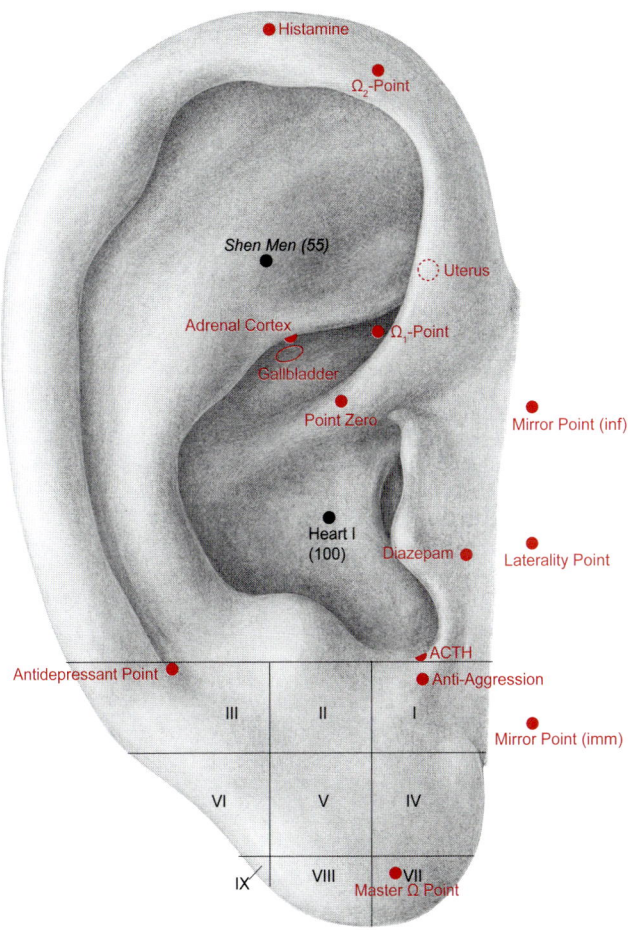

Fig. 10.12-1

Auricular acupuncture based on RAC-palpation

First treatment
- **Right side:** Omega Axis → **2**, Gallbladder → **2**, Point Zero → **1**, Histamine
- **Left side:** Point Zero → **1**, Laterality Point → **1, 2**, Frustration → **2**

Further points used in follow-up treatments
- **Right side:** Immune Axis → **3, 4**, *Shen Men* (55) → **2**, Anti-Aggression → **2**
- **Left side:** Diazepam → **5**, Omega Axis → 2, Antidepressant Point → 2, Heart I (100) → 1, Immune Axis → 3, 4

Body acupuncture

First treatment
LI-11 → **3, 4**, ST-36 → **1, 4**, LR-3 → **2**, LI-4 → **3**

Further points used in follow-up treatments
SP-4 → **1, 4**, GB-14 → **3**, KI-6 → **1, 4**, SI-3 → **3, 4**, TH-3, TH-5 → **4**, BL-40 → **1, 4**

Additional treatment with Chinese herbal medicine

Gypsum fibrosum (*shigao,* drains and disperses Fire), Flos chrysanthemi (*juhua,* cooling, releases the surface), Semen cassiae torae (*juemingzi,* cools the Liver), Radix scrophulariae (*xuanshen,* cools *Xue*), Gelatina nigra (*e jiao,* nourishes *Xue,* stops bleeding, nourishes *Yin,* moistens the Lungs), Rhizoma anemarrhenae (*zhimu,* drains Fire), Cortex phellodendri (*huangbo,* cooling and drying), Fructus forsythiae (*lianqiao,* cooling and disinfecting), Radix glycyrrhizae (*gancao,* tonifies the *Qi*), Fructus cnidii (*shechuangzi,* tonifies and fortifies *Yang*), Spina gleditsiae (*zaojiaoci,* regulates and invigorates *Xue*), Spica prunellae (*xiakucao,* drains and disperses Fire), Cortex moutan (*mudanpi,* cools *Xue*)

Local laser therapy

At the 9th and 8 further treatments affected skin areas were treated with a Twin Laser (Reimers & Janssen) Infrared/red light with an output of 150/20 mW and Nogier frequency A. A 1 cm^2 area of skin was irradiated for approximately 5 seconds. During the further treatment course laser was used occasionally depending on the intensity of the erythema and the scaling.

Treatment intervals

- Once weekly until April 1998
- Every 10–14 days

Summary

After the first acupuncture treatment the plaques improved considerably for one day but then deteriorated again. During the course of the treatments the affected areas continued to improve but there were fluctuations which were exacerbated by both stress and diet (e.g. nitrate in sausages). By July 1998 the psoriatic rash had disappeared. After using a different shampoo it flared up again in March 1999 but it was possible to alleviate symptoms within 4 months. Since then the patient had been free of symptoms until his death on 28/01/2003

10.13 Collagenosis (e.g. Lupus erythematodes)

M.S., 61-year-old female; treatments since 17/10/1998, for collagenosis from 17/03/2004 until 25/05/2004

Primary medical history

- Following tumour treatment regularly increased ESR (approximately 42–54/72–90)
- During a routine check up at the beginning of March 2003: ANA IgG titre of 1:1280 (normal value below 1:80)
- CRP: 17.84 mg/l (below 5 mg/l)
- No skin changes
- Recurrent cervical myalgia
- Occasionally increased sweating
- Secondary findings:
  - History of invasive lobular mamma carcinoma (tumour resection with axillary dissection, dissection, pT1cN1M0G3R0ER+PR-), radiation therapy and adjunctive chemotherapy, tamoxifen for 5 years
  - hypertension (treated with Enalapril comp 10/25)

TCM diagnosis

- Deficiency of the Middle
- Lung deficiency
- Liver stagnation
- Phlegm obstructing the channels
- Weak immune system

Treatment principle

Relieve symptoms by
1. Tonifying deficient Organs/meridians
2. Resolving Phlegm
3. Relaxing tense sections of the (cervical) spine
4. Strengthening the immune system
5. Supporting the Liver

Treatments (› Fig. 10.13-1)

Disposable needles were used for both auricular and body acupuncture. These were retained for 20 minutes.

Auricular acupuncture based on RAC-palpation

First treatment
- **Right side:** Immune Axis → **4**, Kidney I + II → **2**, *Shen Men* (55) → **5**
- **Left side:** Point Zero → **1, 2**, Omega Axis → **3**, Laterality Point → **1**, Thymus → **4**

Further points used in follow-up treatments
- **Right side:** Cervical Spine → **3**, Hypertension (19) → **1**
- **Left side:** Interferon → **4**, Cervical Spine → **3**, Frustration → **5**

Body acupuncture

First treatment
GV-20 → **1**, GB-41 → **1**, LR-3 → **1, 5**, KI-6 → **1**, ST-36 → **1, 3** TH-10 → **2**

Further points used in follow-up treatments
LU-5 → **1, 2**, BL-40 → **1, 3**, GB-20 → **3**, SP-9 → **2**

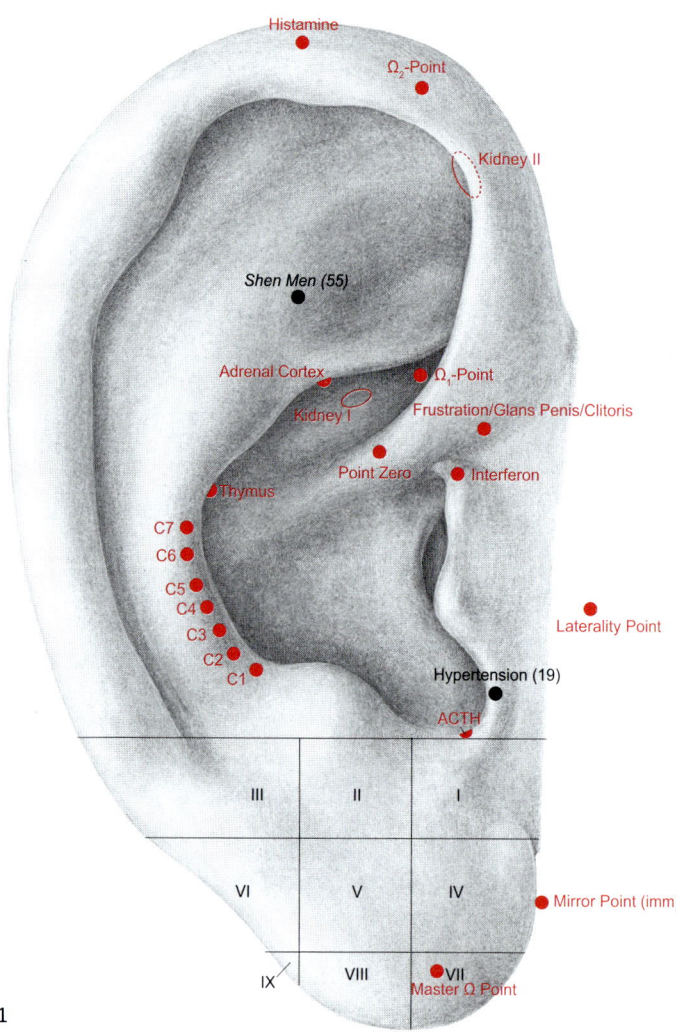

Fig. 10.13-1

Treatment intervals

- Initial treatments approximately every 4 weeks, aftercare following tumour resection
- Due to elevated ANA-titre: treatment intervals reduced, 2 treatments with a 1-week interval
- Then 3 treatments at 2-week intervals
- Treatments for collagenosis concluded on 25/05/2004

Summary

Due to the previous illness (mamma carcinoma) the patient's immune system had been supported for years. Following the diagnosis of an elevated ANA titre this support was intensified for a short period of time, resulting in ANA levels returning to a normal level. Report by the nephrologists: 'Surprisingly, ANA in particular was completely within the normal range during a recent check-up.'

10.14 Prolapsed Disc with Lower Back Pain

W.S., 51-year-old male, treatments: 07/04/1999 to 24/09/1999

Primary medical history

- Recurrent lower back pain since 1996
- At beginning of treatments: acute lower back pain and sciatica on the right-hand side for two weeks
- Altered sensation on the lateral aspect of the right foreleg
- Spinal CT scan of the lumbar spine on 01/04/1999: pronounced mediolateral disc herniation at L5/S1, more pronounced on the right-hand side, suspected sequestrum formation

TCM diagnosis

- Deficiency of the Middle
- Phlegm obstructing the channels
- Wind damage

Treatment principle

Relieve symptoms by
1. Tonifying deficient Organs/meridians
2. Resolving Phlegm
3. Expelling Wind
4. Tonifying local points

Treatments (› Fig. 10.14-1)

Disposable needles were used for both auricular and body acupuncture. These were retained for 20 minutes.

Auricular acupuncture based on RAC-palpation

First treatment

- **Right side:** L5 (muscular) and Vegetative Groove and Disc → **3, 4**, Diazepam → **3**, Frustration
- **Left side:** L3 → **3, 4**

Further points used in follow-up treatments

- **Right side:** L2 → **3, 4**, T6 → **3, 4**
- **Left side:** L2 → **3, 4** L4 →**3, 4**, Diazepam, Laterality Point → **1, 2**

Body acupuncture

First treatment
BL-40 → **1, 4**, ST-36 → **1, 2**

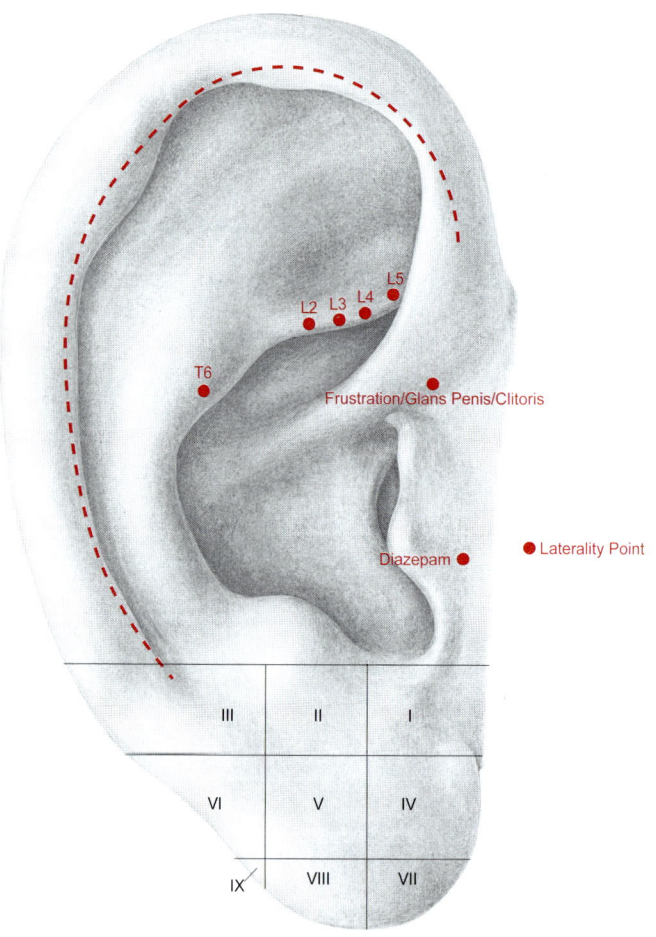

Fig. 10.14-1

Further points used in follow-up treatments

SP-9 → **1, 2**, GB-41 → **1**

For the first 4 treatments 0.1 ml Xylonest 1 % was injected into the lumbar area and the Ω_1-Point on the ear.

Treatment intervals

- First 4 treatments: at intervals of 3 days
- Then 12 treatments at weekly intervals
- 4 further treatments at intervals of 2–3 weeks until symptoms had disappeared

Summary

After the first treatment, symptoms already improved markedly during the day. The patient was able to put weight on his right leg without pain while the sensory disturbances had subsided almost completely. During the night there was still sciatic pain on the right-hand side but the patient was now able to stretch out his legs while lying. After the follow-up treatments there was an initial short-term exacerbation of the pain for a few hours but the diffusely radiating pain continued to retreat to a limited area on the back. Eventually there were days when the patient was free of symptoms but, depending on his activities, the pain would return. Three months after starting treatments the patient was able to go hillwalking for several hours at a time. Since September 1999 the patient has regained his full strength and has no pain at all. To date (December 2006) symptoms have not recurred.

10.15 Alopecia areata

H.S., 32-year-old female; treatments from 26/11/2004 to 10/02/2005

Primary medical history

- Since spring 2004: alopecia areata at the right eyebrow
- Acute onset over a few weeks but no further progression
- Secondary findings:
  - susceptible to colds/flus with chronically recurrent tonsillitis
  - until age 14 migraine attacks, about once a month; no migraines until 2004; renewed attacks in July and October 2004
  - prone to acne, currently minimal
  - surgical scars: appendectomy, tonsillectomy, 2 C-sections (the second one in the previous year)

TCM diagnosis

- Deficiency of the Middle
- Kidney deficiency
- Liver stagnation

Treatment principle

Relieve symptoms by

1. Supporting deficient Organs/meridians
2. Coursing the Liver
3. Supporting the immune systems

Treatments (› Fig. 10.15-1)

Disposable needles were used for both auricular and body acupuncture. These were retained for 20 minutes.

The needled points were also treated with a Physiolaser Olympic (Reimers & Janssen) with an output of 500 mW (infrared, 810 nm). The irradiation of the points was carried out with a surface probe (5–10 Joule per treatment).

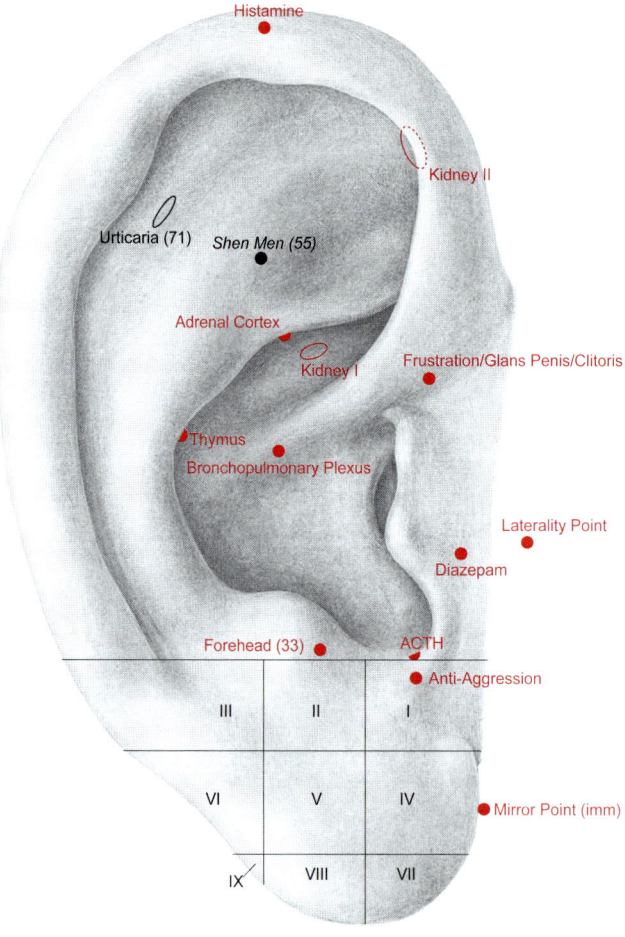

Fig. 10.15-1

Auricular acupuncture based on RAC-palpation

First treatment

- **Right side:** Immune Axis → **3**, Bronchopulmonary Plexus → **1**, Urticaria (71) → **2**, Kidney I + II → **1**
- **Left side:** Frustration → **2**, Anti-Aggression → **2**, *Shen Men* (55) → **2**, Laterality Point → **1**

Further points used in follow-up treatments

- **Right side:** Forehead (33) → **1**, Frustration → **2**
- **Left side:** Diazepam → **2**, Thymus → **3**

Body acupuncture

First treatment

GV-20 → **1, 2**, GB-14 → **2**, LU-5 → **1**, KI-7 → **1**

Further points used in follow-up treatments

LR-3 → **3**

Treatment intervals

- Initially 4 treatments at weekly intervals
- Then 2 treatments at 2–3 week intervals
- By the time of the last treatment symptoms had disappeared

Summary

The patient reported a significant increase in energy after the first treatment ('… after the treatment I cleaned all the windows'). At the time of the first treatment she was also experiencing the early stages of a cold which subsided immediately after receiving acupuncture. The alopecia initially remained unchanged. Only after the 4th treatment there was some hair growth on the affected part of the eyebrow which continued and eventually covered the affected area completely.

10.16 Congenital Adrenal Hyperplasia (CAH)

K. M., 8-year-old male; treatments from 14/07/1999 to 10.11.1999.

Primary medical history

- March 1997: due to a rapid growth spurt suspected precocious puberty; X-ray bone age test confirms an advanced bone age of 13 ½ years (at that time the patient was 6 years old)
- Diagnosis of 21-hydroxylase deficiency, confirming CAH
- Medication: hydrocortisone 3 times daily (7.5–5–5 mg/day)
- Stagnating bone age until 4/1999 with normal testosterone and androstenedione levels but disproportionate weight gain and itchy skin eruptions
- For the above reasons start of acupuncture treatments on 14/07/1999

TCM diagnosis

- Repletion of the Kidneys
- Deficiency and stasis of the Middle
- Impaired *Qi* circulation in the network vessels
- Liver *Yang* rising

Treatment principle

Relieve symptoms by

1. Dispersing repletion
2. Tonifying deficient Organs/meridians
3. Opening the network vessels
4. Coursing *Qi*
5. Calming Liver *Yang*
6. Tonifying local points

Treatments (› Fig. 10.16-1)

The patient was treated with laser (Nogier frequency A); points were stimulated with approximately 0.5 J/point.

Auricular acupuncture based on RAC-palpation

First treatment
- **Right side:** Immune Axis → **2**, Point Zero → **1, 2**, Laterality Point → **2**,
- **Left side:** Infection Axis → **2**, Frontal Sinus → **6**, Maxillary Sinus → **6**, Nose → **6**, Diazepam, Kidney I + II → **2**

Further points used in follow-up treatments
- **Right side:** Testes → **6**
- **Left side:** Testes → **6**, *Shen Men* (55) → **5**, Anti-Aggression → **5**, Desire → **1**, Neural Stomach Point → **1**, Omega Axis

Body acupuncture

First treatment
KI-3 → **4**, LI-4 → **4**, LI-20 → **6**, BL-2 → **6**

Further points used in follow-up treatments
HT-7 → **4**, ST-36 → **2**, LR-3 → **5**,

Treatment intervals

- Once weekly for 3 months
- Then twice monthly for a further month
- Treatments were abandoned at that point.

Summary

The patient came initially for acupuncture to positively influence disproportionate weight gain and inner restlessness. These symptoms could not be explained by taking conventional

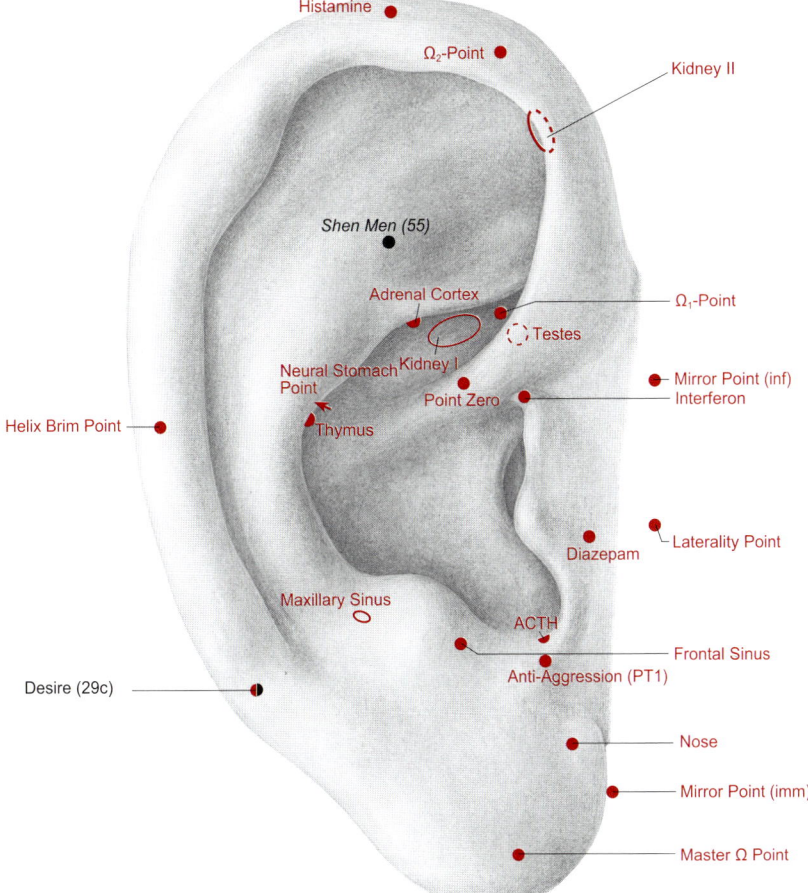

Fig. 10.16-1

medication with glucocorticoids. After the 1st acupuncture treatment the patient felt markedly calmer and had already lost 1 kg, at the 2nd treatment he had lost another ½ kg. The itchy skin rash had also subsided. The Immune Axis was used in order to compensate for the steroid deficiency. However, this resulted in an increased production of the precursor of 17-α-hydroxyprogesterone. After the 3rd treatment symptoms fluctuated considerably. After 2 months there was a progressive androgenisation which had to be compensated for by increasing the cortisone morning dose to 15 mg. For this reason the Immune Axis was not treated anymore with acupuncture, and 17-α-hydroxyprogesterone levels returned to normal. Acupuncture treatments were terminated on 10/11/1999.

> These two case studies (› 10.4.5 and 10.16) demonstrate that treating the Immune Axis can result in elevated blood cortisol levels. In the first example cortisol levels were raised, while in the second example 17-α-hydroxyprogesterone was elevated since cortisol itself could not be synthesised due to the lack of 21-hydroxylase.

11 Current Research Studies

Listed below are the results of a number of research studies about the efficacy of auricular acupuncture. This list does not claim to be systematic nor is it complete; rather it is intended as an incentive for the reader to research further his/her own specific areas of interest with regards to auricular acupuncture. The internet also provides countless sources in this respect.

Semi-permanent needles for Parkinson's disease

Teshmar E (2004) Efficacy and safety of implant acupuncture for Parkinson's disease. Aku MED WISS. 32 (4), 231–234

Anecdotal evidence and a pilot study showed that a specific form of auricular acupuncture (implant acupuncture) resulted in a longer lasting treatment effect for Parkinson's disease. These results demonstrate that treatments with semi-permanent needles are medically advisable, providing a new treatment approach for idiopathic Parkinson's disease.

Evaluation by Prof. Jörg, Klinikum Barmen, Wuppertal; Aku MEDWISS 32 4 (2004) 235:

- This study was neither double-blind nor single-blind.
- The results mention neither the single values nor the calculated mean values so that the statistical significance is not transparent.
- An individual researcher treating 53 patients with several modalities per week is most likely under extreme time pressure. This raises the question who paid for this study and why there were not more researchers involved in it.

Postoperative analgesic requirement with and without auricular acupuncture with semi-permanent needles

Mann C J (1999) Analgesic requirement following total endoprosthesis of the hip and knee with and without semi-permanent needles. Inaugural dissertation, Bochum 1999

Postoperative pain can be effectively treated with auricular semi-permanent needles. For maximum effectiveness it is necessary to regularly stimulate the needles with a small dipole magnet. This procedure saves considerable amounts of analgesic medication. The results of the study show high patient satisfaction with this form of analgesic treatment. Furthermore there was an increase of the patients' general well-being. Postoperative analgesic therapy with acupuncture needles has, among others, the following advantages:

- less postoperative pain
- significantly increased general well-being during the postoperative phase
- considerably higher rate of satisfaction with this form of analgesic therapy
- no risk of overdosing with analgesic medication; stimulating the needles increases the analgesic effect.

Quantifying cerebral effects of auricular acupuncture

Litscher G (2002) Quantifying cerebral effects of auricular acupuncture with innovative computer-aided procedures – comparison with traditional Chinese body acupuncture and Korean hand acupuncture. Europ Z Akup/Der Akupunkturarzt/Aurikulotherapeut. 4, 4–13

According to Paul Nogier and Oriental medicine the ear contains numerous acupuncture points. Nogier hypothesised that the complete human anatomy is represented on the ear. By means of trans-cranial Doppler sonography as well as near-infrared spectroscopy (NIRS) we investigated for the first time the effect of auricular acupuncture on brain function in comparison to traditional Chinese acupuncture and Korean hand acupuncture in 20 healthy subjects in a randomised, placebo-controlled cross-over study.

Conclusion: Innovative biomedical equipment allowed for the first time to demonstrate significant effects of auricular acupuncture on brain functions in humans with objective data.

Acupuncture and anxiety

Anesthesiology (2003) 98, 1328–32

As part of a research study patients were treated with auricular acupuncture, either at the 'relaxation point' or at a sham acupuncture point, prior to being transported to hospital. Patients treated with the 'relaxation point' were markedly less anxious upon arrival at the hospital than patients in the control group. In addition, patients needled at the 'relaxation point' experienced less pain during their treatments, and treatment results were significantly better.

Auricular acupuncture for cancer pain

J Clin Oncol (2003) 15, 4120–26

90 patients with cancer pain not responding to analgesic medication had two treatment courses with auricular acupuncture:

- either at points determined by a point detector, or
- at points not responding to the detector (placebo points), or
- at placebo points to which seeds were fixed.

Two months after the start of the study the pain intensity had decreased by 36 % in the first group, while it had decreased by only 2 % in the two placebo groups.

Auricular acupuncture in the treatment of female infertility

Gerhard I, Postneek F (1992) Gynecol Endocrinol. 6 (3), 171-81.

Following a complete gynaecological/endocrinological workup, 45 infertile women suffering from oligoamenorrhoea (n = 27) or luteal insufficiency (n = 18) were treated with auricular acupuncture. Results were compared to those of 45 women who received conventional hormone treatment. Both groups were matched for six criteria (age, duration of infertility, body mass index, type of infertility, menstrual cycle, and tubal patency). Women treated with acupuncture (results of the control group in brackets) had 22 (20) pregnancies, 11 after acupuncture, 4 (5) spontaneously, and 7 (15) after appropriate medication. 44 % of women with menstrual abnormalities in the acupuncture group remained infertile, compared to 56 % of women in the control group, even though hormone disorders were more pronounced in the acupuncture group. Side effects were observed only during hormone treatment, while various disorders of the autonomic nervous system normalised with acupuncture. Based on our data, auricular acupuncture offers a valuable alternative for the treatment of infertility due to hormonal disorders.

Auricular acupuncture in the treatment of alcohol withdrawal

Shentian S et al (1988) Journal of Traditional Chinese Medicine. 8 (2), 123–124

This clinical report describes the treatment of 310 patients with alcohol addiction who were treated with auricular acupuncture. They were divided into three groups, depending on whether they had come out of their own free will, whether they realised the necessity of undergoing treatment, or whether they were forced into treatment. The authors fixed vaccaria seeds to particular auricular points. The results were good with an overall efficacy rate of 89 %; withdrawal symptoms were mostly avoided.

Auricular acupuncture in the treatment of weight loss in 350 obese patients

Bin X, Jiuzhi F (1985) Journal of Traditional Chinese Medicine. 5 (2), 187–88

A Kuwaiti research study involving 49 obese men and 301 obese women investigated the efficacy of auricular acupuncture for weight loss. During treatment with auricular acupuncture the average weight loss was 4-5 kg per month.

Auricular acupuncture for the treatment of insomnia

J Alter Complement Med 2007, 13 (6), 669–676

After assessing 878 studies about the efficacy of auricular acupuncture for their methodological merit, a Hongkong team evaluated 6 trials. Five commonly treated points included Shen Men (55 cases = 100 %), Heart (100 = 83.3 %), Occiput (29 = 66.7 %), ANS II (34 = 50 %), Kidney I (95 = 33.3 %). The success rate of auricular acupuncture was significantly higher than that of diazepam. While the efficacy of vaccaria seed plasters was also higher than in the control group this did not apply to the use of magnetic pearls.

Auricular acupuncture for the treatment of hot flashes with chemotherapy

Ear acupuncture for hot flushes – the perceptions of women with breast cancer. Complement Ther Clin Pract 2007, 13 (4), 250–57

A British study investigated 16 women with breast cancer undergoing antihormone therapy. Standardised auricular acupuncture was used successfully for the treatment of hot flashes.

Auricular acupuncture for smoking cessation

A randomized controlled clinical trial of auricular acupuncture in smoking. J Chin Med Assoc 2007, 70 (8), 331–38

A Taiwanese study involving 131 individuals investigated the efficacy of auricular acupuncture for smoking cessation. The study group was treated with the points Shen Men (55), ANS II (51), Mouth, and Lung, while the control group received sham acupuncture at ear points not relevant to nicotine abuse. Cigarette consumption in the acupuncture group decreased by 27.1 % and in the control group by 20.3 %. In addition, withdrawal symptoms decreased significantly in the acupuncture group.

Auricular acupuncture in the treatment of acute pain

Auricular acupuncture in treatment of acute pain syndromes: a pilot study. Mil Med 2006, 171 (10), 1010–14

This randomised controlled pilot study investigated A&E patients with acute pain. One group received auricular acupuncture in addition to standard emergency medical care. 23 % of patients in the acupuncture group reported an immediate reduction in pain compared to 0 % of patients in the control group. After 24 hours both groups experienced a similar degree of pain reduction.

Auricular acupuncture for postoperative pain relief after ambulatory knee surgery

Auricular acupuncture for pain relief after ambulatory knee surgery: a randomized trial. CMAJ 2007; 176 (2): 179–83

120 patients were treated with auricular acupuncture prior to ambulatory knee surgery. The control group was needled at the points Shen Men (55), Lung, and Knee while the control group received acupuncture at sham points. The treatments were carried out with semi-permanent needles remaining in situ for one day. The acupuncture group required significantly less ibuprofen to experience the same pain relief as the control group.

Auricular electro-acupuncture reduces histamine-induced itching

Effect of acupuncture on experimentally induced itch. Acta Derm Venereol. 2006, 86 (5), 399–403

Histamine was applied to both forearms of 32 healthy subjects. 5 minutes later one ear was treated with electro-acupuncture. In some cases this completely prevented a reddening of the ipsilateral forearm.

Auricular acupuncture for the treatment of vasomotor symptoms in prostate cancer patients

Auricular acupuncture: a novel treatment for vasomotor symptoms associated with luteinizing-hormone releasing hormone agonist treatment for prostate cancer. BJU Int. 14 August 2008

A British study investigated 60 patients with vasomotor symptoms following LHRH (luteinizing-hormone releasing hormone, gonadotropin releasing-hormone 1) agonist treatment for prostate cancer. The patients received auricular acupuncture once weekly for 10 weeks. Patients reported an average reduction of their symptoms on a six-point scale from a mean 5.0 to 2.1. This corresponds to pain relief equivalent to conventional analgesic medication.

Auricular acupuncture for the treatment of back and pelvic pain in pregnant women

Auricular acupuncture as treatment for pregnant women with low back and posterior pelvic pain: a pilot study. Am J Obstet Gynecol. 25 June 2009 (online-publication)

An American study investigated pregnant women with lower back and pelvic pain. One group received auricular acupuncture, a second group was treated with sham acupuncture, and a further group received no treatments. Compared to the two control groups the study group reported a significant pain reduction and a generally improved ability to function.

Objectification and quantification of laser needle acupuncture

Laserneedle-Akupunktur auf dem Prüfstand der Wissenschaft (Laser needle acupuncture under scientific examination). Schweiz Z GanzheitsMedizin. 2003, 15, 253–259

This study, headed by Prof Litscher (Graz), demonstrated significant laser-induced changes in peripheral microcirculation, blood flow velocity as well as the skin/surface temperature in

22 healthy subjects. There was a significant increase of 0.7 degrees in the tissue temperature at a depth of 1 cm as well as a significant acceleration of the blood flow velocity.

Case study: laser needle therapy for the treatment of mastitis

Laser needle acupuncture in the treatment of mastitis. Schweiz Z GanzheitsMedizin. 2004, 16, 179–180

This individual study describes the case of a woman suffering from mastitis treated with laser needle stimulation. There was a complete recovery after 6 treatments. The first treatment was followed by a short-term exacerbation of symptoms, an additional sign of the effectiveness of this form of treatment.

Laser needle therapy for spontaneous osteonecrosis

Laser-Needle Therapy for Spotaneous Osteonecrosis of the Knee. Photomedicine and Laser Surgery. 2008, 26 (4), 301–306

A 63-year-old patient with spontaneous osteonecrosis diagnosed by MRI scan was treated with laser needle therapy. After 5 weeks there was a significant reduction of bone marrow oedema, a check-up after 35 weeks showed a stable and complete recovery.

12 Appendix

12.1 Anatomical Structures on the Ear and Innervation

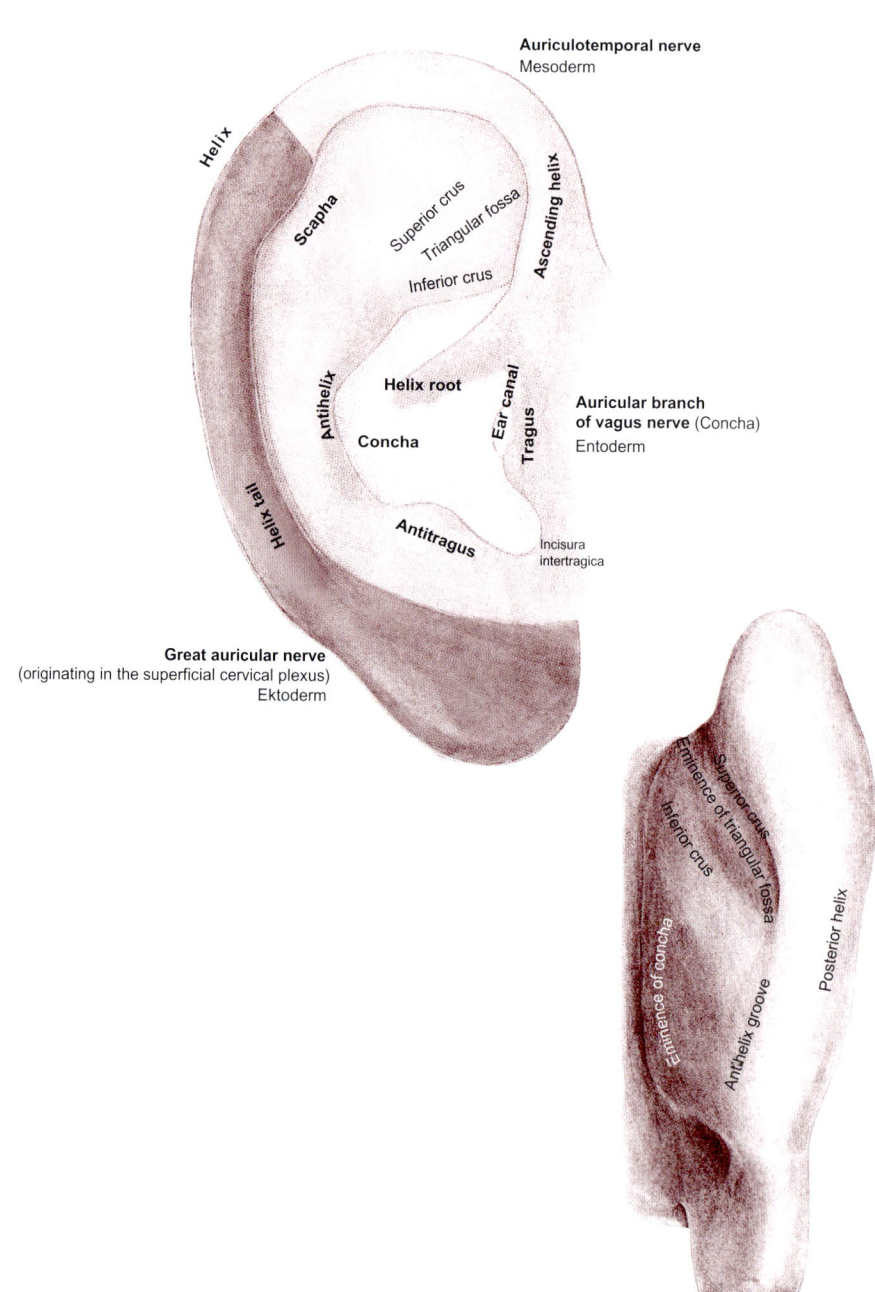

Auriculotemporal nerve
Mesoderm

Helix

Scapha

Superior crus

Triangular fossa

Inferior crus

Ascending helix

Antihelix

Helix root

Ear canal

Tragus

Concha

Auricular branch of vagus nerve (Concha)
Entoderm

Helix tail

Antitragus

Incisura intertragica

Great auricular nerve
(originating in the superficial cervical plexus)
Ektoderm

Eminence of triangular fossa

Superior crus

Inferior crus

Eminence of concha

Antihelix groove

Posterior helix

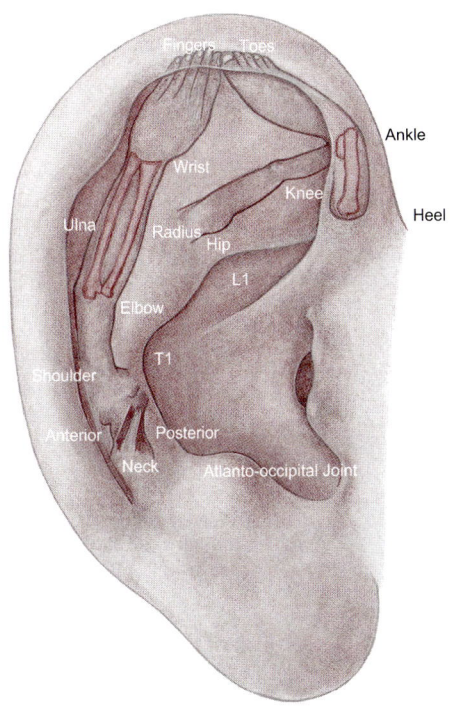

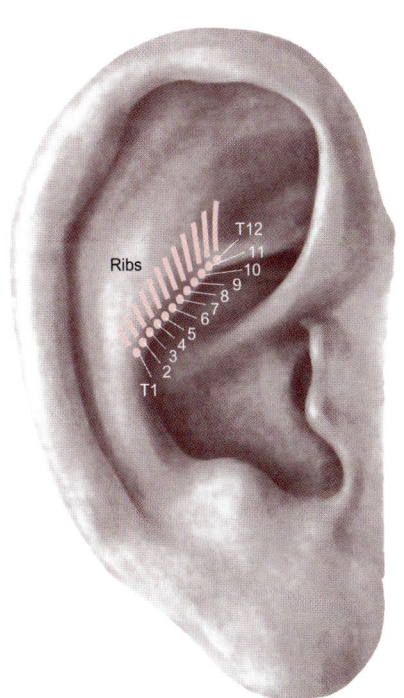

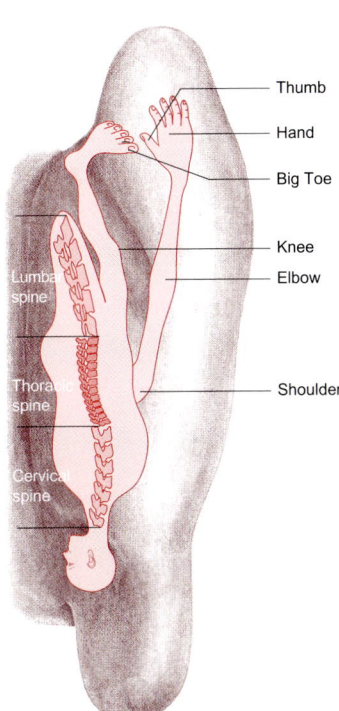

12.3 The Organs Represented on the Ear

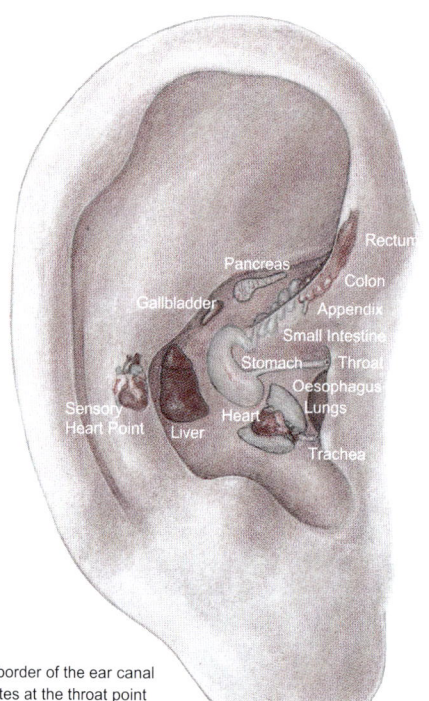

Locations:

Throat:	upper border of the ear canal
Oesophagus:	originates at the throat point
Stomach:	curving around the helix root
Trachea:	lower border of the ear canal
Lungs:	originate at the trachea
Gallbladder:	in the middle third of the superior concha, lateral
Spleen:	left ear only, slightly superior to Pancreas Tail

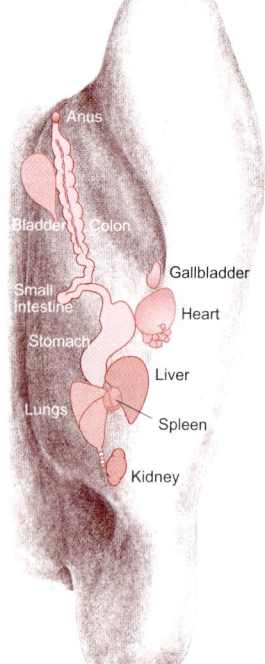

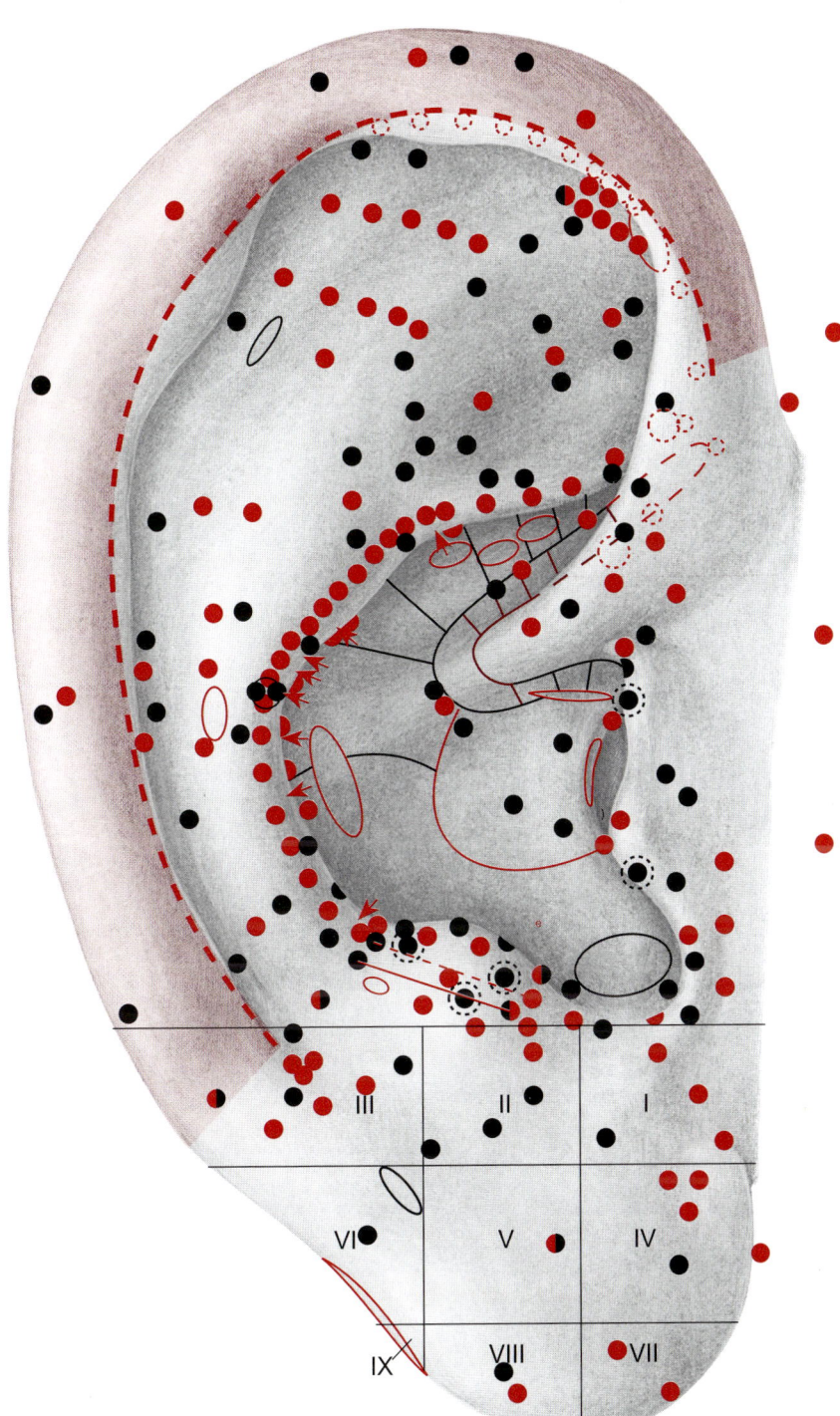

12.5 French Auricular Points

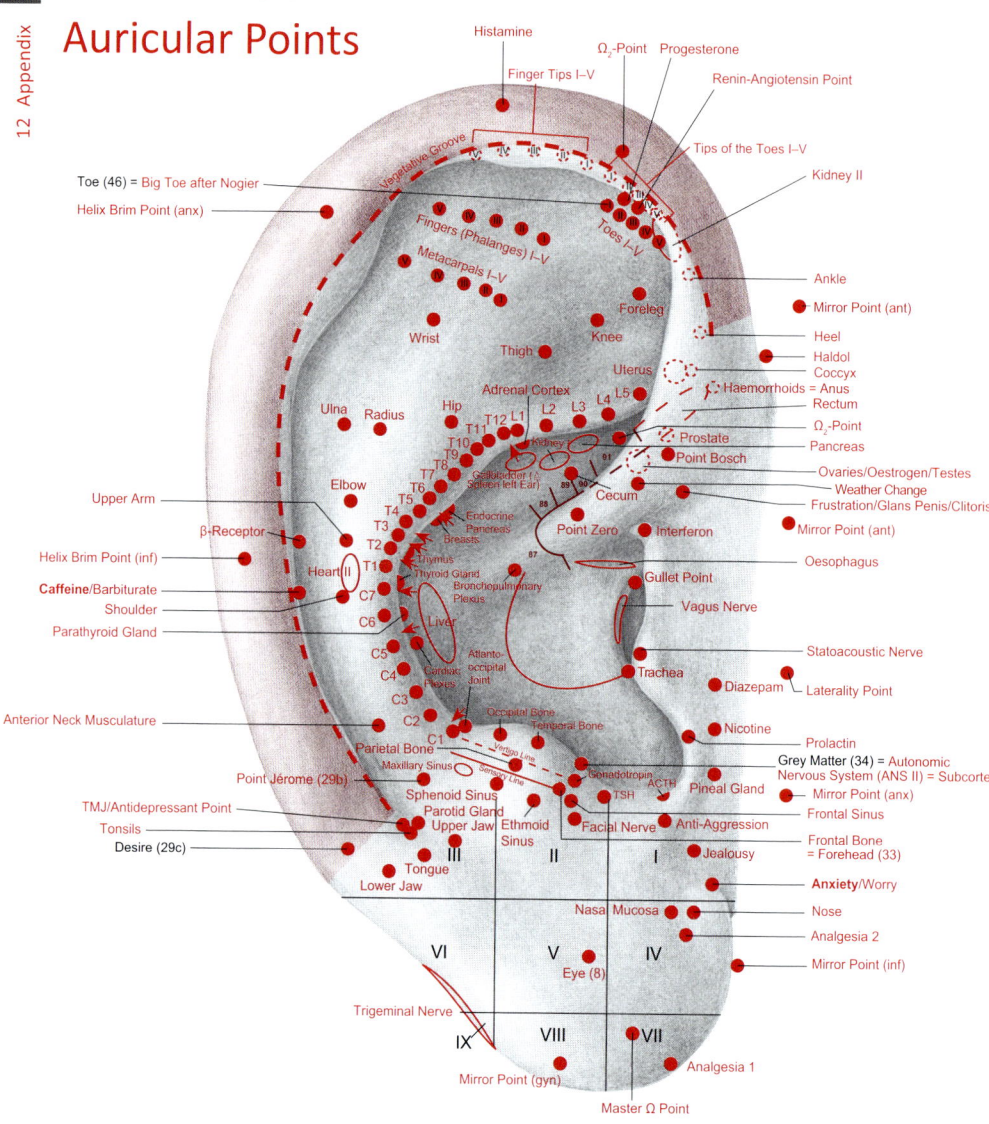

Histamine
Ω₂-Point
Progesterone
Finger Tips I–V
Renin-Angiotensin Point
Tips of the Toes I–V
Vegetative Groove
Kidney II
Toe (46) = Big Toe after Nogier
Helix Brim Point (anx)
Fingers (Phalanges) I–V
Toes I–V
Metacarpals I–V
Ankle
Foreleg
Mirror Point (ant)
Knee
Heel
Wrist
Thigh
Haldol
Coccyx
Uterus
Haemorrhoids = Anus
Adrenal Cortex
L4 L5
Rectum
Ulna
Radius
Hip
L1 L2 L3
Ω₂-Point
T12
Kidney
Prostate
Pancreas
T11
T10
Point Bosch
Ovaries/Oestrogen/Testes
T9
T8
Gallbladder
(Spleen left Ear)
Weather Change
Elbow
T7
Cecum
Frustration/Glans Penis/Clitoris
Upper Arm
T6
Endocrine
Mirror Point (ant)
T5
Pancreas
Point Zero
Interferon
T4
Breasts
β-Receptor
T3
Thymus
Oesophagus
T2
Thyroid Gland
Helix Brim Point (inf)
T1
Bronchopulmonary
Gullet Point
Heart II
Plexus
Vagus Nerve
Caffeine/Barbiturate
C7
Shoulder
C6
Statoacoustic Nerve
Parathyroid Gland
Liver
Trachea
C5
Diazepam
Laterality Point
C4
Cardiac
Atlanto-
Plexus
occipital
C3
joint
Anterior Neck Musculature
C2
Nicotine
C1
Occipital Bone
Temporal Bone
Prolactin
Parietal Bone
Vertigo Line
Grey Matter (34) = Autonomic
Maxillary Sinus
Sensory Line
Nervous System (ANS II) = Subcortex
Point Jérome (29b)
Gonadotropin
Mirror Point (anx)
ACTH
Sphenoid Sinus
Pineal Gland
Frontal Sinus
TMJ/Antidepressant Point
Parotid Gland
TSH
Anti-Aggression
Frontal Bone
Tonsils
Upper Jaw
Ethmoid
Facial Nerve
= Forehead (33)
Desire (29c)
III
Sinus
Jealousy
II
I
Tongue
Anxiety/Worry
Lower Jaw
Nasal Mucosa
Nose
VI
Analgesia 2
V
IV
Mirror Point (inf)
Eye (8)
Trigeminal Nerve
X
VIII
VII
IX
Mirror Point (gyn)
Analgesia 1
Master Ω Point

● Point on the anterior aspect of the ear

◑ Both Chinese and French point

⚬ Hidden point

◌ Point on the reverse side

⊽ Point located on the edge

▢ Point zones

➹ Point on the Sympathetic Groove

⊽ Point on the Hormonal Line

Bold Points on the dominant side are printed in **Bold**

Chinese points representing the inner organs:

84 Mouth
85 Oesophagus
86 Cardia
92 Bladder
93 Prostate
94 Ureter
95 Kidney
96 Pancreas/Gallbladder
97 Liver
98 Spleen

French and Chinese points representing the inner organs

87 Stomach ■
88 Duodenum ■
89 Small Intestine ■
90 Appendix IV ■
91 Colon ■

Points in the Sympathetic Groove (arrows):

C1/2: Superior Cervical Ganglion
C5/6: Middle Cervical Ganglion
C7: Inferior Cervical Ganglion/Stellate Ganglion
T2: Neural Thyroid Point
T2/3: Neural Thymus Point
T3/4: Neural Stomach Point
T5/6: Neural Liver Point/Resentment
T12: Neural Adrenal Cortex Point

12.6 Chinese Auricular Points

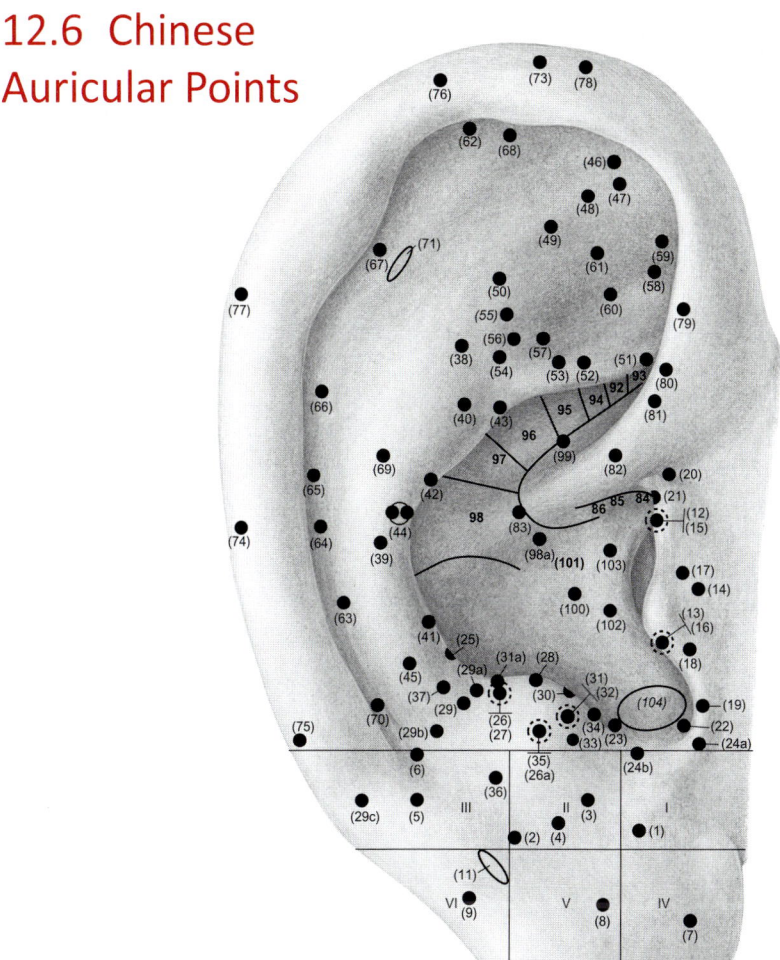

1	Tooth	26	Tooth Ache (on the inside)	46	Toe	75	Tonsil III
2	Palate	26a	Thalamus	47	Heel	76	Liver I
3	Floor of the Mouth	27	Larynx and Tooth (on the outside)	48	Ankle	77	Liver II
4	Tongue	28	Pituitary Gland	49	Knee Joint	78	Apex of the Ear
5	Uppar Jaw	29	Occiput	50	Hip Joint	79	External Genitalia
6	Lower Jaw	29a	Nausea	51	Autonomic Nervous System I (ANS I)	80	Urethra
7	Tooth	29b	Point de Jérome	53	Buttocks	81	Rectum
8	Eye	29c	Desire	55	*Shen Men*	82	Diaphragm
9	Inner Ear	30	Parotid Gland	56	Pelvic Cavity	83	Branching Point
10	Tonsil IV	31	Asthma	57	Hip	84	Mouth
11	Cheek	31a	Cough-Relieving Point	58	Uterus	85	Oesophagus
12	Apex of Tragus	32	Testes	59	Blood Pressure Lowering Point	86	Cardia
13	Adrenal Glands	33	Frontal Bone/Forehead	60	Dyspnoea	92	Bladder
14	External Nose	34	Autonomic Nervous System	61	Hepatitis Point	93	Prostate
15	Larynx/Pharynx		(ANS II)/Grey Matter/Subcortex	62	Fingers	94	Kidney
16	Inner Nose	35	Sun	63	Clavicle	95	Kidney
17	Thirst	36	Vertex	64	Shoulder Joint	96	Pancreas/Gallbladder
18	Hunger	37	Cervical Spine	65	Shoulder	97	Liver
19	Hypertension	38	Sacrum and Coccyx	66	Elbow	98	Spleen
20	External Ear	39	Thoracic Spine	67	Wrist	98a	Muscle Relaxation
21	Heart/Arrhythmia	40	Lumbar Spine	68	Appendix I	99	Ascites
22	Endocrine System	41	Neck	69	Appendix II	100	Heart I
23	Ovaries	42	Thorax	70	Appendix III	101	Lungs
24a	Eye I	43	Abdomen	71	Urticaria	102	Bronchi
24b	Eye II	44	Mammary Glands	73	Tonsil I	103	Trachea
25	Brainstem	45	Thyroid Gland	74	Tonsil II	104	*San Jiao* (Triple Warmer)

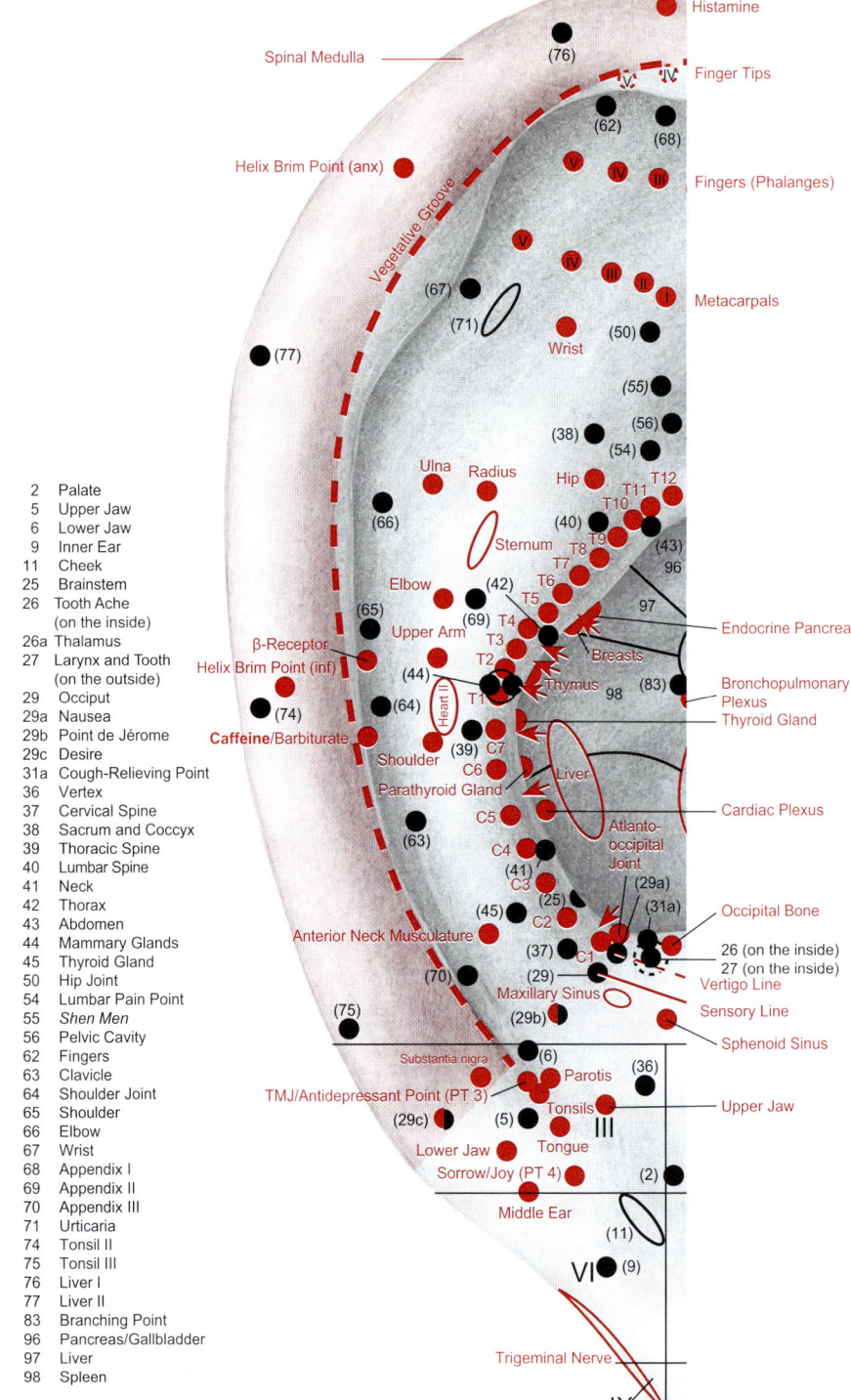

Histamine
Spinal Medulla
(76)
Finger Tips
(62)
(68)
Helix Brim Point (anx)
Fingers (Phalanges)
Vegetative Groove
Metacarpals
(67)
(71)
Wrist
(50)
(77)
(55)
(56)
(54)
(38)
Ulna   Radius   Hip   T12
T11
T10
(66)   (40)   T9
Sternum   T8   (43)
T7   96
Elbow   (42)   T6
T5   97
(65)   (69)   T4   Endocrine Pancreas
β-Receptor   Upper Arm   T3
Helix Brim Point (inf)   T2   Breasts
(44)   T1   Bronchopulmonary
(74)   (64)   Thymus   (83)   Plexus
Caffeine/Barbiturate   Thyroid Gland
(39)   C7
Shoulder   C6   Liver   Cardiac Plexus
Parathyroid Gland   C5   Atlanto-
(63)   occipital   Occipital Bone
C4   Joint
C3   (29a)
(45)   (25)   (31a)   26 (on the inside)
Anterior Neck Musculature   C2   (37)   27 (on the inside)
(70)   (29)   Vertigo Line
Maxillary Sinus   Sensory Line
(75)   (29b)   Sphenoid Sinus
Substantia nigra   (6)   (36)
Parotis
TMJ/Antidepressant Point (PT 3)   Tonsils   Upper Jaw
(29c)   (5)   III
Lower Jaw   Tongue
Sorrow/Joy (PT 4)   (2)
Middle Ear
(11)
VI   (9)
Trigeminal Nerve
IX

2   Palate
5   Upper Jaw
6   Lower Jaw
9   Inner Ear
11   Cheek
25   Brainstem
26   Tooth Ache
       (on the inside)
26a   Thalamus
27   Larynx and Tooth
       (on the outside)
29   Occiput
29a   Nausea
29b   Point de Jérome
29c   Desire
31a   Cough-Relieving Point
36   Vertex
37   Cervical Spine
38   Sacrum and Coccyx
39   Thoracic Spine
40   Lumbar Spine
41   Neck
42   Thorax
43   Abdomen
44   Mammary Glands
45   Thyroid Gland
50   Hip Joint
54   Lumbar Pain Point
55   Shen Men
56   Pelvic Cavity
62   Fingers
63   Clavicle
64   Shoulder Joint
65   Shoulder
66   Elbow
67   Wrist
68   Appendix I
69   Appendix II
70   Appendix III
71   Urticaria
74   Tonsil II
75   Tonsil III
76   Liver I
77   Liver II
83   Branching Point
96   Pancreas/Gallbladder
97   Liver
98   Spleen

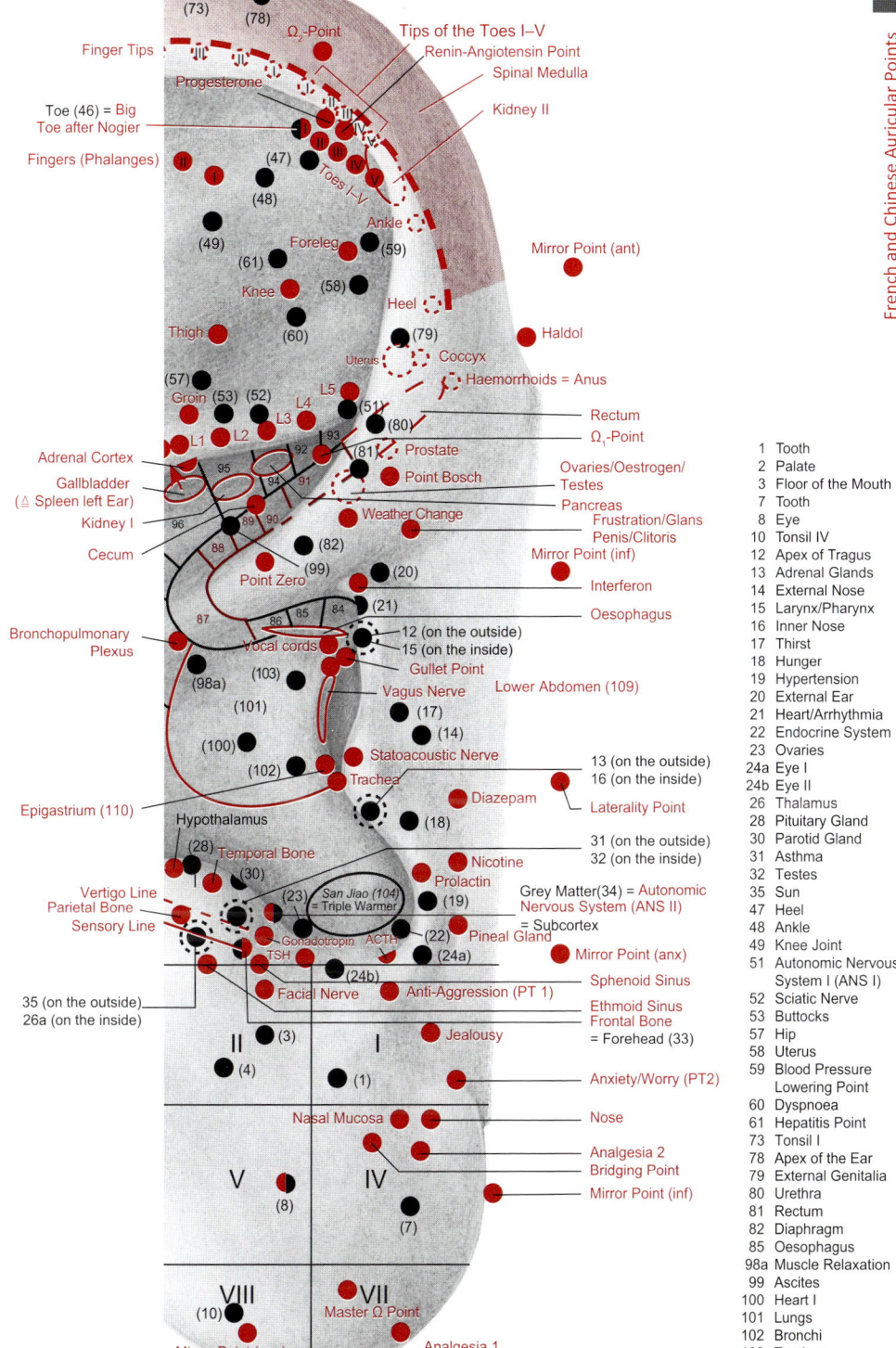

(73)
(78)
Ω₂-Point
Finger Tips
Renin-Angiotensin Point
Tips of the Toes I–V
Spinal Medulla
Progesterone
Kidney II
Toe (46) = Big
Toe after Nogier
Fingers (Phalanges)
(47)
(48)
Toes I–V
Ankle
Mirror Point (ant)
(49)
(61)
Foreleg
(59)
(79)
Knee
(58)
Heel
Haldol
Thigh
(60)
Uterus
Coccyx
Haemorrhoids = Anus
(57)
Groin (53) (52)
L5
Rectum
L4
L3
(51)
Ω₁-Point
L1
L2
(80)
Prostate
Adrenal Cortex
95
92 93
(81)
Point Bosch
Gallbladder
(△ Spleen left Ear)
94 91
Ovaries/Oestrogen/
Testes
Pancreas
Kidney I
96
90
Weather Change
Frustration/Glans
Penis/Clitoris
Cecum
88 89
(82)
Mirror Point (inf)
Point Zero
(99)
(20)
Interferon
87
86 85 84
(21)
Oesophagus
Bronchopulmonary
Plexus
Vocal cords
12 (on the outside)
15 (on the inside)
Gullet Point
(98a)
(103)
Vagus Nerve
Lower Abdomen (109)
(101)
(17)
(100)
(14)
(102)
Statoacoustic Nerve
13 (on the outside)
16 (on the inside)
Epigastrium (110)
Trachea
Diazepam
Laterality Point
Hypothalamus
(18)
31 (on the outside)
32 (on the inside)
(28) Temporal Bone
Nicotine
Vertigo Line
(30)
Prolactin
Grey Matter(34) = Autonomic
Nervous System (ANS II)
= Subcortex
Parietal Bone
(23)
San Jiao (104)
= Triple Warmer
(19)
Sensory Line
Gonadotropin ACTH
(22) Pineal Gland
TSH
(24a)
Mirror Point (anx)
(24b)
Facial Nerve
Sphenoid Sinus
35 (on the outside)
26a (on the inside)
Anti-Aggression (PT 1)
Ethmoid Sinus
Frontal Bone
= Forehead (33)
II
(3)
I
Jealousy
(4)
(1)
Anxiety/Worry (PT2)
Nasal Mucosa
Nose
Analgesia 2
Bridging Point
V
IV
Mirror Point (inf)
(8)
(7)
VIII
VII
(10)
Master Ω Point
Mirror Point (gyn)
Analgesia 1

1 Tooth
2 Palate
3 Floor of the Mouth
7 Tooth
8 Eye
10 Tonsil IV
12 Apex of Tragus
13 Adrenal Glands
14 External Nose
15 Larynx/Pharynx
16 Inner Nose
17 Thirst
18 Hunger
19 Hypertension
20 External Ear
21 Heart/Arrhythmia
22 Endocrine System
23 Ovaries
24a Eye I
24b Eye II
26 Thalamus
28 Pituitary Gland
30 Parotid Gland
31 Asthma
32 Testes
35 Sun
47 Heel
48 Ankle
49 Knee Joint
51 Autonomic Nervous
System I (ANS I)
52 Sciatic Nerve
53 Buttocks
57 Hip
58 Uterus
59 Blood Pressure
Lowering Point
60 Dyspnoea
61 Hepatitis Point
73 Tonsil I
78 Apex of the Ear
79 External Genitalia
80 Urethra
81 Rectum
82 Diaphragm
85 Oesophagus
98a Muscle Relaxation
99 Ascites
100 Heart I
101 Lungs
102 Bronchi
103 Trachea

12.7 Index

12.8 Auricular Points in Alphabetical Order

Auricular points of the French School are shown in red, those of the Chinese School in black.

Abdomen *(fu)* (43)   83
ACTH   89
ACTH   105
Addiction   104
Adrenal Cortex   88, 105
Adrenal glands   89
Adrenal Glands (13)   250
Analgesia 1   91
Analgesia 2   91
Ankle   75
Ankle (48)   75
Anterior Neck   71
Antiaggression point   93
Antidepressant point   79, 93, 108
Anus   83
Anxiety   93
Apex of the Ear (78)   98
Apex of Tragus (12)   91
Appendix I (68)   83
Appendix II (69)   83
Appendix III (70)   83
Appendix IV *(lanwei IV)* (90)   81
Ascites *(hushuidian)* (99)   98
Asthma *(dingchuan)* (31)   85
Autonomic Nervous System (ANS II)
   (34)   91
Autonomic Nervous System I *(jiaogan)*
   (51)   89

Barbiturate   90
Beta-Receptor   90
Bladder   102
Bladder (sensitive bladder) *(pangguang)*
   (92)   86
Blood Pressure Lowering Groove
   (105)   85
Blood Pressure Lowering Point (59)   85
Bourdiol   94
Brainstem (25)   98
Branching point   98

Branching Point (83)   263
Breast   88
Bronchi *(zhiqiguan)* (102)   81
Bronchopulmonary plexus   98, 108
Buttocks (53)   69

Caffeine   90
Cardia *(penmen)* (86)   81
Cardiac plexus   98
Cecum   81
Cervical spine   100
Cervical spine (37)   69
Cervical spine, posterior ear *(zhongerbei)*
   (107)   100
Cheek *(jia)* (11)   79
Clavicle (63)   73
Clitoris   87, 92
Colon   102
Colon (91)   258
Cough-Relieving Point (31a)   85

Darwin's Tubercle   75
Desire (29c)   92
Diaphragm *(ge)* (82)   83
Diazepam   91, 109
Diclofenac   91
Duodenum *(shi'erzhichang)* (88)   81
Dyspnoea *(chuandian)* (60)   85

Elbow   73, 101
Elbow *(zhou)* (66)   73
Endocrine Pancreas   88
Endocrine System *(neifenmi)* (22)   89
Epigastrium *(shangfu)* (110)   121
Ethmoid sinus   77
External Ear (20)   77
External Genitalia (79)   87
External Nose (14)   77

12.9 Chinese Auricular Points

1	tooth 79	37	Cervical Spine 69
2	Palate 79	38	Sacrum and Coccyx 69
3	Floor of the Mouth 79	39	Thoracic Spine *(xiongzhui)* 69
4	Tongue 79	40	Lumbar Spine *(yaozhui)* 69
5	Upper Jaw *(shanghe)* 79	41	Throat *(jing)* 83
6	Lower Jaw *(xiae)* 79	42	Thorax *(xiong)* 83
7	Tooth *(bayamazudian)* 79	43	Abdomen *(fu)* 83
8	Eye *(yan)* 77	44	Mammary Glands *(ruxian)* 83
9	Inner Ear 79	45	Thyroid Gland 89
10	Tonsil IV 79	46	Toe *(zhi)* 73
11	Cheek *(jia)* 79	47	Heel *(gen)* 75
12	Apex of Tragus 91	48	Ankle 75
13	Adrenal Glands 250	49	Knee Joint 75
14	External Nose 77	50	Hip Joint *(kuanguanjie)* 75
15	Larynx/Pharynx 84	51	Autonomic Nervous System I
16	Inner Nose 77		*(jiaogan)* 89
17	Thirst 99	52	Sciatic Nerve *(zuogushenjing)* 69
18	Hunger 99	53	Buttocks 69
19	Hypertension 84	54	Lumbar Pain Point 69
20	External Ear 77	55	Shen Men *(shenmen)* 91
21	Heart/Arrhythmia 84	56	Pelvic Cavity 91, 292
22	Endocrine System *(neifenmi)* 89	57	Hip 75
23	Ovaries 87	58	Uterus 87
24a	Eye I 79	59	Blood Pressure Lowering Point 85
24b	Eye II 79	60	Dyspnoea *(chuandian)* 85
25	Brainstem 98	61	Hepatitis Point 85
26	Tooth Ache 77, 91	62	Fingers 73
26a	Thalamus 91	63	Clavicle 73
27	Larynx and Tooth 77	64	Shoulder joint 73
28	Pituitary Gland 89	65	Shoulder *(jian)* 73
29	Occiput 91	66	Elbow *(zhou)* 73
29a	Nausea 77	67	Wrist *(wan)* 73
29b	Point de Jérome 92	68	Appendix I 83
29c	Desire 92	69	Appendix II 83
30	Parotid Gland 77	70	Appendix III 83
31	Asthma *(dingchuan)* 85	71	Urticaria 98
31a	Cough-Relieving Point 85	73	Tonsil I 76
32	Testes 87	74	Tonsil II 76
33	Frontal Bone/Forehead 77	75	Tonsil III 76
34	Autonomic Nervous System	76	Liver I 83
	(ANS II) 91	77	Liver II 83
35	Sun *(taiyang)* 91	78	Apex of the Ear 98
36	Vertex *(ding)* 77	79	External Genitalia 87

80 Urethra   87
81 Rectum   83
82 Diaphragm *(ge)*   83
83 Branching Point   263
84 Mouth *(kou)*   80
85 Oesophagus *(shiguan)*   81
86 Cardia *(penmen)*   81
87 Stomach *(wei)*   81
88 Duodenum *(shi'erzhichang)*   81
89 Small Intestine *(xiaochang)*   81
90 Appendix IV *(lanwei IV)*   81
91 Colon   258
92 Bladder (sensitive bladder)
   (pangguang)   86
93 Prostate *(qianliexian)*   87
94 Ureter   86
95 Kidney *(shen)*   86
96 Pancreas/Gallbladder *(yidan)*   81
97 Liver *(gan)*   81

98 Spleen *(pi)*   82
98a Muscle Relaxation   70
99 Ascites *(hushuidian)*   98
100 Heart I *(xin)*   81
101 Lungs *(fei)*   81
102 Bronchi *(zhiqiguan)*   81
103 Trachea *(qiguan)*   81
104 *San Jiao* (Triple Warmer)   98
105 Blood Pressure Lowering
    Groove   85
106 Lumbar Spine, posterior ear
    (shangerbei)   100
107 Cervical Spine, posterior ear
    (zhongerbei)   100
108 Thoracic Spine, posterior ear
    (xiaerbei)   100
109 Lower Abdomen *(xiafu)*   121
110 Epigastrium *(shangfu)*   121

12.10 New Auricular Points